Veterinary Dermatology

For Elsevier:

Commissioning Editor: Mary Seager
Development Editor: Rita Demetriou-Swanwick
Project Manager: David Fleming
Designer: Andy Chapman
Illustrations Manager: Bruce Hogarth

Veterinary Dermatology

A manual for nurses and technicians

Frances J M Gaudiano MA VN Dipl Derm

Consultant Editor

Cathy F Curtis BVet Med DVD MRCVS

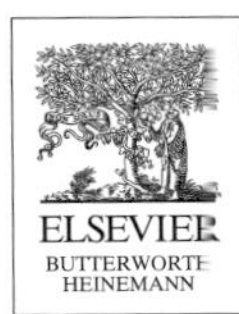

EDINBURGH LONDON NEW YORK OXFORD PHILADELPHIA ST LOUIS SYDNEY TORONTO 2005

ELSEVIER
BUTTERWORTH
HEINEMANN

First published 2005

ISBN 0 7506 8804 1

British Library Cataloguing in Publication Data
A catalogue record for this book is available from the British Library

Library of Congress Cataloging in Publication Data
A catalog record for this book is available from the Library of Congress

Knowledge and best practice in this field are constantly changing. As new research and experience broaden our knowledge, changes in practice, treatment and drug therapy may become necessary or appropriate. Readers are advised to check the most current information provided (i) on procedures featured or (ii) by the manufacturer of each product to be administered, to verify the recommended dose or formula, the method and duration of administration, and contraindications. It is the responsibility of the practitioner, relying on their own experience and knowledge of the patient, to make diagnoses, to determine dosages and the best treatment for each individual patient, and to take all appropriate safety precautions. To the fullest extent of the law, neither the publisher nor the author assumes any liability for any injury and/or damage.

The Publisher

The publisher's policy is to use **paper manufactured from sustainable forests**

Printed in China

Contents

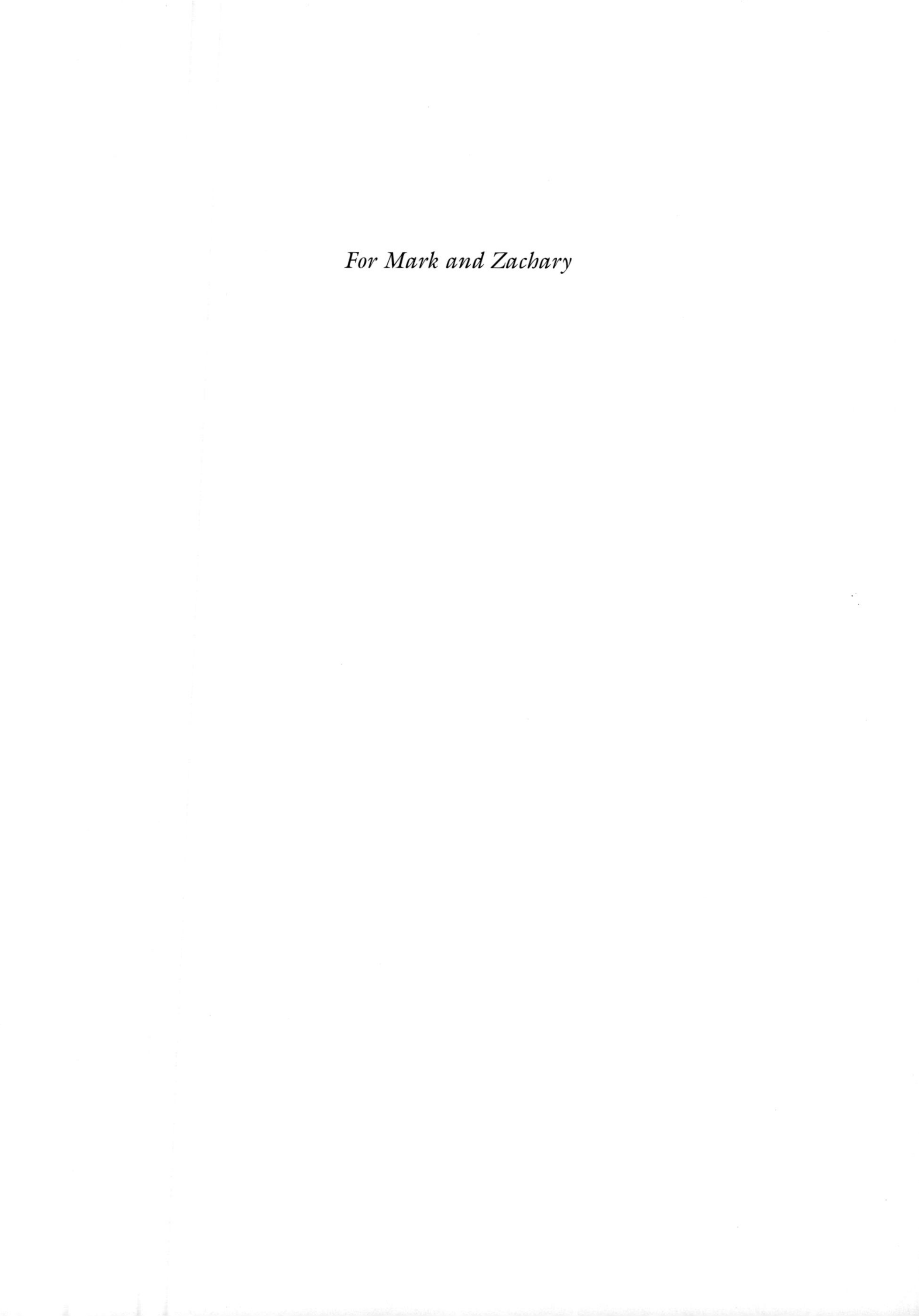

For Mark and Zachary

Acknowledgements

Thank you to Dr Annette Loeffler, who contributed advice and guidance throughout the writing of this book. Particular gratitude is due for her assistance with the chapter on neoplasia and the many photographs she contributed to this book. Thanks must go to Natalie Perrins, who also kindly contributed her photographs to the book.

Chapter 1

Introduction to the skin

CHAPTER CONTENTS

The skin is the largest organ in the body serving a variety of important functions. Anatomically, the skin can be likened to a sandwich of three layers: the hypodermis, the dermis and the epidermis, with the dermis being the 'meat' of the sandwich.

EMBRYOLOGY

Embryonically, the epidermis forms from a ground substance out of which develops a layer of cells called the ectoderm. That divides into two layers, the basale and periderm. A third layer forms between these two, creating the stratum intermedium; this forms another sandwich:

Periderm
Stratum intermedium
Stratum basale

Simultaneously, the dermis develops from precursor cells. These metamorphose into fibroblasts, which produce collagen fibres for strength and elastin for elasticity. Amidst all these fibres, clumps of precursor cells mesh into hair bulbs. These bulbs are situated beneath hair germs, originating in the epidermis. The germs and bulbs grow towards each other and form a hair follicle. Bulges develop on either side of the follicle, and these develop into sebaceous and sweat glands. Blood, nerve and lymphatic systems stretch their vessels and fibres outwards, creating their essential networks throughout the dermis.

During the second half of gestation, the subcutis starts developing, beginning as lipocytes and growing into useful fat storage cells, known as adipocytes.

In the mature skin, each layer has its own anatomy and physiology, serving different facets of the skin's functions.

THE HYPODERMIS

On the bottom layer we have the **hypodermis**, also referred to as the subcutis or the panniculus (see Fig. 1.1). This is largely a layer of fat (adipose) cells suspended in a fibrous mesh that descends down from the layer above. As it is composed of fat, the hypodermis serves as an energy reserve. It also provides insulation and helps to form the contours of the visible body. In areas that receive a lot of wear and tear, such as the footpads, the hypodermis will be thicker, providing some shock absorption. In a few areas of the body, the hypodermis can be the thickest skin layer.

THE DERMIS

Above the hypodermis lies the **dermis**. This area is probably the most active in that it is innervated with a rich blood, lymph and nerve network. Glands and hair follicles populate this section of the skin. As befits its framework function, the dermis is generally the thickest layer of the skin. The primary structure of the dermis is a collection of collagen and elastin fibres subsisting in a ground substance of protein and mucopolysaccharides. The fibres extend down into the hypodermis, giving a skeleton for the adipose cells to cling to.

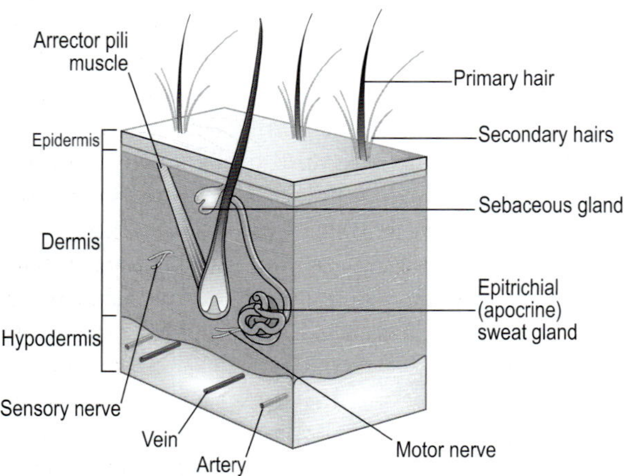

Figure 1.1 Cross-section of the skin.

Within the dermis, the fibres provide the support for the hair follicles, glands and vessels, as well as acting as a storage area for water and electrolytes.

The cellular population of the dermis consists predominantly of fibroblasts (important in wound healing) and macrophages, essential for control of foreign substances that can enter the dermal layer. **Mast cells** are large, round, granular cells which tend to populate the area around blood vessels. These cells become significant during the inflammatory processes associated with insult to the skin. When we see reddened skin, mast cells have degranulated, causing blood vessels to dilate and become more permeable. Mast cells can do this in response to an allergen interacting with certain antibodies coating their surface.

HAIR AND THE HAIR FOLLICLE

One of the most significant structures of the dermal layer is the hair follicle. Dogs and cats have compound hair follicles, providing them with a much denser hair coat than humans or, for that matter horses. For every primary, or guard hair that erupts from a follicle, there will be one to four smaller primary hairs and 5 to 20 secondary hairs. In the dog, the coat density can be measured at 100–600 hairs per cm^2 while in the cat the density is 800–1600 hairs per cm^2. Primary hairs erupt from separate pores and have their own **epitrichial** (meaning, associated with a hair follicle) glands and a muscle (Fig. 1.2 illustrates this arrangement). Secondary hairs come from a common pore and have only one associated gland (the sebaceous gland). The muscle working with hair follicles is the **arrector pili**, a smooth muscle innervated by cholinergic fibres. In other words, the muscle reacts when stimulated by adrenaline and noradrenaline. The purpose of the arrector pili is to raise the hair shaft, thus trapping air between the hair and the skin surface. This serves as a form of insulation to warm the animal. A further use is in the 'raising of the hackles'. The guard hairs along the dorsum and tail lift, making the animal appear larger to potential foe – or a scary veterinary nurse attempting to get an animal out of its kennel!

On either side of the follicle lie the **adnexae**: the sweat and sebaceous glands associated with the hair follicle. The sweat gland is placed higher along the

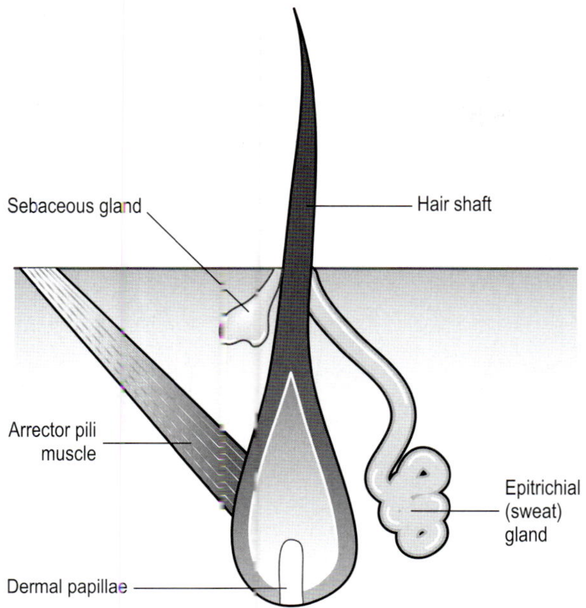

Figure 1.2 The hair follicle and associated structures.

follicle, with the sebaceous gland on the opposite side. The arrector pili muscle originates at the bottom of the follicle. The **sebaceous gland** is a simple gland that empties, via a duct, directly into the hair follicle. Cells lining the interior of the gland die and, mixing with an oily substance, form **sebum**, which is secreted into the follicle. Sebum is a natural moisturiser that also acts in a protective fashion, helping to destroy microbes on the skin layer. Sebum production is promoted by the male hormone androgen, which is why teenage boys often suffer from distressing acne problems more so than teenage girls. In dogs, the males (and sometimes females) experience sebum problems when a sebaceous gland, of pheromonal importance on the mid-dorsal tail, becomes over-productive, causing a greasy, bald patch. This condition is known as tail gland hyperplasia. This is not at all becoming and can be very upsetting to the owner of a show dog! When cats suffer from this condition it is referred to as 'stud tail'. Luckily, for females, oestrogen restrains the production of sebum so they are less prone to its overproduction . The sebaceous gland tends to be larger in areas with less hair, as on the ventrum. A specialised sebaceous gland exists on the eyelid, contributing to the pre-corneal tear film. This gland is known as the **meibomian** gland.

Sweat glands also empty into the hair follicle and assist the sebaceous gland with moisturising and protective duties. Sweat does not serve as a thermoregulator in the dog and cat as it does in man. However, there are **atrichial** (unassociated with hair follicles) sweat glands on the footpads. Sweating can occur here when the animal is frightened – think of those sweaty footprints of cats on the examination table. Footpad sweat can help to reduce friction and protect the pad. Again, specialised glands exist on the eyelid, where the **Moll** gland helps to protect the cornea. Mammary glands and anal sacs are other examples of specialised sweat glands.

Hair grows at an average rate of 2 mm per week, with the photoperiod being the strongest influence on the rate of growth. Thus the fastest growth occurs in the summer with significant shedding in the spring and autumn. Coat length is generally determined by genes, obvious when one considers the appearance of different breeds.

Hair grows in an asynchronous pattern; otherwise, the animal would appear to be bald some of the time and fully coated at other periods in the cycle. There are three main phases in the growth cycle: **anagen**, **catagen** and **telogen**. Anagen is the growing phase in the cycle. A papilla in the dermis gives nutrients to the hair bulb. As the hair begins to grow, it extends upwards, along the length of the follicle, towards the skin surface. As the shaft grows, it pushes the existing hair out of the way, causing it to be shed into the environment. During catagen, the bulb at the bottom of the shaft pinches away from the papilla, thus separating from its nutrient source. Telogen is the resting phase, when the hair can exist for several weeks until a new hair comes along and pushes it out of the way. The three phases are illustrated in Figure 1.3.

The environment (toasty radiator, warmed–house or drafty shed), physiology, nutrition, season, climate and genes all affect hair growth. Male hormones tend to promote growth and thickness of hair shaft while female hormones inhibit growth. The hormone thyroxine is required to initiate anagen. This is why hypothyroid dogs can exhibit bald patches and 'rat tail'. One of the symptoms of hypothyroidism is the predominance of hairs in the telogen phase, leading to easy **epilation** and eventually **alopecia**. Another hormone, cortisol, inhibits anagen.

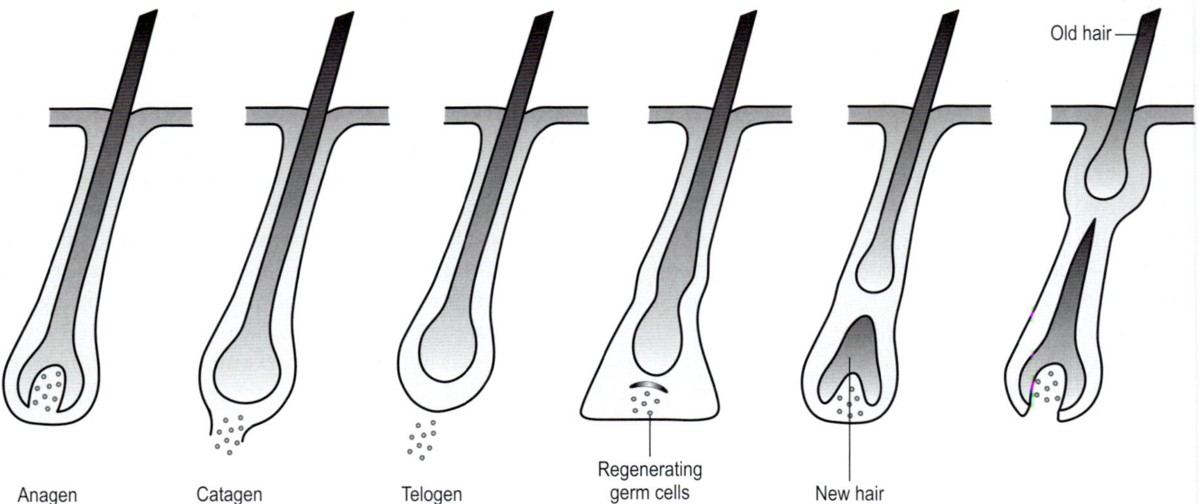

Figure 1.3 Hair growth. 1: *Anagen* is the growing phase of the hair cycle. 2: *Catagen* is when the hair shaft separates from the papilla. 3: *Telogen* is the resting phase in the hair cycle.

Thus, in hyperadrenocorticism, the excess levels of cortisol will cause thinning of hair coat and alopecic areas.

Vibrissae are specialised hairs which work as pressure and touch receptors, giving animals the ability to feel or sense things in the dark. Blood-filled sinuses, riddled with nerve fibres, eg Merkel cells encapsulate the vibrissae. The chin, muzzle, eyelids and, in the cat, the carpal pads, are where the vibrissae are located.

BLOOD, LYMPH AND NERVES

The dermis is nourished by a rich blood supply consisting of three vascular plexi in the superficial, mid and deep dermis. Dilation and constriction of these vessels play an important part of thermoregulation and in the inflammatory processes. Because the outermost layer of the skin, the epidermis, is avascular, the vessels of the dermis also provide nutrients for the epidermis.

The lymphatic vessels exist in the upper dermis and drain into the subcutis/hypodermis, travelling from plexi there to local lymph nodes. Nutrients are carried to the dermis and epidermis via the lymph vessels and debris is carried away along these routes. Sampling cells, for example Langerhans cells, in the epidermis and dermis will travel through the lymphatics, carrying messages about foreign substances in the skin to the lymph nodes. Depending on the nature of the message – 'DEMODEX MITES! WATCH OUT!' or 'just another commensal microbe' – the lymph nodes will mount an immunological response.

The nerve plexi are terminal branches of larger nerve trunks and tend to follow the pattern of the blood vessels. Sensory and motor nerves exist, the motor nerves to control the arrector pili muscle and, in some cases, stimulate contraction of sweat glands. The sensory nerves have special endings, such as Merkel cells, which infiltrate the vibrissae, and also exist freely.

THE BASEMENT MEMBRANE

Directly above the dermis, existing like a sort of sticky sandwich spread, is the **basement membrane**. This is the attachment area between the dermis and the epidermis. Here lie the fibres and **desmosomes** (spiny intercellular attachments) that create a base for the epidermis as well as a protective barrier for the dermis. Certain drugs cannot pass through this barrier, thus ensuring both the safety and efficacy of many topical treatments. Communication between the dermis and epidermis occurs at the basement membrane. Nutrient exchange occurs at this junction and it is here that major cells affecting wound healing interact and develop.

THE EPIDERMIS

Finally, we come to the **epidermis**. The epidermis consists of four or five layers of cells, illustrated in Figure 1.4. At the bottom, the **stratum basale** consists of live cells with nuclei which undergo active mitosis. Reproduction produces daughter cells, which migrate upwards towards the top layer of the epidermis. Skin cells of the epidermis are known as **keratinocytes**, although at each layer the keratinocyte undergoes a series of modifications. At the next layer, the **stratum spinosum**, the keratinocyte takes on a slightly flattened shape and forms strong attachments to its mother and adjoining cells. These spiny attachment points are referred to as desmosomes. As the cells evolve, they become granular cells of the **stratum granulosum**. Two types of granules exist in these cells: lamellar granules, made up of fats and lipids, and keratohyalin granules – protein filaments that help to harden the cell exterior. At the final layer, the keratinocyte loses its nucleus, flattens and dies. The **stratum corneum** is a keratinocyte graveyard. In essence, the journey from basale to corneum is the passage from life to death. The average life span of the keratinocyte is 22 days but can be as short as 15 days when keratinisation disorders exist. Animals with dandruff/seborrhoea have hyperkeratinisation disorders in which the keratinisation process has accelerated to a pathological point and skin is being shed, or **desquamated**, at an increased rate.

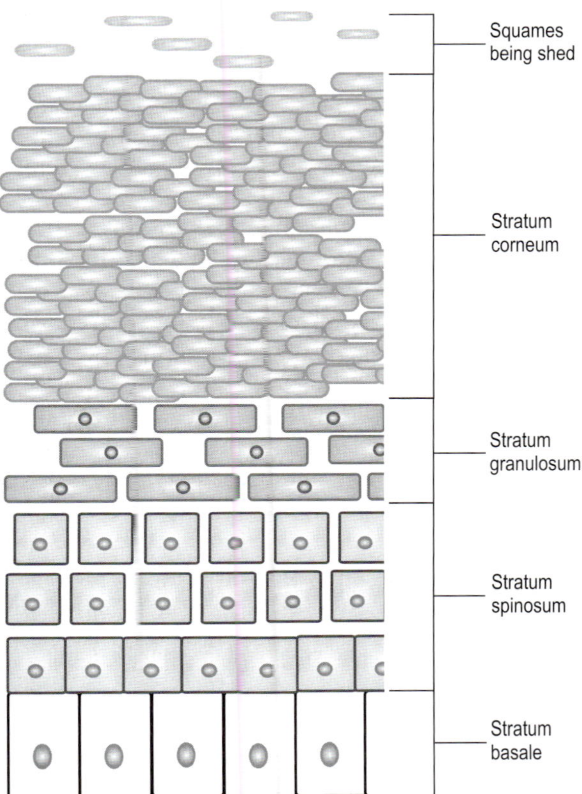

Figure 1.4 The layers of the epidermis.

The entire epidermal structure is usually 0.1–0.5 mm thick in haired areas, increasing in thickness in areas where greater wear occurs. Footpads can be up to 1.5 mm thick. In specialised areas, such as the nose and footpads, a clear, hard layer forms below the stratum corneum. This extra layer is known as the **stratum lucidum**. It can be very thick and provides a protective function. The living keratinocytes are usually only three or four cell layers thick, whereas the cornified layer can be as deep as 50 layers thick. In fact, over half the epidermis consists of the stratum corneum. While once thought of as merely a site for the shedding of deceased cells, it is now evident that the stratum corneum does have protective and immunological functions. The fats and lipids taken from the granulosum layer, mixed with sebum, form a cement between cornified cells. This cement seals in moisture and nutrients and creates a barrier to foreign substances. Additionally, within the cement, there are antimicrobial agents. Keratinocytes, in general, have the ability to phagocytose invading substances and can communicate information about invaders to lymphocytes, thus enabling the beginning of an immune response. Chemical messengers, such as interleukin-1, are produced by keratinocytes and used to relay messages to other cells, regarding the need for immunological defences. Keratinocytes injected with melanin provide protection from ultraviolet rays and give the animal's skin colour.

Cells other than keratinocytes exist within the epidermal layer. The recipe for an epidermis is as follows:

- 85% keratinocytes
- 8% Langerhans cells
- 5% melanocytes
- 2% miscellaneous, for example white blood cells and Merkel cells.

Langerhans cells are dendritic (have long branches) and come from the bone marrow. Langerhans cells cruise around in the epidermis and sample allergens attempting to force the keratinised barricades. Allergens are anything not of the body – parasites, topical medications, carpet powder, grass, pollens, bacteria from another animal's tooth, etc. The Langerhans cells take their samples to the local lymph node and present them to T-lymphocytes. The T-cells react to the presented antigens and proceed to the epidermis to do battle, or not, as the case may be. Over-reaction leads to an allergic response and under-reaction leads to invasion by foreign bodies. But more on this later....

Melanocytes are pigment-producing cells. Melanin is important as it absorbs ultraviolet rays and the harmful metabolites that occur when sunlight interacts with skin cells. Think of white cats with no ear tips due to squamous cell carcinomas. The number of melanocytes and their location determine the colour of the skin and hair in that area, on that animal. Dalmatians, for example obviously, have concentrations of melanocytes in their spots. The pigment melanin is produced in tiny packets called melanosomes. These melanosomes are injected into keratinocytes, in essence, dyeing them. The two major melanins are eumelanin, which is brown/black, and phaeomelanin, which is yellow/red.

Merkel cells are touch receptors. In the Merkel cell, the nucleus is actually in the top section of the cell and the nerve ending rests directly below, communicating eventually with the brain. Merkel cells are found beneath tylotrich pads, slightly thickened areas that are scattered over various parts of the body.

FUNCTIONS OF THE SKIN

So now we know the anatomy of the skin, what function does it serve? It actually has a myriad of functions, a dermatological dozen if you will:

1. The skin forms a watertight barrier which encloses and shapes the body while simultaneously protecting it.
2. The skin provides accommodation for hair follicles, along with sweat and sebaceous glands.
3. Through the use of hair, fat and blood vessels, the skin helps to regulate the body's temperature.
4. Utilising Merkel cells at tylotrich pads, vibrissae and free nerve endings, the skin provides sensory perception.
5. The skin is an external indicator of internal health, very useful for animals that can't tell us how they feel.
6. In the hypodermis, the skin provides a storage area for fat reserves.
7. As part of its protective function, the skin is a site for the first stages of an immune response. Inflammation via mast cells is one such response. Sampling by Langerhans cells and the resulting T-cell reaction is another example.
8. The skin participates in antimicrobial activity, utilising sebum and other chemicals.
9. The skin is an area for secretion and excretion: sweat, sebum, pheromones, etc.
10. Pigmentation in skin cells provides another protective function of the skin, and is involved in sexual displays, camouflage, et cetera.
11. Changes in blood pressure are aided by the vasodilation and vasoconstriction of blood vessels in the dermis.
12. Vitamin D, with the assistance of sunlight, is produced in the skin.

GLOSSARY OF TERMS

Adnexa: Associated glands, such as the sweat and sebaceous glands, associated with the hair follicle.

Alopecia: Baldness.

Anagen: The growth phase of a hair shaft.

Apocrine: A structure adjacent to a hair follicle – synonymous with epitrichial.

Arrector pili: The muscle associated with the hair follicle. When contracted, the hair raises, either to insulate the animal or to create a defensive posture.

Atrichial: Referring to a structure that does not occur in conjunction with the hair follicle. For example, a sweat gland occurring in a footpad.

Basement membrane: The junctional zone between the dermis and the epidermis. The basement membrane serves as both a barrier and a communication site between the dermis and epidermis.

Catagen: The intermediate phase in the hair growth cycle at which the hair shaft separates from its nutrient source.

Dermis: This is the middle layer of the skin. It is highly vascular and carries nutrients to the epidermis. The hair follicle and its associated structures exist within the dermis, as do blood and lymph vessels and nerve plexi.

Desmosomes: Spiny intercellular attachments.

Desquamation: Shedding of the cells of the stratum corneum.

Eccrine: Synonymous with atrichial.

Epidermis: This is a four- or five-layer structure that ends in a thick, horny, protective covering of dead cells. The layers of the epidermis are the: stratum basale, stratum spinosum, stratum granulosum, stratum lucidum (in specialised areas) and stratum corneum.

Epilate: To remove hair.

Epitrichial: Referring to a structure that occurs adjacent to the hair follicle ('tricho' being Latin for hair); for example: a sweat gland emptying into the hair follicle

Hypodermis: This is also known as the subcutis or the panniculus. It is the deepest layer of the skin and is primarily a fat storage area.

Keratinocytes: Skin cells of the epidermis.

Langerhans cells: Members of the immune system which travel mostly in the epidermis, sampling foreign substances and carrying messages about these substances to the lymph system.

Meibomian: A specialised sebaceous gland on the eyelid that contributes to the pre-corneal tear film.

Melanocytes: Pigment-producing cells found within the epidermis.

Merkel cells: Sensory cells in the epidermis, located at specialised pressure points at various locations in the body.

Moll gland: A specialised sweat gland on the eyelid that produces a protective substance for the cornea.

Sebaceous gland: A gland which secretes sebum into the hair follicle.

Sebum: Sebum consists of cells from the lining of the sebaceous gland plus oil. Sebum has moisturising and antibacterial functions.

Squames: The flattened cells of the stratum corneum.

Stratum basale: The deepest layer of the epidermis. This is where active reproduction of keratinocytes occurs.

Stratum corneum: This is the outermost layer of the epidermis. It can be up to 50 cell layers thick and consists of flattened, hard, anuclear cells. It is a protective barrier between the organism and the outside world.

Stratum granulosum: This is the third layer of the epidermis. The cells in this layer contain granules.

Stratum lucidum: This is a special layer of the epidermis that occurs only at the footpads and on the nose. It is a clear, hard, thick layer with a protective function.

Stratum spinosum: This is the second layer of the epidermis, consisting of cells strongly bound to each other by spiky connections known as desmosomes.

Telogen: The resting and final phase of the hair growth cycle.

Vibrissae: Commonly known as whiskers. These are specialised hairs with sensory capabilities.

Further Reading

Ackerman L 1993 Pet skin and hair coat problems. Veterinary Learning Systems, New Jersey, p 1-6

Foster A, Foil C (eds) 2003 BSAVA Manual of dermatology. BSAVA, Gloucester, p 1-10

Nesbitt G, Ackerman L 1998 Canine and feline dermatology. Veterinary Learning Systems, Trenton, New Jersey, p 6-24

Scott D W, Miller W, Griffin C E 2001 Muller and Kirk's Small animal dermatology, 6th edn. W B Saunders, London/NewYork, p 1-70

Chapter 2

Dermatology clinics

CHAPTER CONTENTS

Dermatology is a time-consuming art when performed properly. Taking a thorough history is essential for an accurate diagnosis. Client education is an important facet of treating a dermatological condition, and this can take a lot of time. In a busy general practice it is easy to cut corners in the interests of keeping your appointments on schedule – no one likes a waiting room full of impatient people. On the other hand, clients also want to find the cause of their pets' problems and not just treat the symptoms. Most pet owners want to understand how to carry out treatments properly at home. In the ideal world, every dermatology case should get a 60-minute appointment. This would afford you with sufficient time to get all the background information needed, carry out some in-house testing and then adequately train the client in any procedures that need to be carried out at home. Outside of the referral centre, 1-hour appointments are not feasible. However, if a vet and nurse can work together on dermatology cases, twice the amount of work can be achieved in the limited time available!

There are several different ways to involve the nurse in dermatological examinations. It is best if the veterinarians and nurses at a practice create a system that works for their particular practice. Some methods of approaching skin cases include:

1. Requesting that clients fill out a questionnaire (see the examples in this chapter) regarding the pet's skin condition before attending a consultation. This can be done via the post or directly prior to the appointment while waiting in the reception area.

2. Having the veterinary nurse take a brief medical and dermatological history prior to the consultation with the vet. This can be done in an examination room, or even in the reception area if necessary.
3. The veterinary nurse can do a general health examination, take a medical and dermatological history (sample forms below) and proceed with basic diagnostic tests prior to the consultation with the veterinary surgeon.
4. The nursing staff can run regular 'flea clinics'. These clinics would be open to registered clients. Flea clinics can be free of charge as long as a flea product is purchased. Explaining appropriate flea control can be time consuming and should be done by a knowledgeable member of staff. Most clients don't know about the flea life cycle and don't understand why supermarket insecticides are not effective.

Regardless of the approach taken, it should be assumed by the reception staff that dermatological problems will take longer to deal with than a routine visit. Double appointments should be booked for skin cases and charges should be adjusted accordingly. It may help to explain to clients that one longer, slightly more expensive appointment will increase the likelihood of solving the problem more quickly and, in the long run, less expensively. Practices do need to charge for a nurse's time when a complete history is taken and a dermatological examination is performed as these appointments will take at least 30 minutes. It does not make sense to give away the time of specially trained and qualified personnel! A well-performed preliminary dermatological examination is a valuable service to both the pet and the client and certainly worth a monetary investment. Of course, nurses cannot diagnose or prescribe medications so the animal must always see a veterinarian after a preliminary work-up is completed by a nurse.

It should be pointed out that dermatology cases often require follow-up appointments. Once a diagnosis is established and a treatment plan is organised by the veterinarian, follow-up appointments could be carried out by a qualified veterinary nurse. If progress is not continuing smoothly, the nurse can bring her concerns to the veterinarian overseeing the case and appropriate appointments can be made with the veterinary surgeon as necessary. Again, follow-up appointments carried out by nurses can be charged for, albeit at a lesser fee than consultations with a veterinary surgeon. The loss in revenue can be balanced by the fact that the animal may be seen more often by a nurse than a vet. This will enable closer monitoring of the case and aid the client with any difficulties he or she may be having carrying out the treatments at home. Clients will be more compliant if they receive more frequent feedback and assistance, especially with challenging situations such as food trials and frequent bathing. Telephone contacts are supportive as well, and can easily be carried out by a nurse. All telephone conversations should be logged and the information gathered would be kept with the animal's notes.

Vets are often worried that allowing nurses more responsibility will reduce revenue. Usually the reverse is true. Allowing a nurse to carry out dermatology clinics frees the vet to proceed with other business. With extra time being invested in dermatology cases, more diagnostic tests can be carried out. With increased client compliance, more medication and ancillary products are sold. Finally, putting time into dermatology cases generally results in more accurate diagnosis and more effective treatment plans – in other words, happier clients and healthier patients.

An example of a medical history form is shown in Figure 2.1.

A detailed medical examination should always be done by a veterinary surgeon. However, a nurse is perfectly capable of assessing an animal's overall state of health and whether or not the body systems are functioning in an efficient manner. Some skin conditions will cause a general state of disease with pyrexia, depression and anorexia. Conversely, some systemic disease states will have a dermatological component.

The animal should be observed at rest, before beginning any investigative procedures. Notice how the animal is sitting or laying down. Does it look comfortable? Does respiration seem even and of a normal rate? (Normal is approximately 20–30 breaths per minute.) Are there any signs of increased inspiratory or expiratory effort? How does the animal move? Is it stiff or are there any signs of proprioception deficits? Is there a head tilt?

The body condition score begins at 1 with an emaciated animal, 2 being an obviously thin animal,

MEDICAL HISTORY

Client's Name: Pet's name:

Species: Breed: Sex:

Neutered: Yes/No Vaccination status:

Lifestyle: town/country Working/show/pet

How long in current owner's possession? Imported: Yes/No

Any overseas travel:

Other in-contact pets:

Where exercised:

Where does pet sleep and on what bedding?

What food is fed?

What snacks/treats fed?

Previous, current or chronic health problems:

Behaviour problems and/or any recent changes in behaviour:

Appetite: Consistency of stool:

Level of thirst: Frequency of urination:

Exercise tolerance: Recent changes in weight:

Coughing/sneezing Discharges from any orifice:

Has pet been wormed and with what treatment?

Have flea treatments been used on pet and/or environment? Note product(s) used.

Is the animal on any current medication or supplements?

Figure 2.1 Medical history form.

3 is the ideal state, 4 somewhat overweight, and 5 being obese.

Note the strength of the pulse and whether there is a difference between the heart rate and pulse rate. Irregular sounds and arrhythmias should be looked out for, along with any sounds of rattling or fluid in the chest. Observe the mucus membranes for colour and capillary refill time. The lymph nodes should be palpated and any swelling noted. The abdomen should also be palpated – and the testes as well in intact males.

Starting at the nose and moving caudally, examine the body for discharges, injuries or any abnormalities.

An example of a medical examination form is shown in Figure 2.2.

The questionnaire depicted in Figure 2.3 (dermatological history) can be conducted as an oral interview with the client or given to the client to complete in the waiting room prior to the appointment. Some dermatologists post questionnaires to their clients and ask the client to bring in the completed form when attending the consultation.

A thorough hands-on dermatological examination is the final step in the history-gathering process. It is during the examination that lesions are identified. It is helpful to use a diagram to mark down where the lesions occur on the animal. Various types of lesion are described in a glossary at the end of this chapter. Dermatological terms should be used to describe the skin conditions observed. Begin

MEDICAL EXAMINATION

General demeanour: Body Condition Score: (1–5)

Weight: Temperature: Pulse:

Respiration: Colour of mucus membranes: Capillary refill time:

Comments on chest auscultation:

Palpation of lymph nodes (mandibular, pre-scapular, axillary, inguinal, popliteal):

Any obvious defects/injuries of:

Eyes

Ears

Nose

Dorsum

Ventrum

Limbs

Feet

Genitals and anal region

Figure 2.2 Medical examination form.

DERMATOLOGICAL HISTORY

What is the presenting complaint?

Are any other pets in household affected with a skin condition?

Are any people in the household affected with a skin condition?

When did the problem start?

What was the age of your pet when the problem started?

What did the skin condition look like at the beginning?

Where on the body did the skin problem start?

Has the problem become progressively worse?

Have you noticed your pet rubbing/scooting/chewing or licking itself/scratching/ grooming excessively? (Circle all that apply.)

Was the animal itchy at the beginning of the condition? If so, has it become more uncomfortable over time?

On a scale of 1–5, with 1 being slightly itchy and 5 being tremendously itchy, describe how itchy your animal is:

Does the skin condition get worse at a certain time of year?

Has your pet had recent or chronic digestive problems?

Have you noticed any hair loss? Where on the animal?

Have female pets : (a) been spayed?

(b) had abnormal or irregular cycles?

(c) been pregnant?

Figure 2.3 Dermatological history form.

Have male pets : (a) been neutered?
(b) are other male dogs attracted to your male dog?

Medication:

List any medications or supplements you have used on your pet for this condition, including shampoos and ointments:

Have any of the above treatments helped? If so, which ones?

Please list any current medications, including dosage:

Please list any flea control products you have used recently:

How often do you use flea products?

Have your treated your home and car with an insecticide?

Clinical signs:

Please tick if any of the following are present or have occurred in the past:

Greasy skin or coat __
Dandruff (scurf) __
Scabies (mange) __
Red skin __
Dark patches on skin __
Earmites (canker) __
Light patches on skin __
Ringworm__
Thickened skin __
Pimples (spots) __
Open sores __
Scabs __
Small bumps __
Lumps __
Hair loss __

Scratching __
Chewing __
Licking __
Rubbing __
Scooting __
Overgrooming __
Scratching at ears __
Shaking head __
Hairballs __

Fleas __
Lice __

Any comments you wish to add:

Figure 2.3—cont'd Dermatological history form.

at the nose and work towards the tail, as with any clinical examination.

DERMATOLOGICAL EXAMINATION

Nose: Any crusting or colour changes?
Oral cavity: Observe for lesions – for example, ulcers, blisters, haemorrhages, et cetera.
Eyes: Check for ocular discharge, inversion or eversion of eyelids, alopecia around eyes (the 'spectacled' look).
Muzzle: Examine lip folds for moist dermatitis.
Ears: Note the colour of the inside of pinnae, look for any crusting on the edges of the pinnae, examine any exudate, note smell coming from ear, ascertain whether the vertical canal is inflamed or thickened. Use an otoscope to visualise the tympanic membrane if possible. If scabies is suspected, try a pedal-pinnal reflex test by rubbing the edges of the pinna together. If this action instigates scratching with the hind leg, it is worthwhile taking several skin scrapes for sarcoptid mites.
Dorsum: Move through the hair coat on the back of the pet. Examine the health of the coat as well as observing the skin for lesions, scale, crust and external parasites.
Ventrum: It is sometimes easier to stand the animal on its hind legs to examine the abdomen, although

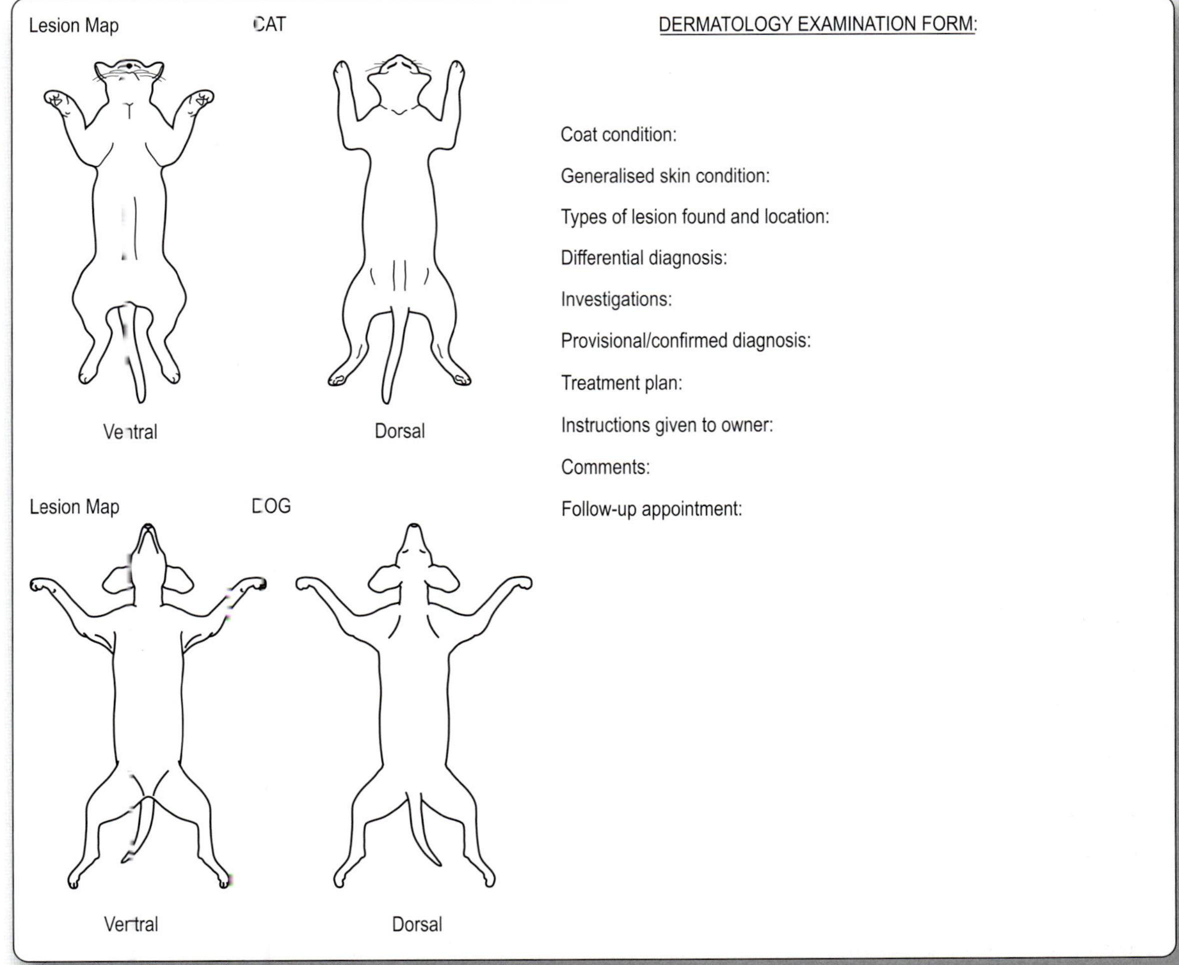

Lesion Map CAT

Ventral Dorsal

Lesion Map DOG

Ventral Dorsal

DERMATOLOGY EXAMINATION FORM:

Coat condition:

Generalised skin condition:

Types of lesion found and location:

Differential diagnosis:

Investigations:

Provisional/confirmed diagnosis:

Treatment plan:

Instructions given to owner:

Comments:

Follow-up appointment:

Figure 2.4 Dermatology examination form.

some pets will roll over and allow you to explore the chest and abdomen. The colour of the skin should be noted, any obvious lesions, thickening of skin and areas of hair loss.

Limbs: Examine for lesions, lumps or swellings.

Feet: Examine the state of the nails: are they brittle, cracked or broken? Is the nail bed inflamed? Look between the webs of the toes to note the colour of the skin, any lesions, parasites or malodour. Examine the pads for fissures and skin thickness. Look between the pads for foreign bodies, lesions, and skin colour, et cetera.

Perianal region: Check for skin colour and signs of self-trauma. Note the state of the anal sacs and the type of discharge from them.

Note any lumps or swellings found on the body.

A form like the one depicted in Figure 2.4 can be used, marking the areas on the diagrams where lesions appear. An example of how this form would be filled in is shown in Figure 2.5.

Figure 2.6 shows a progress report form used for follow-up appointments.

It is recommended that clients be given an appointments card on which to log their visits. The

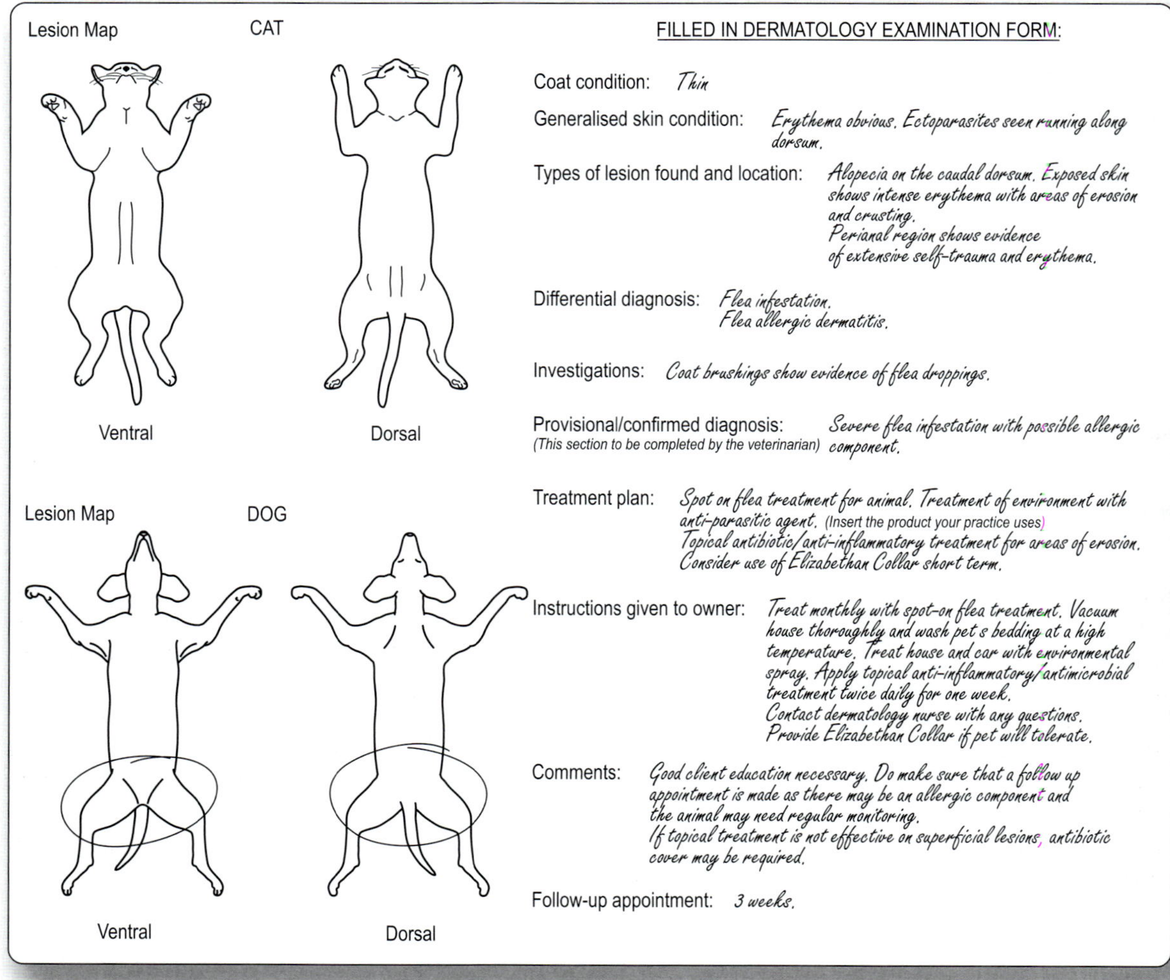

Lesion Map CAT

Ventral Dorsal

Lesion Map DOG

Ventral Dorsal

FILLED IN DERMATOLOGY EXAMINATION FORM:

Coat condition: *Thin*

Generalised skin condition: *Erythema obvious. Ectoparasites seen running along dorsum.*

Types of lesion found and location: *Alopecia on the caudal dorsum. Exposed skin shows intense erythema with areas of erosion and crusting.*
Perianal region shows evidence of extensive self-trauma and erythema.

Differential diagnosis: *Flea infestation.*
Flea allergic dermatitis.

Investigations: *Coat brushings show evidence of flea droppings.*

Provisional/confirmed diagnosis: *Severe flea infestation with possible allergic component.*
(This section to be completed by the veterinarian)

Treatment plan: *Spot on flea treatment for animal. Treatment of environment with anti-parasitic agent.* (Insert the product your practice uses)
Topical antibiotic/anti-inflammatory treatment for areas of erosion.
Consider use of Elizabethan Collar short term.

Instructions given to owner: *Treat monthly with spot-on flea treatment. Vacuum house thoroughly and wash pet's bedding at a high temperature. Treat house and car with environmental spray. Apply topical anti-inflammatory/antimicrobial treatment twice daily for one week.*
Contact dermatology nurse with any questions.
Provide Elizabethan Collar if pet will tolerate.

Comments: *Good client education necessary. Do make sure that a follow up appointment is made as there may be an allergic component and the animal may need regular monitoring.*
If topical treatment is not effective on superficial lesions, antibiotic cover may be required.

Follow-up appointment: *3 weeks.*

Figure 2.5 Filled-in dermatology examination form.

PROGRESS REPORT

Overall condition of coat and skin:

Types of lesion found and locations:

Level of progress: Regressed/Static/Improved

Investigations:

Revised treatment plan:

Advice to owner:

Next appointment:

Figure 2.6 Progress report form.

appointments card should have room to write down the treatments required, as shown in Figure 2.7.

Thorough client education is essential in order to gain good owner compliance and thus success in treatment. Many of the pharmaceutical companies produce helpful leaflets that can be given to clients. Leaflets on how to clean the ear, shampoo your dog and treat the home for a flea infestation are all available. Alternatively, a practice can devise it's own leaflet to give to clients. Don't just hand out literature though, explain the procedure, have the client demonstrate on his/her pet how to do the procedure and then send home the leaflet for reinforcement purposes only.

It is necessary to learn the dermatological terms in order to describe the lesions accurately. In this way, you can record your findings in the history in terms that any future reader will be able to interpret correctly. The glossary below should be of use.

Appointment card

Date	TREATMENT PROGRAMME – MEDICATION/DOSAGE/FREQUENCY (please bring all medications with you to every appointment, including shampoos, dips)	Next Appt.

Figure 2.7 Appointment card.

GLOSSARY OF TERMS

Location

Generalised: A skin condition that is affecting the entire body, or most of the body of the animal. Generalised alopecia would be a bald dog.

Focal: This is a lesion that has a specific location. One ringworm lesion can be focal. Multi-focal is a term used to describe lesions that occur in several specific locations, such as an animal with several epithelial tumours.

Localised: The skin condition is contained within one area of the body, for example, a dog with demodicosis which only manifests as pododermatitis.

In addition, proper anatomical directions should be given: *cranial/caudal, dorsal/ventral, rostral, plantar/palmar, proximal/distal and medial/lateral.*

Skin character

Erythema: Reddened, as part of the inflammatory process.

Crusty: Dried exudate on the skin. The exudate can be pus, blood or serum.

Hyperpigmentation: Darkened areas of skin, often due to chronic inflammation.

Hyperplastic: Thickening and remodelling of skin due to chronic inflammation. Hyperplastic skin changes are often seen in cases of chronic otitis.

Leukoderma: Areas where pigmentation is less than normal.

Lichenified: Skin is thickened. This is usually seen in response to chronic inflammation.

Pruritic: Itchy.

Scaly: Lots of fragments from the top layer of the epidermis (stratum corneum). When the skin has been insulted, the keratinisation process is accelerated, increasing the amount of shed keratinocytes.

The skin can also be described as *thin* or *fragile*, as is seen in dogs with Cushing's syndrome.

Coat character

Alopecia: Loss of hair.

Dry

Greasy

Leukotrichia: Loss of pigmentation in hair.

The coat can be described as thin, or staring, unkempt, patchy and moth-eaten.

Types of lesion

Bulla: A fluid-filled lesion greater than 1 cm in diameter. These are commonly known as blisters and can be seen in pemphigus vulgaris cases.

Comedo: A hair follicle filled with keratinous debris, better known as a blackhead. Comedos are often seen in cases of demodectic mange.

Erosion: The top layers of the epidermis have been lost but the basement membrane is intact. Erosions can be the result of self-trauma due to pruritus.

Excoriation: This is a linear erosion and is usually caused by scratching due to pruritus.

Fissure: This is a split in the skin that can be of varying depths.

Lentigo: Areas with increased melanin deposits, forming either macules or patches. As a disease, this is known as lentiginosis profusa and is a rare, multi-focal skin disease found primarily in Pugs.

Leukoderma: An area of depigmentation.

Macule: This is a clearly delineated area of altered pigmentation that is less than 1 cm in diameter.

Nodule: A nodule is a raised, well-demarcated area of skin that is greater than 1 cm in diameter. A nodule can extend into the deeper layers of the skin.

Papule: This is a raised, circumscribed lesion less than 1 cm in diameter. Papules are commonly found in cases of pyoderma.

Patch: An area of clearly delineated colour change in a size greater than 1 cm. A scar can be described as a patch.

Plaque: A raised flat swelling greater than 1 cm in diameter. Plaques are sometimes formed in areas of chronic inflammation.

Pustule: A raised, well-circumscribed lesion containing pus. Pustules are often associated with pyoderma. In people, pustules are commonly known as pimples or spots.

Ulcer: This is loss of the skin layers right down to the dermis. An ulcer progresses from an erosion and is a serious break in the integrity of the protective skin layers.

Vesicle: A raised, fluid-filled, well-circumscribed lesion less than 1 cm in diameter. Pemphigus vulgaris has intra-oral vesicles as one of its clinical signs.

Wheal: A raised area caused by oedema. Wheals can be seen in acute allergic reactions and as reactions to insect bites. In people, we usually refer to this as 'hives'.

Descriptive terms for the lesions

Annular: Ring like. Some dermatophytes (the fungi that cause ringworm) will form annular lesions.

Linear: Excoriations are often linear in fashion.

Serpiginous: 'Serpent-like'. A wavy lesion pattern like this can be seen in the disease erythema multiforme.

Symmetrical: Lesions that appear in the same place on both sides of the body are symmetrical. This is often seen in endocrine disease.

Target: This looks like a circle with a target in the middle. This type of lesion can be seen in erythema multiforme.

Terms referring to the feet

As the feet have claws, they have a whole array of problems that do not occur elsewhere in the body. Thus they have their own vocabulary:

Onychogryphosis: Deformity or overgrowth of the nail.

Onychomadesis: Shedding of the nail.

Onychorhexis: Brittle nails.

Paronychia: Inflammation of the nail bed.

Further Reading

Ackerman L 1993 Pet skin and hair coat problems. Veterinary Learning Systems, Trenton, NJ, p 3-5

Hill Peter B 2002 Small animal dermatology. Elsevier Science, Oxford, p 1-15

Mueller Ralf S 2000 Dermatology for the small animal practitioner. Teton New Media, Jackson, Wyoming, p 1-10

Nesbitt G, Ackerman L 1998 Canine and feline dermatology. Veterinary Learning Systems, Trenton, NJ, p 25-71

Chapter 3

Diagnostic tests

CHAPTER CONTENTS

One of the most exciting things about dermatology is how one quick, diagnostic procedure can change an animal's life. For example, sarcoptic mange is probably the most pruritic disease that can affect a canine. Dogs will literally tear themselves to shreds in response to 'fox mange'. Yet, the solution is so simple. One can do a few skin scrapings right on the consult table, look at the material gathered under the microscope and make a diagnosis, all within 10 minutes time. The treatment for sarcoptic mange is straightforward and, in almost all cases, successful.

Many diagnostic tests for dermatological conditions can be done in-house. Often the tests can be done quickly enough to provide answers the same day the animal is seen. This can be immensely gratifying, especially when a pet has been suffering from an extremely uncomfortable condition. Being able to perform these procedures is a real contribution to animal welfare. In addition, successfully and rapidly diagnosing skin conditions can make you very popular with your clients.

Most diagnostic procedures are simple to learn and do not need a lot of costly equipment. The cost of procedures can be included within a dermatology consultation charge, or procedures can be charged for individually. It is well within a qualified nurse's remit of responsibility to perform dermatological diagnostic procedures. A nurse working with a vet can expedite a dermatology consultation by collecting samples and performing necessary tests while the vet gathers history from the client.

The basic equipment list for dermatology must begin with a decent microscope. The microscope should have an adjustable stage and at least three objectives – low power, high power and oil immersion. Most objectives will have low-power lenses of ×4 or ×10, a high-power lens of ×40 and an oil-immersion lens of ×100. Binocular-vision microscopes are preferred over monocular. A good microscope is a practice investment. It is a reasonably costly piece of equipment, but if used regularly it pays for itself rapidly. Naturally, a microscope needs consistent maintenance, as does any piece of practice equipment.

A few basic rules to remember about microscope care should be listed and posted near the microscope so that all members of the practice adhere to these rules. It takes only one uninformed person to create a repair bill for £500. A diagram of a microscope is included in this chapter for further study (see Fig. 3.1).

1. Never leave the light source on after finishing with the microscope.
2. Do not over-use the immersion oil.
3. Never leave a slide in place after finishing viewing, and NEVER, NEVER leave a slide in place with the lamp on!!
4. Clean the lens with proper lens tissue immediately after use.

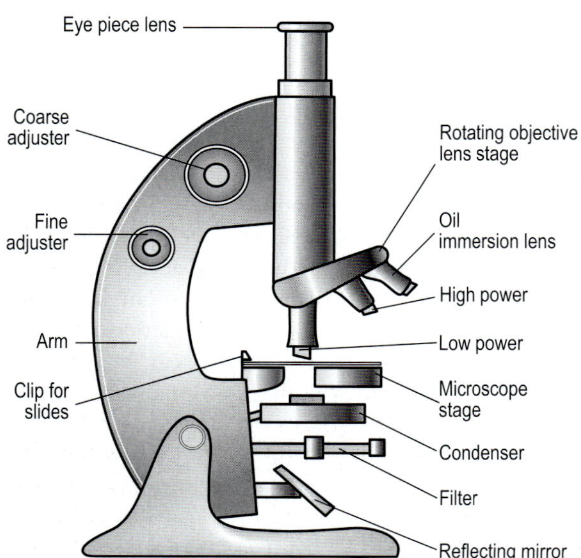

Figure 3.1 Compound light microscope with parts labelled: stage, diaphragm, substage condenser, objectives.

5. Leave the low-power objective in place when finished viewing.
   - Once a day, the microscope should be wiped down with methanol, using lens tissue. The objectives and stage can be carefully wiped with methanol at this time.
   - Once weekly, the objective lenses can be removed and dusted with a soft paintbrush. The lens itself can be wiped with a cotton bud dipped in methanol. Using a circular pattern, the lens should be cleaned from the centre outwards. A cotton bud dipped in methanol can also be used to clean the condensor, the eye pieces and the lens in the base of the microscope.
   - If the bulb needs changing, be sure to avoid touching the bulb directly with fingers, as natural oils from skin will cause the bulb to overheat.
   - An annual service by a professional microscope maintenance person should be booked. Expect to pay £50–£100. University, hospital or professional laboratories can give you the name of a maintenance person that they recommend.

The equipment needed for microscope use and maintenance is as follows:

- oil for oil immersion
- liquid paraffin or mineral oil
- microscope slides
- coverslips
- permanent marker (to label slides)
- acetate tape
- slide holders
- lens tissue
- methanol
- cotton buds
- soft paintbrush
- Romanowsky stains (Diff-Quik, Dade Behring or Rapi-Diff, Triangle Biomedical Services).

So what are we going to look at under the microscope? Certainly insects and arachnids, but much more than that. Just examining shafts of hair can tell us a lot about an animal's skin problem. Yeast may be found in some samples, as may fungal spores. Aspirates from lumps can be examined cytologically. A great deal can be done in-house before it becomes necessary to send samples to professional laboratories. In-house testing can save time as well as money. This is important in busy charity practices and is good for public relations for private practices.

THE TRICHOGRAPH

The simplest material to gather is hair. There are a variety of methods used, all of which will give you slightly different information about the condition of the animal.

Combing

Pulling a flea comb through an animal's coat will gather loose hair, some shed squames (scurf) and perhaps a flea or flea debris. The material from the comb can be pushed onto a slide prepared with a drop of liquid paraffin and then covered with a coverslip. Examine under low power for evidence of ectoparasites. A profusion of dead cells in the sample may be indicative of a keratinisation disorder. An abundance of hair which easily pulls free may hint at an endocrine disorder. The hair can be observed for its stage of development. Lots of hair in the telogen phase may also point towards hypothyroidism. A profusion of broken hairs will indicate self-trauma – the animal has been chewing at its coat. This will tell you that the pet is itchy. So, even if the owner had not seen the pet scratching or rubbing, you will have evidence that the condition the cat or dog is experiencing is a pruritic one – this is an important diagnostic clue!

Coat brushing

Vigorously rub the animal's coat while the pet is standing on the examination table. (You will find that most dogs love this technique but cats may have varying opinions.) If you suspect a flea infestation, put down a damp white paper towel before rubbing the animal. Flea droppings falling onto the damp towel will become red – and the blood-stained towel is an excellent way of convincing an owner that his or her pet truly does have fleas. Taking a clean slide, the debris gathered can be swept onto a slide prepared with a drop of liquid paraffin. Both combing and brushing will yield information about the health of the hair coat, i.e. its stage of development, ease of epilation, presence of ectoparasites and whether or not there are broken shafts.

Hair plucks

Using a pair of epilating forceps (tweezers), pluck hair and place it on a slide prepared with liquid paraffin. This method will tell you about the ease of epilation and the age of the shaft. You will not have epithelial debris to examine but you will be able to identify follicular casts, which can indicate some problem in the hair follicle itself. One disease that affects hair follicles is demodectic mange. It is also possible with the hair-pluck method to pluck a *Demodex* mite right out of its domicile in the hair follicle. If you suspect *Demodex*, pluck hair from affected areas. This may be around the eyes and between the toes. Louse eggs (or nits) are cemented to hair shafts so pluckings can also aptly diagnose a louse infestation. In addition, plucked hair can be examined under a higher power (×40) objective for fungal spores. This does take a lot of practice but can be a useful test for identifying dermatophytes. (See Fig. 3.2 below.)

Materials needed for trichology

- Flea comb
- Microscope slides
- Coverslips
- Liquid paraffin
- Epilating forceps
- White paper towel.

SKIN SCRAPINGS

Skin scrapings are commonly performed to identify either *Sarcoptes scabiei* (mange mites), *Cheyletiella* mites or *Demodex canis/cati*. To catch a scabies mite you will need to do three to five scrapes in areas favoured by these mites: the edges of the pinnae, the chest, and the carpal, the tarsal and elbow regions. Apply one drop of liquid paraffin to a number 10 scalpel blade and one drop of paraffin to a microscope slide. Scrape the skin area chosen at a 45° angle until capillary ooze is created. Scrape the debris gathered on the blade onto a slide and examine under low power. It is best if the condenser on the microscope is partially closed as this

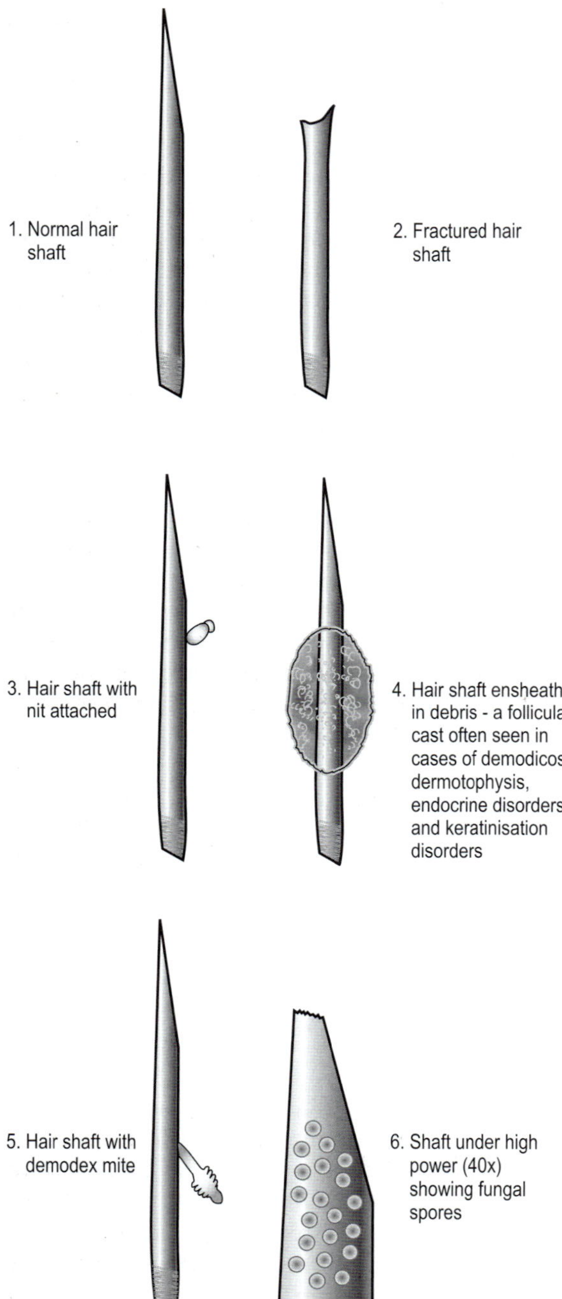

Figure 3.2 Trichography: hair shafts. A: A normal hair shaft. B: A fractured hair shaft. C: A hair shaft with nit attached. D: A hair shaft ensheathed in debris – a follicular cast, often seen in cases of demodicosis, dermatophytosis, endocrine disorders and keratinisation disorders. E: A hair shaft with *Demodex* mite. F: A shaft under high power (40×) showing fungal spores.

creates better lighting for the visualisation of mites. Finding one mite or an egg is diagnostic for sarcoptic mange. However, scrapings are not always successful and scabies should not be eliminated as a diagnosis if clinical signs are consistent with the disease. Serology can be done for evidence of antibodies to *Sarcoptes scabiei* saliva. If scrapes are negative but the dog is pruritic with alopecia and crusting in typical areas of infestation, proceed to a blood test.

For *Demodex canis/cati*, deep scrapes are necessary. The same materials should be prepared but the site locations are different. *Demodex* mites proliferate between the digits and around the eyes. These can be difficult areas to scrape so you should also do hair plucks if *Demodex* is suspected. The skin chosen should be squeezed and scraping should continue until a decent area of abrasion with capillary ooze is created. Scrape at least five sites, if possible. The material gathered can be placed onto a slide with liquid paraffin and examined under low power, with the condenser partially closed. Discovering one mite or egg is diagnostic. Again, one may not be lucky enough to catch these parasites. Currently, there is no blood test available for identifying demodectic mange, and the treatment for demodicosis is much more demanding and extensive than that for scabies, i.e. regular dips versus a spot-on treatment. Choosing to diagnose by clinical trial is, therefore, a difficult decision. Some vets will opt for a biopsy to identify suspected demodicosis before committing an animal and its owner to several weeks of amitraz dips.

Materials needed for skin scrapes

- Number 10 scalpel blades
- Microscope slides
- Coverslips
- Liquid paraffin.

Health and safety tip: Sarcoptic mange is zoonotic! If you suspect it, wear gloves and an apron when examining the animal. Scrupulously clean the examination room after the consultation.

TAPE STRIPS

Tape strippings are commonly used to identify infection with the yeast *Malassezia pachydermatis*. A piece of acetate tape (3M Scotch tape is the best as it holds up well in the stains) is stuck to the areas of skin in question. *Malassezia* likes to grow in warm, moist places so try skin folds, interdigitally and inside the pinnae. Press the tape several times to the area in order to gather as much material as possible. The tape is then secured to one end of a slide, looped and then attached to the opposite side of the slide. The loop of tape is dipped in modified Wright's stain ('Diff-Quik' or 'Rapi-Diff'). Dip the tape five times in each stain, starting with the fixative (light-blue stain), moving on to the red eosin stain and then the dark-blue thiazine stain. Be sure to count out a full second with each dip, so that the tape gets 5 full seconds in each stain.

When you have finished dipping, peel off one end of the loop and fasten the tape flat to the slide. Rinse the back of the slide and then pat the slide dry in a paper towel. When dry, apply one drop of immersion oil and examine under the oil-immersion objective. *Malassezia* yeasts have been described as peanut or dumbbell-shaped. They are dark blue after staining by the method described. The yeast is a commensal organism so one or two found on a full slide examination would not indicate a problem. However, more than one yeast per high-power field can be defined as a *Malassezia* infection and warrant treatment. A photograph is included in this book to help with identification (see Chapter 5, Fig. 5.6).

Materials needed

- Acetate tape
- Microscope slides
- Immersion oil
- Romanowsky stains
- Paper towels.

Do remember to clean the oil objective after viewing and be sure to put the low-power objective back in place. Remove oil from the stage if necessary. *Health and safety tip*: Dispose of all microscope slides in a glass bin once they have been viewed. Broken glass can be dangerous, and live mites can escape from slides! If you wish to save a slide, clearly label it with a permanent marker and place it in a slide holder.

OTOSCOPY

Otoscopic examination is a necessary part of every skin examination. The dermatology nurse should be familiar with the use of an otoscope and should be able to look down an ear canal and identify the tympanic membrane. When examining the ear, the colour of the pinna, as well as the auditory meatus and the vertical and horizontal canals should be noted. The type and quantity of exudate are important observations to record. A swab may need to be taken from the ear canal, and occasionally tape strippings are taken from the pinnae. Bacterial and yeast infections of the ear are common. Ear infections can exist in isolation or be part of a greater disease picture, such as atopy or food sensitivity.

A different otoscope head should be used to examine each ear canal because the left canal may contain different organisms to the right canal. This should also be remembered when dispensing ear drops and cleaners. If different organisms are identified in different canals, a different bottle of medication will need to be dispensed for each ear.

It is handy to keep a bowl of disinfectant in the consulting room. After the head of the otoscope has been wiped down with spirit it should soak in a disinfectant for 10 minutes. Be sure that the disinfectant is effective against Gram-negative organisms and fungal spores.

Materials needed

- Otoscope
- At least two otoscope heads
- Disinfectant.

CYTOLOGY FROM A SWAB

Cytology can reveal the microbial milieu of the ear canal. Bacteria and yeast may be identified. Additionally, you may gain an idea about what type of bacteria are prevalent in the area swabbed. Commonly, the ear is swabbed, utilising a cotton bud. Do not dig deep into the canal – a gentle circling of the inner rim of the auditory meatus is adequate. Roll the contents of the swab onto a clean glass slide and then stain with Diff Quik/Rapi-Diff, as described above. Examine your findings with the oil-immersion lens.

Neutrophils tend to stain violet to purple and are relatively large cells. You may also find cocci (round bacteria) singly, in groups, or in strings, as with streptococci. Round, dark brown/black objects inside an epithelial cell are likely to be melanin, not cocci. This can be confusing at first, but as you look at more slides it becomes easier to distinguish between cocci and melanin granules.

Cocci are Gram-positive bacteria are, on the dog, usually *Staphylococcus intermedius*. This is a commensal bacterium that overgrows only when the skin is in a diseased state. Rod-shaped bacteria are Gram-negative and do not normally appear on the skin. Rods can exist only on unhealthy skin – a moist, dirty ear is a favoured breeding ground for Gram-negative bacteria such as *Pseudomonas* spp. Identifying the type of bacteria can help you choose appropriate antibacterial agents. Many antibacterials are not effective against Gram negatives and would thus be a waste of time and money for an ear infested with *Pseudomonas* spp. In-house cytology is not a substitute for culture and sensitivity testing however. If Gram-negative bacteria are sited on a slide, it is best to take a sterile swab sample and send it to a professional laboratory for bacteriology, culture and sensitivity. In this way, the correct treatment can be implemented from the start and the animal is not left suffering with inappropriate antibiotic coverage.

Materials needed

- Cotton buds
- Glass slides
- Romanowsky stains
- Immersion oil
- Sterile swabs with transport medium.

IMPRESSION SMEAR

Another way of studying the cellular make-up of a lesion is by gathering material for an impression smear. Pustules can be pricked with a 20 gauge needle and then a glass slide pressed to the pustule. Another glass slide is then placed at a perpendicular angle onto the material sampled. Press down and then slide off the top slide. This action should spread the material enough to form a thin layer of cells. Stain and examine as above.

Findings should, in most cases, include neutrophils and bacteria. A sterile pustule is a rare finding and would indicate the need for further testing, possibly a biopsy.

FINE-NEEDLE ASPIRATE BIOPSY

Fine-needle aspirate biopsy (FNAB) is a technique used to gather material from inside a raised lesion. Cutaneous masses can be investigated using a 23 gauge needle and a 5 ml syringe. Wipe the area with surgical spirit and then insert the needle and pull back to aspirate two or three times. Without completely removing the needle from the skin, readjust the needle several times, repeatedly drawing back on the syringe. When you feel that you have aspirated something, remove the needle from the skin and detach the syringe. Fill the syringe with air and re-attach it to the needle. Then spray the contents of the needle onto a slide. Stain and examine under oil immersion (See Fig. 3.3.).

The finished slide may reveal fat cells, or serum, or possibly even mast cells. Multiple mast cells may indicate that the animal is developing a malignant neoplasm. A biopsy must be harvested as soon as possible!!! Mast cell tumours can grow very quickly. If caught in the early stages, mast cell tumours can be controlled and the prognosis is good. If left for even a few weeks, the tumour may metastasise, then the prognosis can be guarded to grave. With any lump or bump it is ALWAYS worth doing an FNAB. It is a simple test that takes very little time and costs the client little money. The one time you feel the lump and decide it is only a lipoma may be the one time you are wrong. Most clients do worry about lumps and want to know what is growing on their pets. It is always better to know rather than guess. However, cytology is no substitute for biopsy and histopathology. A definitive diagnosis should be made from a biopsy sample rather than an aspirate.

Materials needed

- 22 gauge needle
- 5 ml syringe
- Slides
- Romanowsky stains
- Immersion oil.

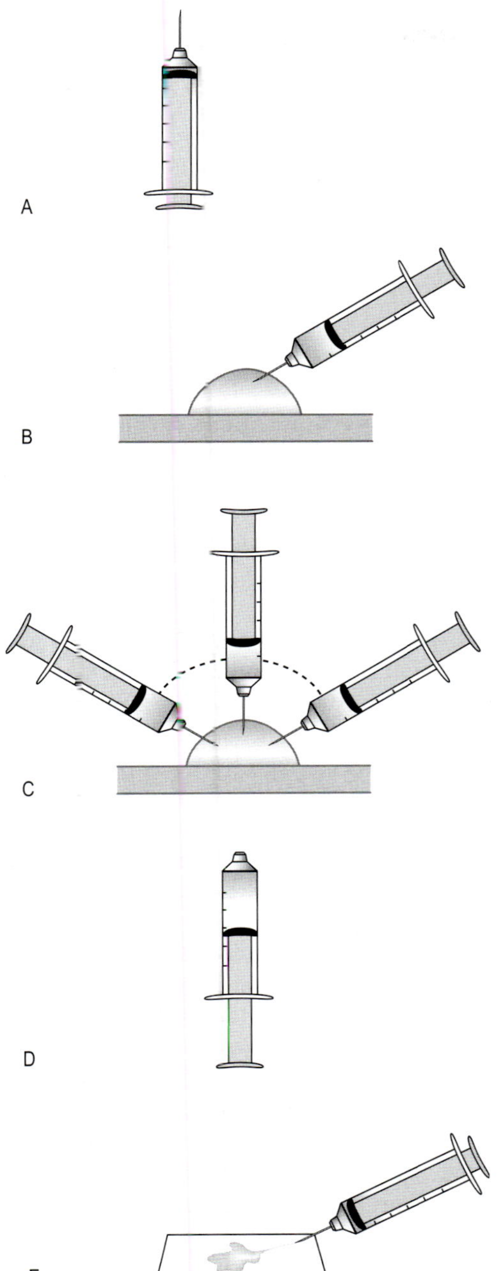

Figure 3.3 Fine-needle aspirate biopsy technique. A: Select a 5 ml syringe and a 23 gauge needle. B: Insert needle into the mass and pull back on the syringe plunger two or three times. C: Re-direct the needle within the mass several times, aspirating repeatedly at each re-direction. D: Remove needle from syringe and fill syringe with air. E: Re-attach needle, and express sample onto a glass slide. Stain with cytological stain (e.g. Diff-Quik or Rapi-Diff).

Health and safety tip: Make sure that your practice has adequate waste containers for sharps and glass. These items need to be disposed of separately.

BIOPSY

It may be necessary to excise a section of skin for a variety of reasons. One, of course, is to identify a suspected neoplasm; however, fungal disease, demodicosis and autoimmune diseases can also be diagnosed via biopsy. Two types of skin biopsy technique are commonly used in dermatology: punch and simple excision. Both usually require general anaesthesia or heavy sedation. Only in very compliant animals can biopsies be harvested under local anaesthetic. Regardless of the control method, most dermatologists prefer to inject around the site to be excised with a local anaesthetic, such as lignocaine. In preparation, the area is clipped and cleaned with surgical spirit. Note that a full surgical scrub may not be indicated as the vet may be interested in the organisms growing on the skin and may not want them eradicated by a thorough preparation.

If performing a punch biopsy, a variety of punches are available, including 4 mm, 6 mm and 8 mm. The size needed will depend on the size of the animal and the site chosen for sampling. Excision biopsies require a scalpel. The size of margin chosen in the excision sample is partially dependent on the suspected diagnosis. Excisional biopsies usually include samples of both healthy and diseased tissue for comparison. See Figure 3.4 for an example of the

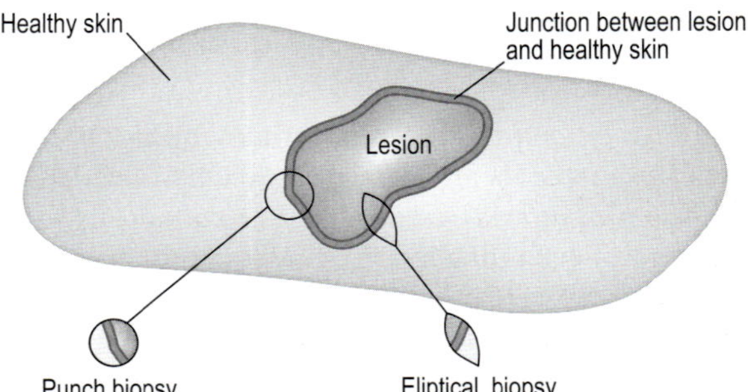

Figure 3.4 Excisional biopsy technique. A punch biopsy contains all three types of skin. (In practice, this can be difficult to achieve with a punch biopsy.) An eliptical biopsy contains lesional, junctional and healthy skin for comparison.

technique. The sample should be placed in a pot of formalin, at least ten times the volume of the sample, and clearly labelled with the animal's name and the site from which the sample was taken. Pathologists are really happy when the submission forms are filled in accurately and in detail. Add as much information about the animal's condition that you feel may be helpful. Be sure to pack the sample securely and according to postal regulations. Taping the pot shut and wrapping it in absorbent layers is courteous to postal staff and will safeguard your precious sample. Mark the envelope as a pathological sample and ideally post during the week and not over the weekend.

The site should be closed with suitable skin suture material, depending on the preference of your practice. If necessary, stitches can be removed when discussing the biopsy results with the owner.

Materials needed

- Some means of sedation/anaesthesia and monitoring
- Biopsy punches in a variety of sizes
- Scapel and blade holder
- Suture material and needles
- Needle holders/Gillies
- Local anaesthetic
- Needle and syringe
- Swabs
- Surgical spirit
- Drape
- Scissors
- Formalin pots
- Padded envelopes
- Packing material
- Laboratory forms.

It can be helpful to put together a biopsy box so that the materials are always ready when needed. *Health and safety tip*: Formalin is a dangerous substance and even inhaling the fumes can be harmful. Purchasing pre-filled sample pots from a laboratory is one way of avoiding risk. If you choose to fill your own pots be very wary of spills and wear protective clothing during the procedure. Placing a urinary catheter attached to a syringe in the bottle is a much safer way of obtaining the solution than pouring! Make sure you are using a 10% formalin solution for biopsy samples.

THE WOOD'S LAMP

The Wood's lamp is an instrument that is sometimes useful in diagnosing dermatophytosis. The lamp must be warmed up for at least 5 minutes and the animal needs to be examined in a darkened room. When shining the lamp over the animal, concentrate on areas with suspicious lesions (annular rings of alopecia with crusting edges). Also, remember that ringworm often (but not always!) likes to grow nose to tail, so be sure to examine the facial region carefully. Ringworm is more prevalent in younger animals who have not yet developed an immunity to the disease. In the likely event that you will be examining a kitten, do clean it up first. Bits of food and milk can distract you and lead to false positives.

A positive reading will show an apple-green fluorescence. HOWEVER, only one type of common dermatophyte, *Microsporum canis*, will fluoresce, and even this type will not always fluoresce. Some authors quote a percentage as low as 60% for *M. canis* fluorescence. Cats are more prone to *M. canis* than to other types of dermatophytes, and among cats Persians seem to be genetically prone to *M. canis*. Therefore, if you have a young cat that happens to be Persian and has lesions that might be indicative of ringworm, the Wood's lamp may give you a definitive diagnosis. Otherwise, it is preferable to do a fungal culture to double-check your findings. Treatment for dermatophytosis can be lengthy, expensive and has potentially toxic side-effects.

FUNGAL CULTURE

Samples for a fungal culture should be gathered from the edges of the lesion(s) as this is the area where the fungi are actively growing. Pluck hair from the edges and place the hairs in a dermatophyte medium – modifed Sabouraud's dextrose agar. Alternatively, you can use the 'Denman brush method' which involves brushing over the entire coat with a hard rubber brush and then pressing the brush into the agar plate. Another method, the 'Mackenzie coat-brush technique', uses a new toothbrush to collect material from the edge of a lesion, which is then pressed into the agar. Regardless of your collection technique, the plate needs to be carefully labelled and stored properly for accurate analysis. A warm, dark corner or cupboard is ideal.

except that you might forget to check the plate every day. It is absolutely necessary to examine the plate daily for 10 days for colour changes. The yellow-to-red change is caused by alkaline metabolites from the dermatophytes affecting the phenol red pH indicator. After 10 days, environmental fungi can cause colour changes. It is a good idea to have one person assigned to the daily task of checking the fungal plates and recording the status of each plate.

Materials needed

- Dermatophyte test medium (DTM) such as 'Dermafyt', by Kruuse
- Toothbrush, epilating forceps or rubber brush (or all three)
- Daily tick sheet for examining DTM.

Health and safety tip: Ringworm is zoonotic. Wear gloves and an apron when examining a suspected case. Clean the examination room from top to bottom after a consultation. Spores can live in the environment for 18 months.

BLOOD SAMPLING

Blood sampling is performed in dermatology in order to establish the general health of the patient and also for the diagnosis of specific diseases. Serum can be analysed for antibodies to *Sarcoptes* mites and some companies also offer analysis for IgE responses to a variety of allergens. Consult your laboratory for the amount of blood needed for each test and collect in a plain or brown-topped serum tube. It is best to take the sample from the jugular vein if more than two millilitres (2 ml) of blood are required.

Biochemistry can be useful in helping to diagnose endocrine disorders such as hypothyroidism and hyperadrenocorticism, although further tests are needed to confirm both of these diagnoses. For hypothyroidism a total thyroxine level (T4) plus a thyroid-stimulating hormone (TSH) assay should be requested. A TSH stimulation test can also be used to diagnose hypothyroidism. Usually, 2 ml, taken in a serum tube, is adequate for this test. For hyperadrenocorticism, an adrenocorticotropic hormone (ACTH) stimulation or low- or high-dose dexamethasone suppression tests may be requested. These tests involve a basal sample and then a second (and sometimes a third) sample post-injection of either synthetic ACTH or dexamethasone. The protocol for these tests will be discussed in more detail in the chapter on endocrine disorders.

INTRADERMAL ALLERGY TESTING

This test is usually done only at specialist centres. Once an animal has been diagnosed with atopic disease the owner can elect to have intradermal skin testing (IDST) done in order to establish the specific allergen–IgE responses which are causing the atopic reaction. IDST is performed only if the owner wishes to have a hyposensitisation course made up for his or her animal. When the substances the animal is allergic to are identified, a unique course of immunotherapy can be made solely for the treatment of the animal named.

Most test kits include dust mites and storage mites as allergens along with grass, tree and weed pollens appropriate to the country the animal is living in. Dermatologists may test for only a few allergens or for as many as 50. The animal is prepared by being heavily sedated and then a large rectangle is clipped on the lateral chest wall. Rows of dots are marked in the clipped area and the allergens are injected fastidiously along the rows so that an accurate record can be made of which allergen is injected where. After 15 minutes the animal is inspected for reactions. A 'control' injection of histamine is always injected, along with a neutral injection of saline. The difference between the diameter of the histamine and saline wheals is measured and an average is found. For example, the histamine wheal may measure 15 mm, while the saline measures 5 mm. Thus, the average is 10 mm. Any other wheal measuring greater than 10 mm in diameter is considered to be a positive result and indicative of a sensitivity to that allergen. The allergens causing wheals greater than 10 mm are recorded and used as the components of the hyposensitisation course. An intradermal allergy test is shown in Figure 3.5.

Materials needed

- Clippers
- Marking pen

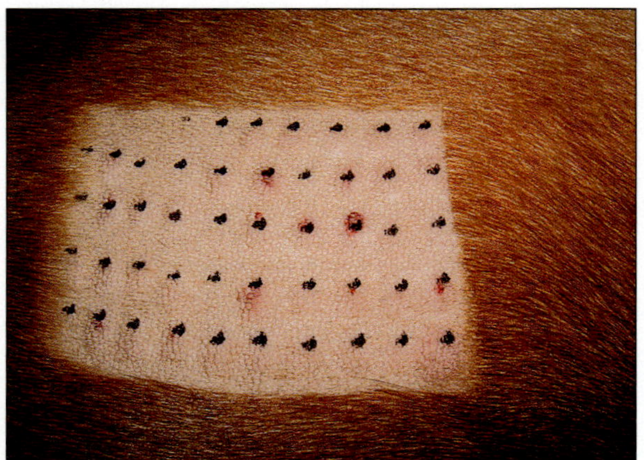

Figure 3.5 Intradermal skin test: The large, erythematous wheals are positive reactions to the allergen injections. Photo by Natalie Perrins, with permission.

- Up to 50 micro-fine insulin syringes
- Allergen test kit
- Chemical sedation
- Monitoring tools for sedation (e.g. a stethoscope).

Health and safety tips: Do not attempt to recap 50 needles. Place the sharps bin next to the examining table and dispose of each syringe directly after use.

Do not place the test kit on the examination table with the animal. Even under sedation, the animal may move unexpectedly, causing the glass vials in the kit to be broken.

Further Reading

Hill Peter B 2002 Small animal dermatology. Elsevier Science, Oxford, p 148-185

Mueller R 2000 Dermatology for the small animal practitioner. Teton New Media, Jackson, Wyoming, p 21-43

Chapter **4**

Ectoparasites of the dog and cat

CHAPTER CONTENTS

Ectoparasites are responsible for the majority of dermatological problems seen in the pet animal. Therefore, it is essential to become thoroughly familiar with the most commonly seen parasites, their life cycles and life styles.

There are two major groups of ectoparasites seen in dermatology: the insects and the arachnids. Within the insect group the ubiquitous flea and the louse cause the most problems. In exotic pets and, occasionally in the dog and cat, flies can also be a nuisance. In the arachnid group, it is ticks and mites which are of dermatological interest.

Beginning with the basic insect, we have a three-segmented creature consisting of a head, thorax and abdomen. There are six legs connected to the thoracic region and each of these six legs has six segments, modified according to the needs of the species. For example, the flea has legs adapted for jumping while the louse has legs more useful for clinging to hairs. Similarly, the mouthparts are specialised in the different species according to the diet and eating habits of that particular insect. This can be clearly seen in the extremely different eating apparatus afforded to the sucking, versus the biting louse.

The head of the insect is the attachment area for the sensory organs such as the antennae and the compound eyes. The thorax consists of three fused segments while the abdomen is composed of 9–11 fused segments.

FLEAS

A good flea-control programme is essential for skin health in the domestic pet. It is pointless to embark on a course of diagnostic tests without ascertaining the level of flea control being practiced by the owner. You will be told, repeatedly, that the pet does not have fleas. If it is not on a flea-control programme and it is pruritic, it probably does have fleas, despite the owner's protests to the contrary. This can be a very difficult issue to deal with as many owners equate a flea infestation with a dirty home. Sometimes it is helpful to prove the presence of fleas by wetting a paper towel and placing some coat brushings onto the damp towel. As the flea faeces reddens the towel, you have your proof. Another method is to use the drug nitenpyram (Capstar, Novartis). The animal can be given an oral dose of the drug and then kennelled on a white towel for 30 minutes. The resultant carnage of dead fleas can be carried out to the owner. However, this test can backfire if the owner accuses your kennels of being flea-ridden! A third method is to tape strip along the dorsum and hope to gather some flea dirt.

The typical flea-infested animal is pruritic, often extremely so. If a cat or dog is particularly sensitive to flea saliva, dermatological signs will develop. Erythema may be present, along with alopecia and secondary pyoderma. The pattern of lesions in the cat is usually dorsal and can extend from the neck to the tail base. Small, crusted papules appear which have been likened to millet seeds, hence the name miliary dermatitis. In the dog, the dorsal lumbar area extending to the tail base is the particular area for reaction to flea bites. In the dog, the papules are larger, erythematous and not typically crusted.

Fleas cause irritation due to their feeding patterns and their progression across the animal's skin. Pets allergic to flea saliva tend to have more serious dermatological problems. Heavy infestations can cause anaemia in young animals. Unchecked, such infestations can be fatal. The flea is a vector for the internal parasite *Dipylidium caninum*; thus, any flea-infested pet should also be properly wormed. It is possible that the flea can act as a vector for haemobartonellosis or feline infectious anaemia, so a heavily infested cat should be tested for this blood parasite. Fleas can do a lot of damage and owners need to understand the importance of a rigorous flea-control programme utilising effective veterinary, as opposed to store-bought, products.

Laterally compressed and wingless, the flea is light brown to black in colour and can range in size from 1 to 6 mm, with the female being the larger of the sexes. One of the reasons that fleas pose such a problem to both man and beast is that there are over 2000 species of flea and most are happy on a variety of hosts. This polyxenous nature makes the flea very adaptive and thus very successful as a parasite. The most common type of flea found in the United Kingdom is *Ctenocephalides felis felis*, or the cat flea. It is distinguished from other species of flea by the unique comb pattern found on its mouthparts.

While the cat flea reigns supreme in Britain, the dog flea (*Ctenocephalides canis*) can also be found, particularly in large kennels. Hedgehog fleas (*Archeopsylla erinacei*), rabbit fleas (*Spilopsyllus cuniculi*), the burrowing chicken flea or 'stick-tight flea' (*Echidnophaga gallinades*) and the human flea (*Pulex irritans*) are among the species also found in these isles.

The life cycle of the flea (see Fig. 4.1) begins with a blood meal taken by the adult flea. One to 2 days after feeding, the female is able to lay eggs. She can lay 50 eggs per day, but her peak production period will be days four to nine. She can live 50 days, laying continuously, if she has a good blood supply. However, she will die within 4 days if she becomes separated from her host.

The eggs fall to the ground, taking 1 to 10 days to develop into larvae. Larvae are positively geotropic and negatively phototropic. That is, they like to burrow deep into warm, dark places like carpets and pet bedding. They feed on organic matter and flea faeces, curling up protectively when they feel vibrations approaching. During the larval stage, the flea will moult three times, eventually reaching a size of 5 mm. This stage can take 5 to 18 days, depending on conditions. Ideally, the flea likes a temperature of about 75° Fahrenheit/22° Centigrade with a humidity factor of 75%. In the ideal climate, the flea cycle can take as little as 12 days in total. If conditions are less favourable, the cycle can last up to a year.

The final stage of development is the pupa. The pupa has a sticky cocoon and is able to cover itself in protective debris. This is the one stage in the life cycle resistant to all current flea treatments and environmental controls. It is also the stage with the

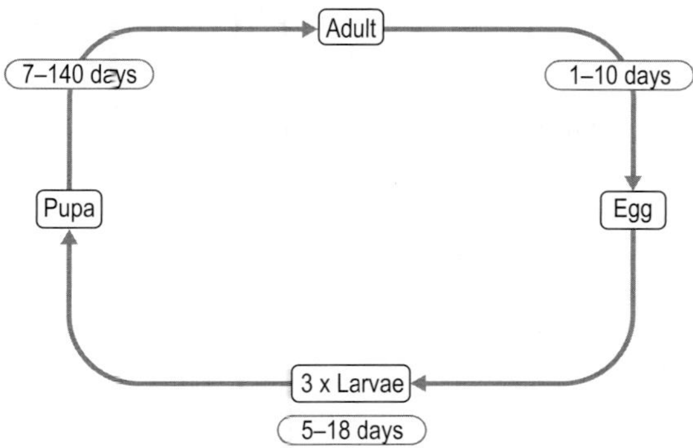

Figure 4.1 Life cycle of the cat flea (*Ctenocephalides felis felis*).

greatest flexibility in terms of waiting for ideal conditions to emerge as an adult. The pupa can take 7–140 days to metamorphose. When the time is right, that is, when a host passes by giving off heat, carbon dioxide, and vibrations as it approaches, the adult flea gets ready to emerge rapidly from the cocoon and leap on the host to begin feeding.

Treatment of a flea infestation does not need to be complicated; it just needs to be regular. A veterinary adulticide should be chosen. Some examples of the adulticides available include: selamectin (Stronghold, Pfizer), imadicloprid (Advantage, Bayer) and fipronil (Frontline and Frontline Combo, Merial). Whichever preparation is chosen, the most important point is to use it correctly and as often as the manufacturer recommends. Secondly, environmental control is almost always necessary. Studies have shown that pets living in a home with environmental control have significantly fewer fleas than other pets treated with the same spot-on adulticide. A premise spray with an insect growth regulator as well as an adulticide decreases the number of treatments needed. Two products which both offer 12 months of environmental control are available. Both products contains permethrin, an adulticide, and either methoprene, or pyiproxyfen, which are insect growth regulators. Both of these growth regulators are designed to target insects only and should not have a detrimental effect on the mammals living in the home. An alternative to premise sprays are environmental powders that act by dehydrating the flea (Fleaban, Animal Care). Vacuuming prior to spraying or spreading powder can increase the efficacy of treatment and simultaneous washing of the pet's bedding is advisable.

Faced with the client who cannot or will not use an environmental spray, a different route of flea elimination is required. It is possible to treat the environment by using an insect growth regulator that is administered to the pet. Thus, any flea feeding on the pet will ingest the insect growth regulator, which will effectively sterilise it. As no viable eggs will subsequently be dropping into the environment, the 'off-pet' flea population will eventually be dramatically reduced. This sort of control does need to be coupled with an adulticide as well to control any current flea infestation on the pet. Lufenuron (Program, Novartis) is an insect growth regulator that can be given as a liquid or injectable form to cats and in tablet form to dogs. Some owners do seem to comply well with the 6-monthly injections given to cats and there is the added advantage that reminders can be sent out to these clients. Nitenpyram (Capstar, Novartis) can be the adjunctive adulticide therapy given in these instances. New developments in flea control occur continuously. (See the formulary near the end of this chapter.)

Obtaining client compliance is crucial for the successful treatment of a flea infestation. First, a client must be convinced that fleas are the problem. Coat brushings to prove the presence of fleas/flea dirt may be necessary for some clients. With the indoor cat that has been grooming excessively, demonstrating the existence of fleas may be impossible. It is still necessary to convince the client that a 'clinical trial' for the presence of fleas is important. Explaining the life cycle and the vast number of eggs that just one flea can lay is one place to start. Supportive leaflets, created by the practice or those distributed by drug companies, can help to back up the advice given by the nurse. Scheduling follow-up meetings to monitor the progress of the pet will go a long way towards showing the client how much better the pet is feeling once the fleas have been eradicated. Follow-ups can help the client to remember to administer the additional treatments and renew their prescriptions. Once fleas are no longer visible, or the summer has ended, many clients will cease to administer treatment and the animal may deteriorate.

Some points to communicate to clients verbally and in a leaflet format:

1. The flea's life cycle requires regular treatment of the pet and the environment.
2. Apply the pet's treatment as often as the manufacturer recommends. Do not skip treatments or your pet may become re-infested.
3. Modern pet treatments for flea infestation are designed to act on fleas only and should not harm your pet, yourself or your children.
4. Frequent bathing of the pet may reduce the efficacy of some flea treatments.
5. Wash the pet's bedding at a high temperature once weekly.
6. Vacuum the home thoroughly before applying an environmental spray.
7. Spray the entire home, even rooms the animal does not frequent. It is possible that you have unwittingly carried the mature or immature fleas to other areas of the house. Don't forget to treat the car if the animal travels with you from time to time. Outside sheds and garages should be treated if the animal frequents these locations.
8. The house spray needs to be used only once a year if used correctly. Be sure to use enough spray for the size of your house.
9. Fleas can cause other health problems. Control of an infestation will make a significant difference to your pet's quality of life. Be sure to obtain a worming tablet from your veterinarian if your dog or cat has had a flea infestation.
10. Store-bought flea (and worm) control products are not as effective and may not be as safe as veterinary products.
11. Please contact the veterinary nurse if you need any advice on the use of flea control products.

Key points to remember about *fleas:*
Clinical signs: Obvious fleas, pruritus, especially to caudal-dorsal trunk in dogs and dorsum in cats, papular lesions. May be a complaint that other animals or the client have been bitten.
Diagnostic tests: Coat brushings, tape strip, and clinical trial with flea products.
Treatment: Veterinary Spot on or spray + environmental spray or powder.

LICE

The louse is a dorsoventrally flattened insect. It is wingless and has three body segments and six legs. Claws appear on the end of each leg. Lice are usually of a light brown to yellow colour and either sucking or biting varieties. The biting suborder is known as '*Mallophaga*' and it contains a louse that can be found on dogs, *Trichodectes canis* (see Fig. 4.2). This creature of 1–2 mm is visible to the naked eye. Under the microscope, *T. canis* is distinguished by its helmet-shaped head and a thorax that is small in relation to the head. The eggs, or nits, can also be clearly seen by microscopic examination. Eggs are white and operculated (have a cap on top) and are found cemented to hair. Infestations with lice are known as 'pediculosis'.

The louse has a life cycle of 14–21 days (see Fig. 4.3), consisting of adult, egg and nymph stages. Three moults, or ecdyses, occur during the nymphal stage. Lice are host-specific and spend their entire life cycle on the host. However, lice can live for 3–7 days off the host so environmental treatment is indicated with an infestation.

Trichodectes canis is a very mobile parasite and its constant travelling through the coat is one source of irritation for the dog. The primary source of nutrition for *T. canis* is epithelial debris. The infested dog will be pruritic, with mild to severe erythema. Infestation is generally on the dorsum but can spread to any area. Hot spots, or moist dermatitis, can occur with infestation. *T. canis* is

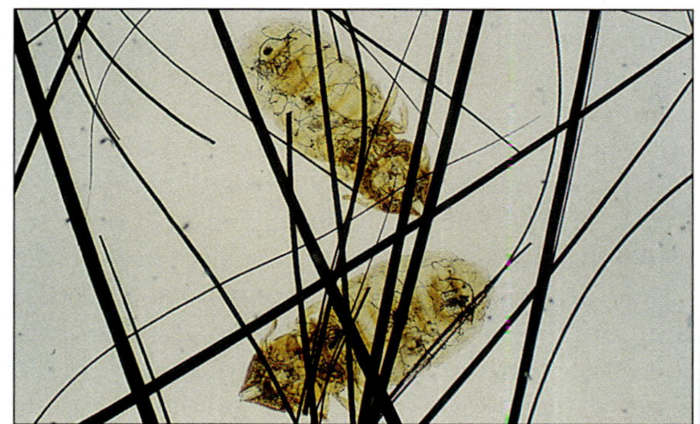

Figure 4.2 *Trichodectes canis*: the biting louse of the dog. Note the helmet-shaped head. Reproduced with permission from Medleau L & Hnilica KA, Small animal dermatology, W B Saunders, London, 2001. Photograph by D Angarano.

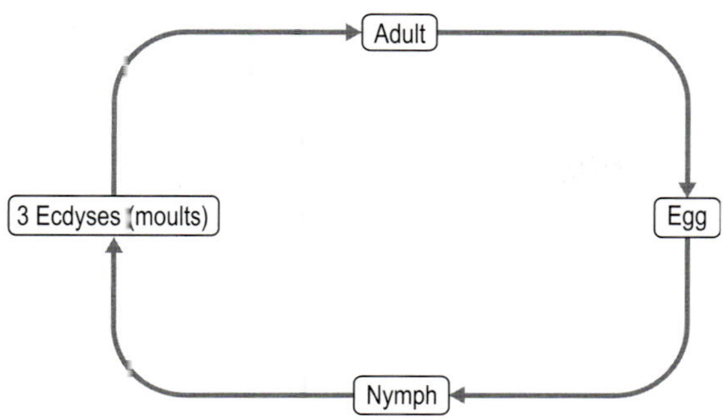

Figure 4.3 Life cycle of the louse.

more prevalent in winter months as heat has an inhibitory effect on its life cycle. Severe infestations can lead to anaemia in the young or debilitated animal. Additionally, *T. canis* is a vector for the canine tapeworm, *Diplydium caninum*.

Felicola subrostrata is the feline biting louse (Fig. 4.4). It is a beige or yellow insect with brown, transverse bands. *F. subrostrata* is 1–1.5 mm in length, with a triangular head. The head is larger than the thorax, a feature typical of biting lice. This louse prefers to infest the head and shoulder regions of the cat, causing pruritus and erythema. Self-trauma is not uncommon with this infestation.

The sucking lice belong to the order *Anoplura*. *Linognathus setosus* (Fig. 4.5) has mouthparts specially adapted for sucking blood from its host, the dog. This louse has a long, thin cephalic region to house its elongated mouthparts. The thorax is wider than the head, helping to differentiate this species from the biting lice. *L. setosus*' preferred sites of attachment are pendulous ears such as spaniel or basset hound pinnae. Severe infestations may cause anaemia.

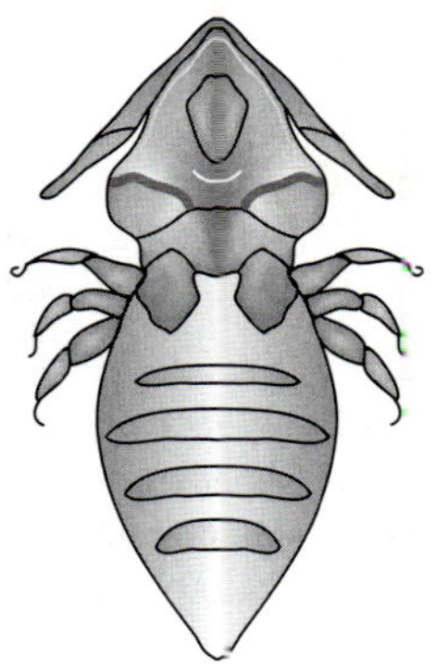

Figure 4.4 Cat louse (*Felicola subrostrata*). Note the triangular head.

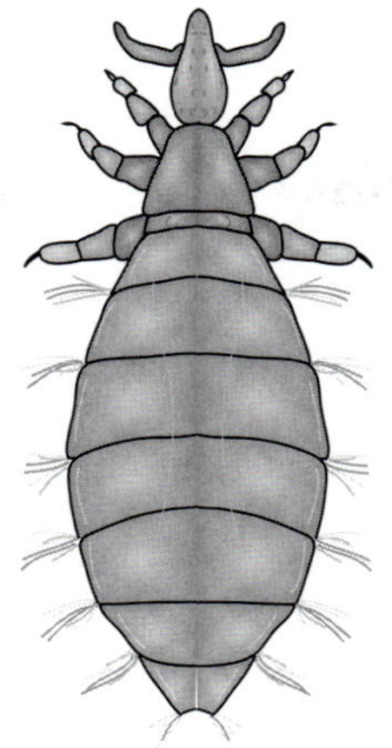

Figure 4.5 Canine 'sucking louse' (*Linognathus setosus*). Notice the elongated headpiece.

Diagnosis of a louse infestation can be achieved through coat brushings, tape strippings or hair pluckings. As lice are surface dwellers, there is no need for skin scrapings. The adults and eggs can be readily identified under low-power magnification.

Selamectin is licensed for the treatment of lice. However, most dermatologists feel that fipronil spray is a better option for eliminating surface-dwelling parasites (see the formulary near the end of the chapter). Also, as lice can infest quite young animals, fipronil is a safe choice in animals less than 6 weeks of age. Two applications, 1 month apart, of either selamectin or fipronil are required to eliminate all stages of the life cycle. Shampoos containing selenium sulphide are a further treatment choice. One shampoo weekly for 3 weeks is sufficient to eradicate all stages of the life cycle. This shampoo is only licensed for use in dogs, however.

As lice can live off the host for a short period of time, environmental treatment is advised. At the very least, all bedding should be washed at hot temperatures and grooming equipment should be cleansed. Lice are host-specific, but co-habiting animals of the same species may become transiently infected. Therefore, all in-contact animals will require treatment.

It should be noted that lice are rarely seen today as ectoparasiticides are so effective. If an animal is infested with lice, the owner is in need of pet care education. The dangers of parasite infestations should be explained and the pest control programme needs to be demonstrated fully, with a follow-up appointment. Worming medication should also be administered because *T. canis* is a vector for *D. caninum*.

Key points to remember about *lice:*
Clinical signs: Obvious lice, pruritus, especially of trunk region.
Diagnostic tests: Tape strip, hair plucks, coat brushings.
Treatment: Fipronil spray or selamectin spot on.

FLIES

Flies are insects (three body parts and six legs). Adult flies feed on blood, sweat, tears, skin secretions, saliva, urine and faeces. Depending on the species, feeding is either via scavenging on the host or puncturing the host's skin. The bites themselves can be very painful and flies are notorious vectors of disease. Additionally, cats can suffer hypersensitivity reactions to fly bites. Papules, crusted papules, plaques and ulcers can appear on the nose and pinnae. Mosquitoes are also responsible for similar hypersensitivity reactions in cats, but tend to be a minor problem in Great Britain.

Although a more familiar problem in rabbits, myiasis (fly strike) can also affect dogs and cats. *Diptera* is the order of flies with one set of wings. There are 120 000 species in this order but two genera are principally responsible for myiasis as we deal with it in veterinary practice. *Cuterebra* spp lay large numbers of eggs on a host or on vegetation, which the host brushes against. The egg stage of the life cycle lasts only 24 hours and then the fly goes through its growth cycle in the host's subcutaneous tissue, each larva dwelling within its own tunnel in the host's axilla, inguinal area or rump. Feeding takes place during three larval stages. Occasionally larvae can migrate up the external orifices of the skull and adversely affect the brain.

The *Calliporidae* genus, commonly known as 'blowflies', has 80 species that are known to cause traumatic cutaneous myiasis in veterinary patients. These species are drawn to body areas damaged by urine scald or poor perineal hygiene. Elderly, incontinent patients are at particular risk of myiasis. Tissue damage, bacterial infection, dehydration and even toxaemia can be the end result of an uncontrolled infestation. Prevention is the best cure. Incontinent patients must be kept clean. Daily grooming and bathing may be necessary, and bedding must be changed regularly. Insecticides for the premises, as well as for the pet, are definitely worthwhile.

Unfortunately, it is likely that the nurse will have to face maggots during the summer season. There is no avoiding the fact that the maggots (the larvae of the fly) have to be removed. The area should be clipped and flushed with copious amounts of saline or dilute chlorhexidine. Individual maggots will need to be plucked out with forceps. In serious cases, debridement of necrotic tissue may be necessary. Keep in mind that the flyblown animal is generally debilitated to begin with so strictly monitor body temperature. Intravenous fluids are required in many cases. Prognosis can rarely be good in flyblown patients. There are pre-existing factors which predispose an animal to myiasis, and whether these be poor husbandry or the incontinence of old age, these factors do not work in the animal's favour.

Once all maggots have been removed, a dose of ivermectin (Ivomec, Merial) can be given as a subcutaneous injection. However, this product is not licensed for use in small animals and is contraindicated in collies and collie-crosses. The efficacy of selamectin (Stronghold, Pfizer) for myiasis has not been documented but as a related molecule to ivermectin, it may be a useful tool in overcoming the infestation. The animal will need to be re-checked daily for at least 3 days to remove any newly hatched maggots. The client should be educated regarding pet hygiene and the products available to help prevent infestations.

Key points to remember about *myiasis:*
Clinical sign: Maggots on animal.
Diagnostic tests: Not needed.
Treatment: Manually remove, clean and debride wound as needed. Discuss husbandry with owner.

ARACHNIDS

Mites and ticks fall within the arachnid family. These creatures have eight legs, an anterior region and a body that is not obviously divided into a thorax and abdomen. The anterior region, known as a 'gnathosoma', is basically a food-carrying tube and attachment area for the mouthparts. These parts consist of claw-like 'palps' and segmented cheliocerae between the palps. The cheliocerae are used to tear, grasp or pierce, depending on the species. Cheliocerae fit within a cone and can extend or retract as needed. Rudimentary eyes can exist in the gnathosoma but are not present in all species.

The posterior region of the body is the 'idiosoma' and is the area of attachment for the eight legs as well as the housing for the vital organs.

Ticks

There are over 800 species of tick with two major genera being of veterinary significance – the *Ixodidae* (hard ticks) and the *Argasidae* (soft ticks.) Ixodid ticks are between 2 and 20 micrometres (μm) in length. Their dorsum is covered by a hard shield known as a 'scutum'. The scutum is used in sexing as the female only has a small scutum, allowing her abdomen to engorge immensely when feeding. The male's scutum will cover its entire dorsum.

Ixodid ticks are not very mobile and are thus forced to wait for a host to arrive. Questing is a popular pastime in this family. Questing involves climbing up a blade of grass and waving their legs when they feel a host approaching. Hosts are detected by vibration, heat, shadow and the expulsion of carbon dioxide. The ixodid tick prefers to attach to ears, which can conveniently dip through the grasses of forests and countryside. Because hard ticks have to make such an effort to attach to a host, they don't let go easily and may stay attached for several days. Unfortunately this gives them plenty of time to pass pathogens on to the host.

The life cycle of the ixodid tick (see Fig. 4.6) begins as vast numbers of eggs are laid on the ground. The eggs will gestate for 2 to 7 weeks before becoming larvae. The larvae may quest for days to weeks before attaching to a host and feeding for 4 to 6 days. They then drop off and moult a few days after their meal. Larvae can survive in the environment for 3 to 8 weeks before entering the nymphal stages. There is one nymphal stage, which can extend in length from 1 to 13 weeks, involving feeding periods on the host of 3 to 10 days. It is not unknown for ticks to regurgitate while feeding, adding to their potential as disease vectors.

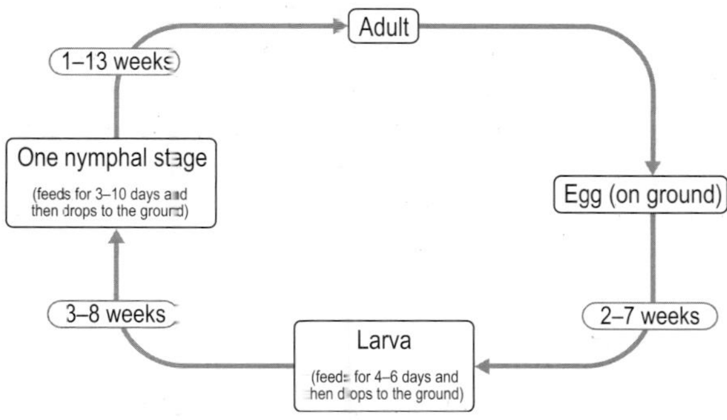

Figure 4.6 Life cycle of *Ixodes* species (ticks).

Altogether, it can take up to 3 years for a tick to complete its life cycle. In that period of time it will have fed on a variety of hosts, although ticks are quite capable of surviving long periods of time with no food at all. Some ticks may start their life cycle on small creatures, such as mice, and move up in size through rabbits, dogs and right up to cows.

Argasidae ticks have a leathery, textured surface. The gnathosoma is not visible from a dorsal view as it is hidden in a ventral recess. There is little sexual dimorphism. These ticks are most prevalent in warm, dry climates and enjoy living in close proximity to their hosts. Chicken coops and pig stys can be great habitats for members of the *Argasidae* family. Because there are so many hosts to choose from in such locations, soft ticks will feed only for a few minutes before moving on to a new host. In this way they can pass diseases on to many hosts in a short period of time, usually feeding while the host is sleeping. The life cycle of the soft tick is different only in that the nymph period may involve from two to seven stages (see Fig. 4.6).

The cutaneous signs of a tick infestation are, firstly, the attached ticks. These can be removed with forceps or by dousing the tick with fipronil. The longer the tick is left in situ, the longer it has to pass on pathogens. The site of attachment will display an inflammatory response with erythema, slight haemorrhage and possibly focal necrosis. Hypersensitivity reactions, such as granulomas, do occur. An abscess may form at the site so thorough cleansing post-removal is highly advised. Forceps can be used to remove a tick by pulling straight out. Using one's fingers is a health and safety risk as several tick-borne diseases are zoonotic. A heavy tick burden can cause anaemia, and even a moderate infestation may lead to bacterial infection. Staphylococcal infections may be serious enough to lead to bacteraemia or septicaemia.

The many serious diseases which can be spread by ticks, with their multi-host life style and extended feeding behaviour, is a great cause for concern. While Britain is largely free from the ravages of tick-borne diseases, one should be aware that animals entering from other countries may have been exposed to tick-borne disease. The law requires that flea and tick treatment be applied prior to entry into the United Kingdom to prevent ticks passing through immigration, however, pets may already have been exposed to disease at that point. Travelling pets that later develop systemic illness should have tick-borne disease included in their differential diagnosis list. A few of the diseases which can occur in areas that are now travel zones within the pet passport scheme are worth mentioning:

Louping illness is caused by a flavivirus that attacks the central nervous system, causing encephalomyelitis. Clinical signs include ataxia, torticollis and paralysis. The disease is associated with sheep via the *Ixoides ricinus* tick; however, dogs and people can be affected. Areas of infestation include France, Norway and the UK.

Ehrlichiosis is caused by a *Rickettsia*-like organism found in Western Europe. It is carried by the brown dog tick, *Rhipicephalus sanguineus* and is spread via wild canids to the domestic dog. Clinical signs of the disease include anaemia, thrombocytopaenia, leucopoenia and pyrexia.

Rocky Mountain Spotted Fever is caused by the organism *Rickettsia rickettsii*. It is spread by the American dog tick, and, not surprisingly, is found on the East and West coasts of the United States. *Dermacentor andersoni* is the West coast tick vector and *Dermacentor variabilis* infects the East coast population. Dogs show signs of lethargy and pyrexia while humans complain of rash, headache, fever, aching joints, and can even develop haemorrhage and die. A similar spotted fever occurs in Southern Europe where dogs are the reservoir for the disease via transmission from *R. sanguineus* or *Haemaphysali leachi*.

Lyme borreliosis is caused by the spirochaete *Borrelia burgdorferi* and occurs in the USA; it is now spreading to Europe. *I. ricinis* (the sheep tick) is responsible for spreading this disease in Europe, which can manifest in the dog with pyrexia, lethargy, anorexia, lymphadenopathy and arthritis. *I pacificus* is the vector for the Western USA and *I. scapularis* infests the North-Eastern USA. In humans the disease can cause flu-like symptoms and rash. More severe cases develop polyraducloneuritis leading to impaired hearing and vision and possibly meningitis.

Babesiosis is caused by the protozoan *Babesia* and is known to occur in the canine population of Southern Europe. Affected dogs suffer from malignant jaundice after having been infected by either *R. sanguineus* or *Dermacentor marginatus*.

Tick paralysis is caused by *D. andersoni* in the Western states of America and *D. variabilis* in Eastern American states. It is known to affect dogs, cats, humans and a variety of other species. Toxins from a single tick's saliva are adequate to cause infection. The toxins cause a disruption to motor nerve synapses in the spinal cord and block neuromuscular junctions. Clinical signs occur about 5 days after a female tick has fed. Respiratory and cardiovascular difficulties ensue. Vomiting, variable body temperatures and eventual paralysis lead to death. Paralysis, which begins with the limbs, can become complete within hours.

If a client is planning to travel with his pet, do remind him or her to practice parasite control throughout the journey and not just 48 hours prior to re-entry. Fipronil is licensed for tick control in the spray form.

Mites

The typical mite is a small creature of usually less than 1 mm in length. As with the tick, there is an anterior or gnathosoma region and a posterior/idiosoma region. The four pairs of legs are arranged in two anterior and two posterior pairs. The first pair of legs is generally the longest pair and carries sensory organs for capturing prey. Each leg is broken into six segments and the last segment can finish in a claw, pad, sucker or filamentous hair. The final segment can be useful in identifying the species; for example, *Otodectes* mites have suckers on the ends of their legs.

The idiosoma is usually soft and wrinkled and in many species adorned with concentric rings (for example, *Notoedres cati*). Two or more dorsal and ventral shields protect the vulnerable idiosoma.

Cheyletiella

Cheyletiella (see Fig. 4.7) is a very mobile surface mite that travels over the pet, feasting on epithelial

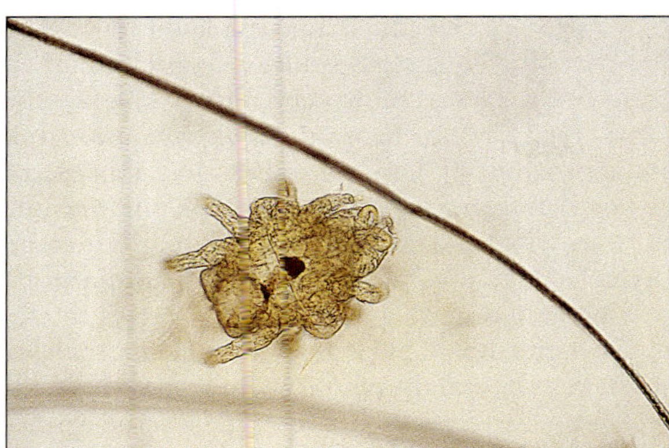

Figure 4.7 *Cheyletiella* species. Different species of this mite affect cats, dogs and rabbits. The piercing mouthparts are distinctive. Reproduced with permission from Medleau L & Hnilica KA, Small animal dermatology, W B Saunders, London, 2001.

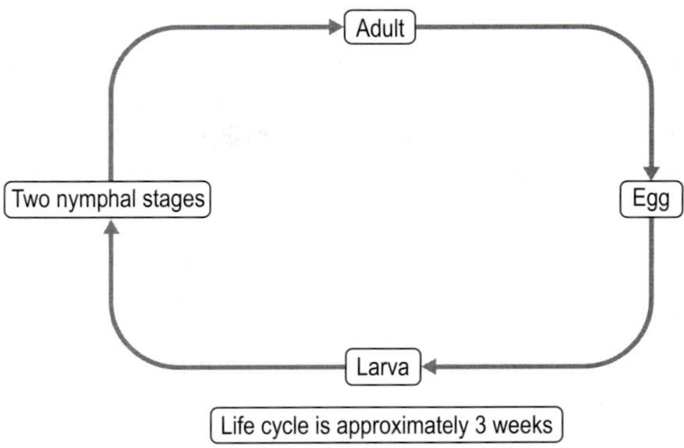

Figure 4.8 Life cycle of *Cheyletiella* species (mites). The life cycle is approximately 3–5 weeks.

debris and even other mites. Occasionally it will use its stylet-like chelicerae to pierce the skin and drink lymph fluid. These stylets appear as hook-like mouthparts under the microscope.

The eight legs of this mite are adorned with combs, which are another identifying point under microscopic examination. *Cheyletiella* also has an indentation on either side of the idiosoma, which can be likened to a waist.

The whole life cycle is completed on the host, but this mite is not host-specific. Owners can and do become infested but these infections are, while very pruritic, self-limiting. Adult mites can, if necessary, live off the host for up to 1 month but the immature stages of the life cycle can survive for only 48 hours off the host. The entire life cycle takes 3 to 5 weeks. The adult lays eggs, which develop into larvae within 4 days. There are two nymphal stages before metamorphosis into the adult form (see Fig. 4.8). It is important to remember the length of the life cycle and the fact that adults can survive in the environment when treating for an infestation.

Three species of *Cheyletiella* which we see most commonly are: *C. yasguri* on the dog, *C. blakei* on the cat and *C. parasitovorax* on rabbits. It should be noted that *C. parasitovorax* can be a vector for myxomatosis (Wall & Shearer 2001). In the dog, clinical signs include what appears to be heavy shedding of cornified skin cells, i.e. scurf or dandruff. In reality, this is 'walking dandruff' – a mix of white, 400 μm mites and scale. Hair may shed more easily and there may be an inflammatory reaction with erythema and pruritus, especially along the dorsal spine. A hypersensitivity reaction and hyperaesthesia may develop, possibly due to the constant stimulation from the movement of the mites. This disease is more common in young and shorthaired dogs.

In the cat, the infestation is placed primarily on the head and trunk and can lead to miliary dermatitis. An appearance of a dandruffy coat and pruritus are the major signs of infestation. Again, the disease is more common in young animals. Asymptomatic carriers exist among both dogs and cats.

Owners who have close contact with their pets may develop papular lesions in groups of three or four papules per site. Favoured sites are the arms and abdomen and 80% of in-contact owners will experience infestation. Thus, lesions on the owner can be very helpful in making a diagnosis!

Diagnosis of *Cheyletiella* infestation is by coat brushings, tape strippings, skin scrapings or even hair pluckings. Live mites and their eggs can be easily visualised under low magnification. Many owners are interested in viewing the findings and certainly this is a dramatic mite to view, with its pincer mouthparts and hairy legs.

Treatment for the dog and cat should be with an acaricidal spray. This is a surface mite and it can be killed more quickly with sprays rather than spot-ons. Fipronil (Frontline Spray, Merial) at 3 ml per kilogram should be applied three times at 1- to

2-week intervals. Eggs are resistant to treatment so repeated treatments are needed to eradiate mites as they develop through the life cycle. As cats resent sprays, an alternative treatment plan can be utilised with ivermectin (Ivomec, Merial) at 200–300 mg/kg three times at weekly intervals. Ivermectin is not licensed for use in small animals and requires written agreement from the owner for off-label use. Use of ivermectin in sheepdogs and sheepdog crossbreeds can have fatal consequences. Selenium sulphide 1% shampoo (Seleen, Sanofi) can be used in dogs, but is not licensed for use in cats. Bathing should occur three times at 1-week intervals. If necessary, bathing can continue for up to 6 weeks. Shampooing aids in removing the excessive scale and debris, providing a less welcoming environment for the mite. Eggs are also removed during bathing. If possible, at least one bath should be part of the treatment programme, even if fipronil is chosen as the major treatment modality. Be sure that the bathing takes place a few days prior to spraying as the efficacy of fipronil is reduced by washing. (Consult the formulary near the end of the chapter.)

All in-contact pets must be treated as cross-infestation is highly likely. Due to the adult mite's ability to survive off the host for a lengthy period of time, environmental treatment with a premise spray is essential in order to avoid re-infestation. As a further note, the consultation room where the animal was seen must be thoroughly cleaned and sprayed with a pesticide.

Key points to remember about *Cheyletiella:*
Clinical signs: Walking dandruff, pruritus of truncal region, and communication to other pets and humans.
Diagnostic tests: Tape strips and coat brushings.
Treatment: Fipronil spray + environmental spray.

Neotrombicula autumnalis

This mite is also known by the common names 'berry bug' and 'harvest mite'. It is a reddish/orange mite of about 200 μm in length. It is parasitic only in its larval stage, so we know it as a six-legged creature, but as an adult it is a free-living eight-legged mite. The legs are relatively long in comparison to the body and all the legs are covered in minute hairs or 'setae'. These long legs enable harvest mites to crawl up stalks of grass from which they can reach out and attach to passing hosts. The life cycle (Fig. 4.9) starts with a 4-day development from egg to larva, followed by 3 to 10 days for the larva (Fig. 4.10) to become a nymph. Larvae feed for approximately 3 days and then have a quiescent period before moving onto the nymph phase. There are two nymphal stages before adulthood. The entire cycle can take 50–70 days and the life span can be as long as 1 year.

Favourite sites of infestation are in Henry's pocket in the ear, the eyelids, ventral abdomen, genital folds and even between the digits. Often several mites will attach in clusters and can be visualised as small

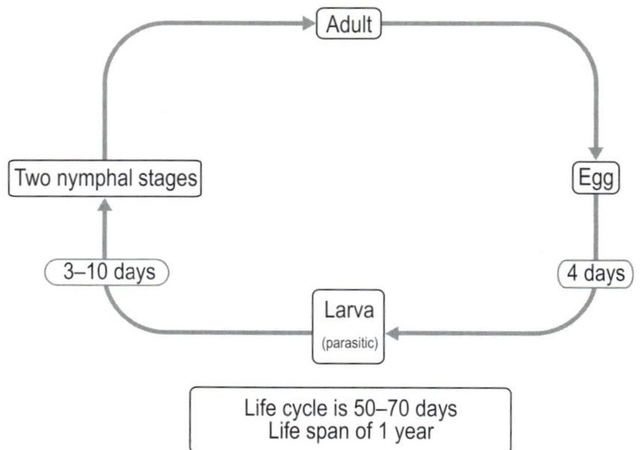

Figure 4.9 Life cycle of *Neotrombicula autumnalis*. The duration of the life cycle is 50–70 days. Adults can survive for 1 year.

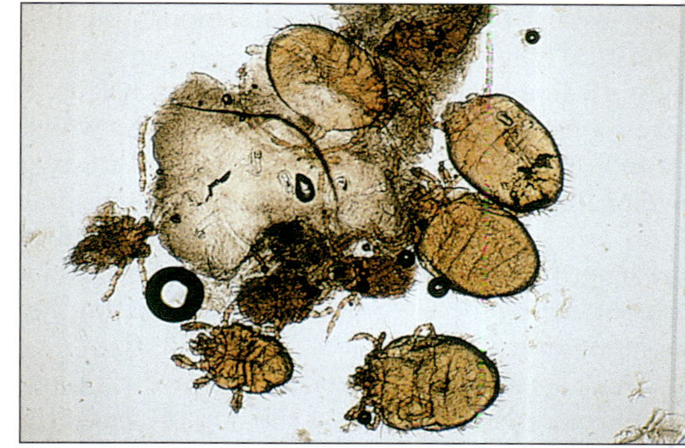

Figure 4.10 *Neotrombicula autumnalis*: This larva is the parasitic stage of the mite. As a larva, it has only six, elongated legs. Reproduced with permission from Medleau L & Hnilica KA, Small animal dermatology, W B Saunders, London, 2001. Photograph by R Malik.

orange dots at the point of attachment. Harvest mites are most active in late summer (hence their name) preferring dry sunny weather along well-drained chalky cliffs and hills. Therefore, this mite has a seasonal and locational prevalence, which can be useful in diagnosis. Clinical signs include pruritus and erythema. Dogs, cats, humans, wild rabbits and foxes are subject to harvest mite infestation. Some hosts exhibit hypersensitivity reactions with papules, wheals and self-trauma leading to excoriation and alopecia. A heavy infestation can even cause pyrexia. Behaviour associated with an infestation would include feet chewing and scratching at the ears.

Diagnosis is often attained by simple observation with the naked eye because the mites are clearly visible. However, skin scrapings can be used to remove the mites from the site and observe them under a microscope. Fipronil is the treatment of choice. Weekly application to the feet and ears can be utilised if needed. Re-infestation is common as hosts that exercise in the chalky downs will repeatedly encounter fresh mites.

Key points to remember about *Neotrombicula autumnalis*:

Clinical signs: Tiny orange dots between toe webs and in Henry's pocket, absent to severe pruritus.

Diagnostic tests: Observation of mite attached to skin, skin scrapings and microscopic examination.

Treatment: Fipronil spray as needed. (Apply to cotton wool and wipe on to affected areas if spray not tolerated).

Otodectes cynotis

Being a surface mite, *Otodectes* (Fig. 4.11) has long legs. In the female the first two pairs of legs have suckers at the final segment, while males have suckers on all four legs. The two anterior pairs of legs are much stronger than the posterior pairs and the fourth pair of legs is by far the shortest. *Otodectes* is just visible to the naked eye as a whitish mite and is easily identified under low-power magnification.

The life span is 2 months with a 3-week life cycle (see Fig. 4.12), including a 4-day period from egg to larval stages, 3–10 days to the nymphal stages and two nymph stages before adulthood. The final nymph stage is the 'deutonymph' stage. At this point, sexual dimorphism has not taken place but adult male *Otodectes* will attach to deutonymphs. If the deutonymph evolves into an adult female, mating can take place. If the deutonymph turns out to be a male, obviously, they are out of luck. Mating is frequently caught on a microscope slide and can be interesting to show to pet owners.

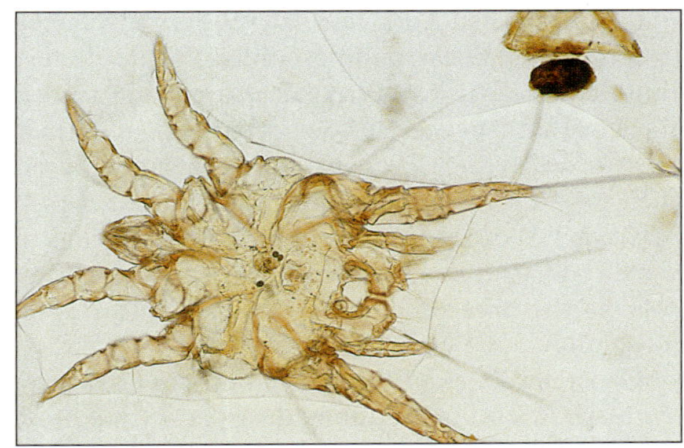

Figure 4.11 *Otodectes cynotis*: This ear mite infects dogs, cats and ferrets. It is identified by the suckers at the distal end of its legs and the forward thrust of the first pair of legs. Reproduced with permission from Medleau L & Hnilica KA, Small animal dermatology, W B Saunders, London, 2001.

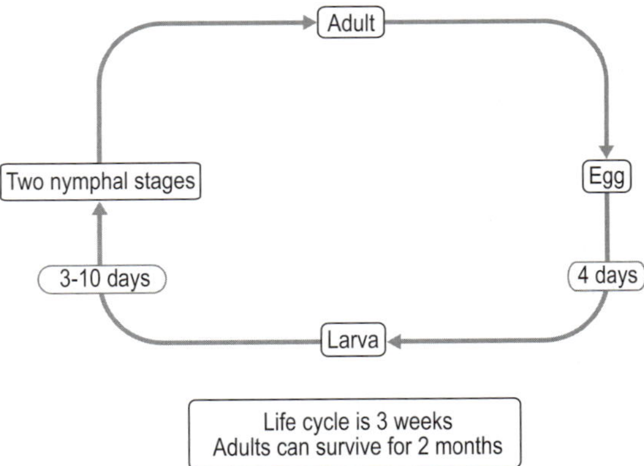

Figure 4.12 Life cycle of *Otodectes cynotis*. The life cycle is 3 weeks. Adults can survive for up to 2 months.

Otodectes feeds on the debris found in the ear canal. Feeding takes place primarily in the morning and evening (breakfast and dinner) and can apparently be very noisy – humans who have experimented with purposeful infestation complain of the din. Clinically, there may be a grey to coffee-grain-type aural discharge, accompanied by much self-trauma to the ear. Aural haematomas are a frequent end result of *Otodectes* infestations. While preferring the ear canal, *Otodectes* can also spread to infest the head and neck. Cats, who curl up into their tails to sleep, may even have infestation sites on their tails. Humans who curl up with infested pets may, rarely, become infected but in humans clinical signs tend to take the form of a papular, pruritic rash at the area of contact rather than an aural infestation.

Generally, *O. cynotis* occurs in puppies or kittens. With age, a level of immunity develops so that most dogs and cats can resist major infestations. However, hypersensitivity reactions can occur and immunocompromised animals are not able to keep a commensal population at bay. Severe infestations can lead to ulceration of the ear canal, secondary bacterial infections, and potentially circling and convulsions if inner ear disease is a sequela.

The diagnostic test for *O. cynotis* is an ear swab examined under the ×40 objective. Material can be gathered on a cotton bud and spread onto a glass slide to then be examined at low magnification. Adult mites, deutonymphs and eggs should be visible. The heat of the microscope lamp will enhance activity levels and the mites should be motile. Coverslips are recommended otherwise the mite may move out of range. Tape strips can also be used to capture mites and secure them on a slide for identification.

Cleaning the ear thoroughly should be the first step of treatment. It is not necessary to use a strong cleanser – any of the veterinary ear-cleaning products would be appropriate, for example: Dog or Cat Ear Cleaner (Leo Animal Health) and Epiotic (Virbac) are both suitable. Debris should be wiped away with cotton wool; cotton buds should be used sparingly, if at all. Cleansers with cerumenolytics will break up the earwax and help the dirt rise to the auditory meatus, where it can be wiped away. Using a cotton bud may cause you to force the wax and mites further into the ear causing a plug – this just sets the ear up for infection deeper inside the ear.

Once the ear is cleaned, eardrops with acaracidal activity can be used. Canaural (Leo Animal Health) and Auroto (Arnolds) are both useful products (see the formulary near the end of the chapter). Most treatments should be given twice daily for 7 days and then there can be a rest period of 7 days. This should be followed by a further 7 days of treatment. In this way, the entire life cycle can be eliminated. Stopping treatment before the end of the 3-week period may lead to a re-infestation. In cats, the product selamectin (Stronghold, Pfizer) is licensed for the treatment of *O. cynotis*. The manufacturers claim that one treatment is adequate to eliminate the problem. Selamectin is not licensed for the treatment of ear mites in dogs but anecdotal evidence supports its use as an aid in control of ear mites in dogs. In many cases, environmental treatment may be necessary as the mite can survive off the host for several months. In-contact pets should be examined for infestations and treated as needed. All grooming equipment and bedding should be disinfected.

Key points to remember about *Otodectes:*
Clinical signs: Coffee-grounds-type exudate in ears, variable pruritus.
Diagnostic tests: Ear swab and microscopy.
Treatment: Clean ears and apply miticidal eardrops for 3 weeks or selamectin spot-on for cats.

Notoedres cati

This is a sarcoptid mite – a type of mite that lives in burrows and nourishes itself on the deeper epidermal skin layers. Sarcoptid mites are not very mobile so they have no need for long legs. Their short, stubby legs are much better suited for burrow dwelling. Their bodies are rounded and their mouthparts are adapted for cutting and sucking.

Notoedres cati sports a pattern of concentric rings on its dorsum. There are four stout pairs of legs with suckers on pairs I and II. At 150–225 μm, this mite is smaller than the more familiar *Sarcoptes scabiei*. The life cycle, however, is very similar to that of *S. scabiei*, lasting 3 weeks and involving egg, larval, two nymphal and adult stages.

Infestations with this mite are rare in England but can occur in cats with immunocompromising conditions, such as feline immunodeficiency virus (FIV). The head and ears are the most common sites of infestation. Initially, the cat will show signs of erythema. However, as the infestation progresses, the skin will develop a yellow-grey crusting. In advanced stages of the disease, the skin will show a chronic inflammatory pattern of thickening, hyperpigmentation and alopecia.

This is a disease causing intense pruritus so self-trauma is unavoidable. Secondary lesions due to self-trauma are to be expected. Without treatment, *N. cati* can lead to death within 4–6 months.

Diagnosis is achieved via skin scrapings. Apply a small amount of liquid paraffin to a number 10 blade and perform superficial scrapes. Multiple scrapings are necessary in order to adequately test for this parasite. At least five sites should be scraped and the slides examined under both low and high power. One mite or an egg is a positive diagnosis for *N. cati.*

Selamectin is not licensed for *N. cati*; however, it is a viable treatment option. As selamectin is effective and licensed for the treatment of *S. scabiei* in dogs, it should be adequate for the elimination of *N. cati*, a related mite, with a similar life cycle and feeding pattern. Two treatments, 1 month apart, should control the infestation. Underlying causes should be investigated. At the very least, an infected cat should be tested for feline leukaemia virus (FeLV) and FIV.

Sarcoptes scabiei and sarcoptic mange

Sarcoptes scabiei (Fig. 4.13) is a mange mite of the dog. This mite is 200–400 μm long. It has two anterior pairs of short, stout front legs and two pairs of vestigial hind legs, decorated with numerous setae. The body is spherical. *S. scabiei* burrows into the epidermal cells, with the female laying its eggs within these burrows. She is capable of laying for 60 days, with the eggs having a 10% chance of becoming larvae. After 3–5 days, larvae emerge into moulting pockets of the burrow. After 3–7 more days, the larvae become nymphs (protonymphs and then deutonymphs) and after a further 3 days transform into adults. The entire life cycle (Fig. 4.14) takes 2–3 weeks, with the nymphal stages and the adult males living on the surface of the skin.

Figure 4.15 shows a dog with a severe infestation of *S. scabiei*.

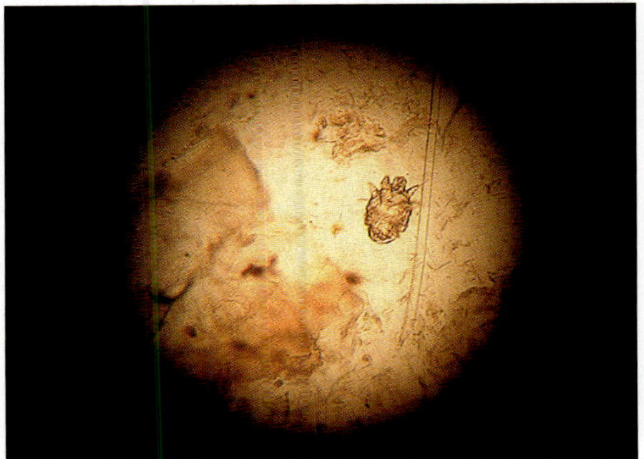

Figure 4.13 *Sarcoptes scabiei:* notice the round body and stubby legs of this mite. Photograph by Natalie Perrins, with permission.

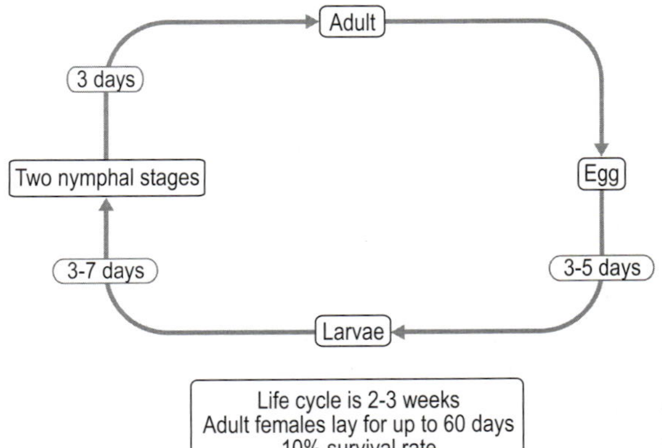

Figure 4.14 Life cycle of *Sarcoptes scabiei.* The life cycle is 2–3 weeks. Adult females lay for up to 60 days with a 10% survival rate.

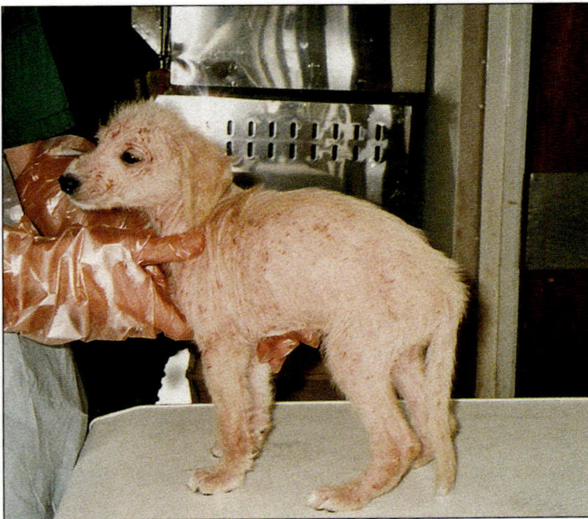

Figure 4.15 This is a puppy with a severe *Sarcoptes scabiei* infestation. Notice the characteristic scale, crust, alopecia and erythema. Photograph by Mark Martin, with permission.

The primary clinical sign of this disease is severe pruritus. The mites' burrowing nature and its method of feeding on skin cells is intensely irritating to canine skin. Due to the overwhelming need to scratch, the dog will create secondary lesions ranging in severity from excoriations to ulcers. Alopecia will almost certainly occur in an uncontrolled infestation and there will be profuse yellowish scale and crust. Erythema and papules will be present and secondary pyoderma is a very common sequel.

Initial signs of the disease often begin on the pinnal edges but will rapidly spread to the face, ventral trunk and legs – with elbows and hocks being the target areas on the legs. *S. scabiei* mites prefer areas with less hair. However, generalised mange will occur if the infestation is allowed to progress unchecked. Internal health will deteriorate, with the dog showing weight loss, depression and lymphadenopathy.

Sarcoptic mange is easily confused with many other skin problems. A differential list can include: *Cheyletiella* infestation, *Otodectes* infestation, pediculosis or dermatophytosis. Flea and food allergies, atopy or even contact dermatitis can show similar lesions. The importance of thorough diagnostic testing cannot be emphasised enough. Sarcoptic mange is an incredibly distressing disease that is really fairly easily treated. If misdiagnosed, the dog could be given corticosteroid treatment, which would not solve the problem and could worsen the situation.

One useful clue towards diagnosis is the transmission of the disease to the owner. Sarcoptic mange is quite contagious so an owner in close contact with an affected dog is very likely to have a papular, pruritic rash, often on the arms and abdomen. Do advise the owner to see his or her GP if he/she complains of a rash! While taking the history, ask about other in-contact pets. If one dog is affected it is almost certain that any other in-contact dogs will also be experiencing pruritus with scaling and crusting, although the diagnosis should not be excluded if this is not the case.

During the initial examination, a pinnal–pedal reflex test can be done by rubbing the edges of the pinna together. This is not a method of diagnosis; however, an itch–scratch reflex to the test should prompt investigation for sarcoptic mange.

Diagnosis of sarcoptic mange can be performed by two standard methods. Multiple skin scrapes is historically the test of choice. As mites are not that easy to collect, the choice of sites should be chosen carefully. Avoid areas where lesions have been created by self-trauma. An area of excoriation or erosion will probably have no intact burrows left. Do choose thinly haired areas in one of the favoured infestation sites mentioned earlier. Gently scissor away the coat and perform superficial skin scrapings. Wipe the acquired debris off the blade onto a slide prepared with liquid paraffin. Examine under low power. Repeat this process at least five times from different likely sites. Inability to find a mite does not mean that the dog does not have mange. If the clinical signs are strongly suggestive of a *S. scabiei* infestation a clinical trial is very worthwhile. Treating for an infestation will do no harm and may cure the animal.

The second diagnostic approach to sarcoptic mange is blood testing for IgG antibody to *S. scabiei*. Blood samples (in the amount specified by the laboratory being used) should be sent in brown-topped serum pots. If the results are positive, you can proceed with treatment.

As this disease is both zoonotic and contagious to other pets, the consultation room will need a good scrub and spraying with an environmental pest control product before introducing your next appointment. Ideally, you should re-locate to another consultation room.

The treatment protocol for sarcoptic mange has been greatly simplified by the advent of selamectin (Stronghold, Pfizer). Two applications of this product, 1 month apart, will control the disease, providing all other in-contact dogs are treated at the same time. Some clinicians choose to apply the doses of selamectin 2 weeks apart. This is extra-license use of the drug; however, anecdotally, there is a quicker rate of recovery with more frequent application of selamectin. As this disease is often contracted from foxes, it is advisable that dogs which exercise in areas frequented by foxes use selamectin monthly as a preventative measure.

Fipronil spray is licensed as an aid in control of sarcoptic mange. Two applications of this product, given 3–4 weeks apart, are necessary to kill at the egg to larval stage of the life cycle. In pups less than 6 weeks of age, this treatment is the safest option.

Amitraz (Aludex, Intervet) is also licensed for the treatment of sarcoptic mange. It is effective against *S. scabiei* at a dilution of 0.025%, i.e. 25 ml in 5 litres of water. It is best to shampoo the dog prior to treatment with amitraz to remove excess scale and crust. The solution should be sprayed onto the dog in a well-ventilated area and protective clothing should be worn. The dip must not be rinsed off after application. This treatment needs to be repeated at 1-week intervals for 2–6 weeks. Skin scrapings should be taken after the second rinse and then every 2 weeks to assess the length of treatment needed. Once negative scrapes are obtained, treatment can be stopped. Clipping will increase the efficacy of the amitraz. Please note that amitraz cannot be applied to Chihuahuas. Do consider that client compliance tends to be better with monthly spot-ons as compared with weekly dips.

Ivermectin has also been used but an extra-license product should be a last resort when there are effective licensed products. Any collie or related breed cannot be given ivermectin as it could prove fatal.

As the pruritus is so severe with this infestation, corticosteroids may be needed until the acaricidals take effect. Any secondary bacterial or yeast infection must be treated also or the pruritus may not be controlled.

Key points to remember about *Sarcoptes:*
Clinical signs: Extreme pruritus, crusting lesions on ventrum, elbows hocks and pinnae. Transmission of infestation to other pets and humans.
Diagnostic tests: Pinnal–pedal reflex, superficial skin scrapings, serology
Treatment: Selamectin spot-on for two doses, fipronil, amitraz dips.

Demodex canis and demodectic mange

Demodex canis (Fig 4.16) is a prostigmatid mite. It is adapted to live deep in hair follicles and sebaceous and meibomian glands. As a commensal, these demodex mites are normal inhabitants of skin, with species specific to their particular hosts. (For example, *Demodex follicuarium* and *D. brevis* are human demodex mites.) Certain elements in an animal's immune system can cause this mite to overpopulate and become a pest.

D. canis is 100–400 μm long and has a tapered 'cigar-like' body, although shorter subspecies have been identified. It is difficult to distinguish between

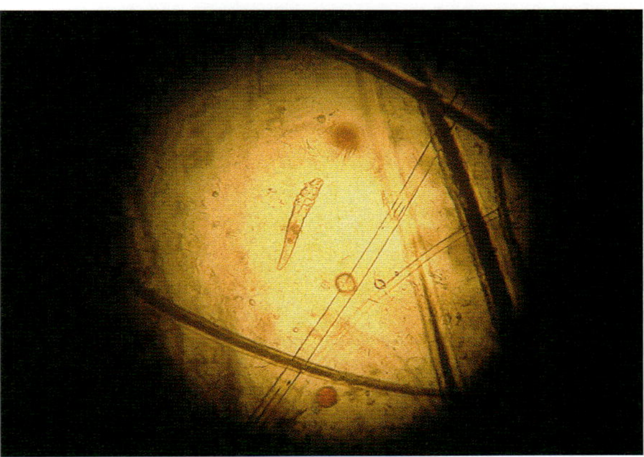

Figure 4.16 *Demodex canis*. This mite is often referred to as 'cigar-shaped'. Its shape is ideal for living within hair follicles. Photograph by Natalie Perrins, with permission.

the anterior and posterior segments of *Demodex*. The posterior segment is greater than half the body length and is covered in striations. There are four stubby pairs of legs with blunt claws on the anterior segment.

The entire life cycle of *Demodex canis* occurs within the hair follicle or glands (see Fig. 4.17). A subspecies of *Demodex* is said to inhabit the stratum corneum. The subspecies tends to be much stubbier in appearance. With both types, if removed from the host, the mite will die in the environment. The female mite lays 20–24 eggs, which will develop through their entire life cycle of 18–24 days within the hair follicle. The egg/larva/nymph/adult cycle that is typical of mites is followed.

Favoured locations of infestation include, firstly, lesions above the eye. Infestation can then occur on the head, forelimbs and trunk. Usually the mite is passed from the dam to the pups during suckling. Most pups will maintain a commensal population, but some immature immune systems will not be able to overcome the infestation and the mites will reproduce excessively. Juvenile demodicosis is often a benign disease that will regress as the pup's immune system develops. Common clinical signs will appear when the pup is between 3 and 15 months of age. The process is self-limiting unless corticosteroid therapy is given. If corticosteroid treatment is prescribed, the immune system will be further suppressed and the demodicosis will become generalised, rather than localised, and cure

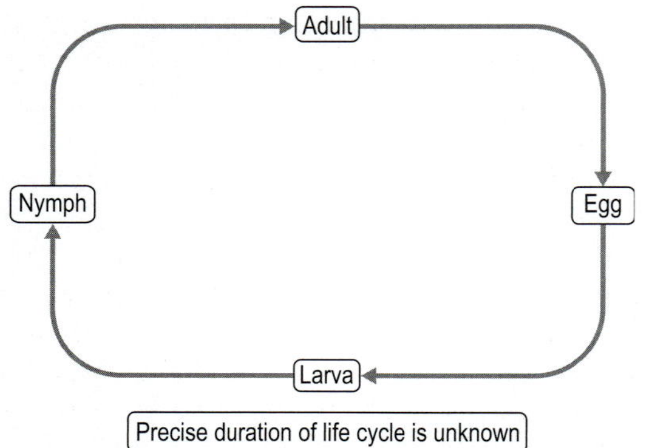

Figure 4.17 Life cycle of *Demodex* species (mites). The precise duration of the life cycle is unknown.

will be much more difficult, or even impossible, to achieve.

Clinical signs in both the puppy and the adult dog include erythema and alopecia with variable pruritus. The variant, shorter form of *Demodex*, which lives more towards the surface, can cause some pruritus. *Demodex canis* lives in hair follicles and creates debris and plugged follicles, i.e. comedones are common signs of demodicosis. In severe cases, confluent comedones will give the skin a bluish tone. Eventually lesional sites may become pustular and hyperpigmentation may result as a sign of chronic inflammation. If the sites show signs of pyoderma along with demodicosis, pruritus may become an issue. Some dermatologists refer to demodicosis with secondary pyoderma as the 'pustular' form of the disease.

Adult-onset demodicosis is a much more serious problem with a more guarded prognosis. Adult-onset demodicosis can be generalised or localised. *D. canis* is three times more common in pure-bred dogs, suggesting that the tendency to develop demodicosis may be genetic in nature. Shorthaired breeds are more likely to be prone to demodicosis, as are Afghans, Collies and German Shepherd dogs. It is believed that affected dogs have suppressed T-cell and lymphocyte function. The dog is able to cope with the commensal populations of *D. canis* and *Staphylococcus intermedius*. However, if any of these organisms begins to multiply, the dog's immune system is not able to respond appropriately. If the mite population increases, hair follicles are damaged, creating debris. This is a hospitable environment for overgrowth with the other commensal, *S. intermedius*.

With susceptible animals, demodicosis will often occur hand in hand with a secondary pyoderma, caused by the *S. intermedius* population. The dog's immune system becomes over-taxed in the attempt to fight off both the pyoderma and demodicosis. Treatment of the pyoderma is essential to help control the demodicosis.

Because of the genetic factor, affected animals should not be used for breeding. Female dogs with adult-onset demodicosis should be spayed as the oestrus cycle may also contribute to increased populations of mites.

Localised demodicosis will often start with the feet and pododermatitis will be the end result of the combined demodicosis and staphylococcal infection. Sometimes the problem will remain localised. In other cases it will generalise. In very complicated cases, adult-onset demodicosis can begin as a generalised disease. It is always prudent to look for underlying causes such as hypothyroidism, hyperadrenocorticism disease or neoplasia. When taking a history, it is essential to ask about any medication that the animal is currently receiving or has received in the past year. Some medications can cause immunosuppression that can instigate a case of demodicosis. Corticosteroid therapy is one drug that can cause immunosuppression but there are many others, especially chemotherapeutic, cytotoxic and immunosuppressive drugs, such as azathioprine (Imuran, GlaxoWellcome).

Diagnosis of demodicosis can be obtained by hair pluckings (as the mite lives in the hair follicle, this method can be effective), deep skin scrapings and biopsy. Acetate tape strips can be useful in identifying stratum-corneum-dwelling subspecies of *Demodex*. Hair pluckings can be placed in one drop of liquid paraffin for examination. Skin scrapes should be taken from multiple sites, and scraping with a number 10 blade must continue until capillary ooze is seen. The collected debris should be wiped onto a slide prepared with liquid paraffin and examined under both low and higher power. If neither of these collection methods is successful, biopsy can be carried out as needed.

The only currently licensed treatment for demodicosis is amitraz (Aludex, Intervet) washes. It is recommended that the dog be thoroughly clipped to enhance the efficacy of treatment. In addition, bathing with a keratolytic shampoo prior to treatment will remove debris and allow the medication easier access to the follicles. (Sebomild, Virbac is one of many choices.) Amitraz must be mixed to a stronger dilution than that used for the treatment of sarcoptic mange. In demodicosis, the dilution is 0.050% or 50 ml in 5 litres of water. The applicant should wear an apron, gloves, goggles and protective footwear such as wellington boots. Dipping should be done in well-ventilated area. Owners or veterinary personnel carrying out the dips should be warned that people on monamine oxidase-(MAO)-inhibitor medication and diabetics can be prone to side-effects from amitraz. Dogs on MAO inhibitors such as the behaviour-modification drugs clomipramine (Clomicalm, Novartis) and selegiline (Selgian, CEVA) cannot be given amitraz dips until they have been off medication for several weeks. Diabetic pets should not be treated with amitraz as they can become unstable. Chihuahuas cannot be given amitraz dips, nor can pregnant or nursing bitches or puppies younger than 12 weeks of age.

The solution should be poured over the dog, carefully avoiding the eyes. It must be allowed to dry on the dog and cannot be rinsed off. This needs to be done once weekly for at least 5 weeks or until you have achieved two negative skin scrapings. Multiple scrapes should be carried out at five different sites at least once a month. Record the ratio of live:dead mites at each scraping. Treatment should continue 2–4 weeks past cure. To achieve this result may take much longer than 5 weeks. In severe cases, 6 months of rinses may be required. In some instances, life-long treatment may be required. Localised, persistent demodicosis can be treated with a 5% solution of amitraz, diluted with mineral oil and applied daily to the lesional areas.

If the owner is unwilling or unable to use amitraz, there are alternatives, although their use is not well documented. Treatment with oral ivermectin has shown some positive results. This is a simple treatment to give; however, it can be difficult to convince the owner to continue with treatment well beyond clinical cure. Additionally, ivermectin is not licensed for treatment in small animals and cannot be used with collie breeds or collie crosses. Moxidectin, used in the United Kingdom as a large-animal wormer, has been used by some clinicians in the treatment of demodicosis. Again, use in small animals is off-license and this should be discussed with the owners.

Milbemycin is a drug that is used in France for the treatment of demodicosis. At present, it is not available in the United Kingdom but can be imported on a named patient basis. A poor response to amitraz or reasons contraindicating the use of amitraz, for example, concurrent diabetes mellitus, are considered appropriate reasons for requesting importation of milbemycin.

It needs to be explained to the owner that demodicosis in the adult canine can have severe complications which may require euthanasia if aggressive treatment is not given as directed. The owner should also be informed that treatment can easily last 6 months, if not longer, and that relapse is common. The expense that will be incurred, the ability of the owner to comply with treatment and, most importantly, the quality of the animal's life must be evaluated when planning a treatment programme. Client education is paramount and written information, such as the sample leaflet below, as well as supportive follow-up appointments, are important.

Information leaflet on demodicosis *Demodex* mites are a natural inhabitant of your dog's skin. People have their own forms of this mite too! However, your dog has a larger than normal population of this mite, resulting in skin disease. Your dog may have a problem with the mite *Demodex canis* because of a depressed immune system and/or some underlying disease. Therefore, it is essential that you do everything you can to assist your dog's overall wellbeing. High-quality nutrition in ample quantities, warm bedding and fresh air and exercise will help your dog's general health. Any concurrent diseases, such as skin infections, will need to be treated along with the *Demodex* infestation. If you are asked to give antibiotics, please make sure you complete the course. If you are worried that your dog is not tolerating the antibiotics well, please contact your veterinarian for an alternative treatment.

Clipping your dog will assist in the efficacy of the dip preparation. You may prefer to have your dog completely clipped by a professional groomer as she will probably do a more aesthetically pleasing job! Do let your groomer know that *Demodex* will not contaminate her grooming parlour. If you are worried about your dog getting cold, do invest in a jacket or jumper for your dog.

Your dog will need to be bathed in a special de-scaling and de-greasing shampoo prior to treatment. This shampoo is necessary to remove the debris the mites have created and allow the dip to penetrate deeply into the hair follicles where the mites live. Please follow the instructions on the shampoo carefully. You may be required to leave the shampoo on your pet for 10 minutes before rinsing. Make sure your dog is comfortable in the bath. Laying on old towel or using a rubber mat inside the bath will prevent slipping. Use mildly warm water. Avoid getting water into the ears by placing cotton wool balls in each ear. Rinse the eyes thoroughly if any shampoo gets into them. Speak soothingly to your dog while bathing it and offer treats if your dog is food-oriented. Be sure to rinse well. Any shampoo left on the skin can be very drying and irritating to your dog. If you are worried about shampooing your dog, a groomer or a vet nurse can do the job for you.

Please make sure you mix the amitraz (Aludex, Intervet) dip according to the dilution instructions. Fifty millilitres (one bottle) in 5 litres of water is appropriate for the average dog. Very large breeds will need 100 ml (two bottles) in 10 litres of water. Consult your vet or vet nurse if you are unsure of how much to use.

Wear gloves and an apron and make sure that you are working in a well-ventilated area. Some people also like to wear goggles and wellington boots for full protection. If you are diabetic or are taking MAO-inhibitor medications (monoamine oxidase inhibitors), you may want to consult your GP before using amitraz to dip your dog.

Once you have poured the dip over your dog, avoiding the eyes, leave the dip to air-dry. Do not towel dry your dog or the dip will be removed.

Dips need to be repeated weekly until your dog is completely free of disease. Your veterinarian will continue to take skin scrapes on a monthly basis. Once your dog's skin scrapings have been free of mites for 2 months you may be able to complete treatment. However, do be aware that relapse is common in this disease. Contact your vet early on if you suspect a relapse. Some dogs will need life-long treatment. Consult your veterinarian if you have any concerns about the treatment, side-effects or length of treatment.

Important points to remember about *Demodex:*
Clinical signs: Alopecia around eyes ('spectacle appearance') later occurring on head, forelimbs, trunk, beet red skin in adult onset.
Diagnostic tests: Hair plucks, deep skin scrapes.
Treatment: Amitraz dips weekly for 5 weeks or until two negative skin scrapes.

FORMULARY OF TREATMENT OF ECTOPARASITE INFESTATIONS IN DOGS AND CATS

Non-licensed products are marked with an asterisk.

Adulticides for use on pet

Fipronil – Frontline spray and spot-on (Merial Animal Health)

The spray is licensed for the treatment of fleas, ticks, lice and in aid of treatment for *Cheyletiella* spp, *Neotrombicula autumnalis* and *Sarcoptes scabiei*.

Can be given to puppies and kittens as young as 2 days of age.

Application at a dose rate of two to four pumps per kilogram (3–6 ml/kg) depending on length of coat and type of infestation. (Smaller pump dispensers will require additional pumps to equal 3–6 mls)

Treatment effective for fleas with a 98% efficacy within 24 hours. Effective for 3 months in dogs and 2 months in cats.

Treatment effective within 48 hours for ticks and lasts 4 weeks in dogs and cats.

Effective within 48 hours for louse species *T. canis* and *F. subrostrata*.

Spot-on licensed for treatment of fleas, ticks and lice (*T. canis, F. subrostrata* and *L. setosus*).

Can be used on puppies and kittens from 8 weeks of age; also licensed for use on breeding bitches, queens and lactating bitches and queens.

Kills 98% of fleas within 24 hours. Efficacy lasts approximately 2 months in dogs, 5 weeks in cats.

Kills ticks within 48 hours and lasts 1 month.

Kills lice within 48 hours and lasts 1 month.

Must wait 48 hours after application of spray and spot-on before bathing animal. Applicators of spray or spot-on should wear gloves and/or wash hands after application. Do not smoke while applying product. Apply in a well-ventilated room.

Sprays available in 100 ml, 250 ml and 500 ml bottles.

Spot-ons available in cat size, puppy application, kitten application and four sizes for adult dogs: 2–10 kg, 10–20 kg, 20–40 kg and 40–60 kg.

Fipronil and Methoprene – Frontline combo (Merial)

This is also a spot-on for dogs and cats. The fipronil component acts on the adult ectoparasites while the insect growth regulator, methoprene, acts on the larval and egg stages of fleas. This combination should help to control environmental as well as pet infestations.

The product is available in four sizes for dogs and one size for cats. Puppies and kittens must be at least 8 weeks of age before application. The product is designed to be effective for up to 8 weeks on adult fleas and 4 weeks on adult ticks. Fleas are killed within 24 hours and ticks within 48 hours.

Imadicloprid – Advantage spot-on (Bayer)

Licensed for the treatment of flea control with nearly 100% efficacy within 12 to 24 hours. Residual activity of 4 weeks. Bathing does not affect efficacy.

Can be given to puppies and kittens from 8 weeks of age.

Skin debris from the treated animal is eaten by larvae. Through this process, the larval population in the environment is controlled.

Spot-on should be applied between the animal's shoulder blades, and the person applying the product should wear gloves and/or wash hands directly after use. Do not smoke while applying agent.

Spot-ons available in two sizes for cats – less than 4 kg and greater than 4 kg.

Dogs sizes: up to 4 kg, 4–10 kg, 10–25 kg, 25–40 kg. Large dogs can use combinations of doses to add up to the correct body weight.

Imadicloprid and Permethrin – Advantix (Bayer)

This product is used for the control of fleas and as a repellent for ticks, mosquitoes and sand flies. Due to its repellent property, it is helpful in the prevention of the tick-borne diseases borreliosis (Lyme disease), babesiosis and ehrlichiosis. Additionally, it is advised for help in prevention of heartworm disease and leishmaniasis due to its repellent activity against mosquitoes and sand flies.

The spot-on product is available in four sizes for dogs only (1.5–4 kg, 4–10 kg, 10–25 kg and 25–40 kg). Dogs must be 7 weeks of age before Advantix may be used on them. The spot-on should be applied to the back of the neck and the handler should wear gloves. The dog should not be bathed until 2 weeks after application for full efficacy of the product.

**Ivermectin (Ivomec, Merial)*

Cats and dogs: 0.2–0.3 mg/kg subcutaneous, intramuscular as an acaracidal. Doses should be given 2 weeks apart to interrupt the egg-to-larval life cycle of *Otodectes, Sarcoptes* and *Notedres* mites. For demodectic mange, ivermectin is given orally at a dose rate of 0.35–0.6 mg/kg once daily (Scott et al 2001) until two negative skin scrapings, harvested 2 weeks apart, are obtained.

**Milbemycin (Interceptor, Novartis)*

Must be imported from France. Dose according to package instructions. Useful in the treatment of demodectic mange in dogs at a dose rate of 0.5–2 mg/kg PO once daily (Scott et al 2001) until two negative skin scrapings, obtained 2 weeks apart, are harvested.

**Moxidectin (Cydectin, Fort Dodge Animal Health)*

Dogs can be given a dose rate of 0.2–0.4 mg/kg once daily until two negative skin scrapings, harvested 2 weeks apart, are obtained (Scott et al 2001).

Nitenpyram – Capstar tablets (Novartis)

Licensed for treating flea infestations. Begins killing within 30 minutes. Nearly 100% kill rate within 4 hours. Maintains high kill rate for 24 hours in dogs and 48 hours in cats. Can be given daily.

Tablets available in two dose sizes according to weight.

Selamectin – Stronghold spot-on (Pfizer)

Licensed for treatment of fleas, ticks, *Toxocara canis*, lice (*T. canis*) *Sarcoptes scabiei*, heartworm preventative in dogs.

Licensed for the treatment of fleas, ticks, *Toxocara cati*, lice (*F. subrostrata*), *Ancylostoma tubaeformae, Otodectes cynotis.*

Efficacy of 98% against fleas within 24 hours in cats and 99% efficacy against fleas in dogs within 36 hours. Effective as a flea ovicidal for 21 days, larvacidal for 30 days and adulticidal for 30 days.

Two doses 1 month apart for treatment of sarcoptic mange and ear mites. Similar treatment schedule advised for lice infestations.

Monthly treatments required for prevention of other parasites listed.

Licensed for use in puppies and kittens from 6 weeks of age.

Selamectin is carried into flea faeces, which are eaten by larvae. Thus, some environmental control is achieved through the use of selamectin.

Animal can be bathed 2 hours after treatment. Applicator should wash hands after and/or wear gloves to apply product. Do not smoke or eat while using product.

Available in cat size, puppy and kitten size (less than 2.5 kg).

Doses for dogs in sizes 2.5–5 kg, 5.1–10 kg, 10.1–20 kg, 20.1–40 kg. Very large dogs should use appropriate combinations of tubes.

Insect growth regulator

Lufenuron – Program and Program Plus (Novartis)

(Program Plus also contains milbemycin for the control of intestinal parasites.)

Chitin synthesis inhibitor destroys eggs. No viable eggs within 24 hours of ingestion of tablet. Dog dosing required monthly. Cat preparation can be given as an injection on a 6-monthly basis or as an oral suspension once monthly.

Safe for use in puppies as young as 2 weeks/ weight of 1 kg. Kittens must be weaned.

Cat's oral suspension in small cat/kitten size and larger cat dose (greater than 4 kg).

Cat injection for small cat/kitten size and larger cat dose (greater than 4 kg).

Dog doses available in four sizes: up to 2.3 kg, 2.3–6.7 kg, 6.8–20 kg, 21–40 kg. Larger dogs to be given the correct number of tablets for their weight.

Environmental control sprays

Insect growth regulators + adulticides – methoprene and permethrin – Acclaim (Ceva Animal Health)

Designed to kill adult fleas and inhibit the growth of flea eggs and larvae.

One application required per year.

One spray bottle will cover 140 m^2 (167 square yards).

Remove all pets before spraying. Do not use around reptiles and fish. Cover food-preparation areas. Do not use around naked flames. Vacuum prior to use and wash human and pet bedding on warm wash (at least 50°C). Treat car also if animal has access to car.

Ventilate car and rooms 30 minutes after spraying. Methoprene is sensitive to ultraviolet rays, so may have reduced efficacy in sunlit rooms.

Insect growth regulators + adulticides – pyriproxyfen and permethrin - Indorex (Virbac Animal Health)

Designed to kill adult fleas and inhibit the growth of flea eggs and larvae.

One application required per year.

One spray can is adequate for a two-bedroom home.

Remove all pets before spraying. Do not use around reptiles and fish. Cover food preparation areas. Do not use around naked flames. Vacuum prior to use and wash human and pet bedding on 50°C wash. Treat car also if animal has access to car. Ventilate car and rooms 30 minutes after spraying.

Boric acid powder (sodium polyborate) – Fleaban (AnimalCare)

Application instructions must be followed exactly. If used properly it can be effective for 1 year for environmental control. The product works by dehydrating the flea. Vacuuming prior to use and washing pets' bedding enhances efficacy.

Shampoos

Keratolytics – for use in mange cases to clear coat of crust and debris, making it easier for antimiticial dips to penetrate.

Benzoyl peroxide – Paxcutol (Virbac)

Leave on dog for 10 minutes. Rinse thoroughly. Person bathing dog should wear gloves. Can be used on a daily basis.

Suitable for dogs only.

Salicylic acid – Sebomild P (Virbac)

Leave on animal for 5 minutes contact time. Rinse thoroughly.

Can be used on a weekly basis.

Can be used on both dogs and cats.

Selenium sulphide – Seleen (Ceva Animal Health)

Keratolytic shampoo with some efficacy against surface mites such as *Cheyletiella*.

Leave suspension in contact with coat for 5–10 minutes. Rinse thoroughly.

Can be used on a weekly basis.

Licensed only for dog, although use in cats has been reported.

Dips

Amitraz – Aludex (Intervet)

For the treatment of sarcoptic and demodectic mange.

Sarcoptic mange – 0.025% solution, 25 ml in 5 litres of water. Dip weekly. Allow dip to dry on animal. Repeat until clinical cure and two negative skin scrapings, 2 weeks apart, have been obtained.

Demodectic mange – 0.050% solution, 50 ml in 5 litres of water. Dip weekly. Allow dip to dry on dog. Repeat until clinical cure and two negative skin scrapes obtained over a 5-week period.

Only for use on dogs. Do not use on Chihuahuas or dogs receiving MAO (monoamine oxidase)-inhibitor medications. Avoid use in diabetic dogs. Applicator should wear protective clothing. Mix dip and apply in a well ventilated area.

Ear treatments with acaracidal activity

Auroto (Arnolds) thiabendazole, neomycin, amethocaine HCl

For the treatment of ear mites (as well as other otitis externa conditions) in dogs and cats. Thiabendazole is the agent active against *Otodectes cynotis*.

Apply three to five drops twice daily into the external ear canals. Treat for 1 week. Do not use if the ear drum is perforated.

Canaural (Leo Laboratories) diethanolamine fusidate, framycetin sulphate, nystatin, prednisolone

For treatment of microorganisms and *O. cynotis* in the external ear canal of dogs and cats. There is no specific ingredient active against ear mites but the preparation has been shown to be effective against *O. cynotis* in clinical trials. Shake the bottle well before using and apply five to ten drops in both ears. Treat twice daily for 1 week, stop treatment for 1 week and then resume twice daily treatment during the third week. Long-term use can cause side-effects due to corticosteroid component.

Oterna (Schering-Plough) – betamethasone, neomycin sulphate, monosulfiram

For treatment of otitis externa caused by (among other things) ear mites. Monosulfiram is the ingredient active against mites. Licensed for use in cats and dogs. Two to eight drops into the external ear canals twice daily until control of the infestation is achieved. Do not use if the tympanic membrane is perforated. Long-term use can cause side-effects due to corticosteroid component.

References and Further Reading

Ackerman L 1993 Diagnosis and management of parasitic skin disease. In: Ackerman L (ed) Pet skin and hair coat problems. Veterinary Learning Systems, Trenton, NJ. p 33–72

August John R 1986 Disease of the ear canal. In: August JR (ed)The complete manual of ear care. Solvay Vet, Inc. Veterinary Learning Systems, Trenton, NJ, p 39–40

Curtis C 1999 Use and abuse of topical dermatological therapy in dogs and cats, Part 2. In Practice September: 448–454

Georgi J, Georgi M 1992 Canine clinical parasitology. Lea and Febiger, London, p 1–17, 35–58

Grant D 1991 Parasitic skin disease. In: Grant D (ed) Skin disease in the dog and cat, 2nd edn. Blackwell Science, Oxford

Grant D I, Thoday K L 1991 The skin. In: Gorman N (ed) Canine medicine and therapeutics, 3rd edn. Blackwell Science, London, p 387–388

Guthrie Arlo 2003 Staying one jump ahead. Veterinary Nursing Times April:21–22

Kristensen F, Jacobsen J, Eriksen T 1996 Otology in dogs and cats. Leo Laboratories, Denmark/Princes Risborough, England, p 30–31

Paterson S 1998 Parasitic skin diseases. In: Paterson S (ed). Skin diseases of the dog. Blackwell Science, London, p 83–117

Scott D W, Miller W H, Griffin C E 2001 Parasitic skin disease. In: Scott D W et al (eds) Muller and Kirk's Small animal dermatology, 6th edn. W B Saunders, London, p 423–516

Wall R, Shearer D 2001 Veterinary ectoparasites. Blackwell Science, Oxford, p 23–49, 55–81, 114–139, 143–156, 162–177

CASE STUDY

Adult canine demodicosis

Signalment

Female, neutered Lurcher, aged 4 years. This bitch was the shorthaired type of Lurcher.

Complaint

Recurrent pyoderma, with pustules and crusting. Violent red colour to limbs, tail and ventrum with nearly complete hair loss in these regions.

History

The bitch was treated for scabies 2 years earlier by another veterinarian. The treatment used was phosmet (Vet-Kem Sponge-on; Sanofi Animal Health) and later selamectin (Stronghold; Pfizer Animal Health). Neither treatment had been successful and the owner had requested a referral to a homeopathic vet. Further treatment at a standard veterinary surgery reported pododermatitis, treated with amitraz (Aludex; Hoechst Roussell) along with sulphadiazine/ trimethoprim tablets (Tribrissen 80; Schering-Plough). None of the follow-up appointments had been kept.

More recently, the bitch had been exhibiting generalised dermatitis, and cephalexin (Ceporex; Schering-Plough) was prescribed at a dose rate of 750 mg per day, divided into two doses. A blood sample was taken for allergy screening (Topscreen, Axiom Laboratories). The bitch tested positive for the indoor panel. In a follow-up appointment, 1 week later, the owner complained of the bitch's pruritus so prednisolone (Prednicare; Animal Care, Ltd) at a dose rate of 5 mg b.i.d. was prescribed, along with essential fatty acids (Efavet 660, Schering Plough) at the dose rate of two capsules per day. A third follow-up visit was recorded, reporting an improvement in the generalised dermatitis.

Physical examination

The owner presented the dog because of a sudden flare up of pyoderma. On examination the bitch was underweight at 20 kg and showed a depressed demeanour. Most alarming was the extreme erythema and alopecia of the limbs, entire ventrum, head, pinnae and tail (see Fig. 4.18). Macules and patches of various sizes, along the limbs and facial region, suggested a long-standing inflammatory process. Pustules and crusting were evident, especially on the ventrum, along with signs of self-trauma.

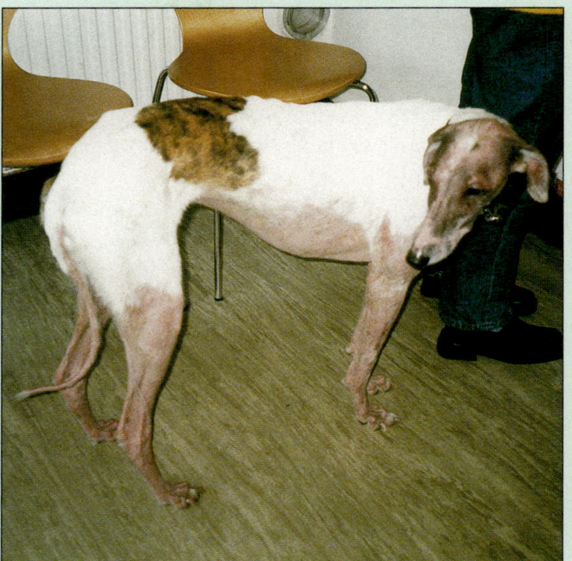

Figure 4.18 Adult onset demodicosis. The beet red skin of this dog can be seen in chronic demodicosis. Photograph by Frances Gaudiano.

Differential diagnosis

- Demodicosis
- Sarcoptic mange
- Dermatophytosis
- Pyoderma
- *Malassezia* dermatitis
- Atopy
- Food sensitivity
- Drug eruption
- Hypothyroidism
- Keratinisation disorder
- Pemphigus complex.

Diagnostic procedures

The bitch was admitted for a thorough dermatological work-up in order to get a definitive diagnosis and begin an appropriate and structured treatment programme. A blood sample was taken for haematological and biochemical analysis. The only abnormality detected was a slight lymphopaenia, which can be seen in cases of demodicosis.

Premedication was administered and then the bitch was induced with propofol (Rapinovet; Schering-Plough) and intubated with a size 10 tube. She was maintained on 2% halothane (Halothane; Merial Animal Health) while multiple skin scrapings were taken. Tape strips were also taken along with six biopsies. The biopsy sites included the dorsal rostral region, periocular region, lateral neck, lateral toe of the left forefoot, medial right thigh and the dorsal mid-tail region. The biopsy sites were sutured closed with polymide 2/0 (Supramid; SMI). The sutures were to be removed in 10 days time. A swab was also taken from a punctured pustule and sent to a laboratory for analysis.

Demodex canis was identified on the skin scrape slides so amitraz washes were prescribed to begin 3 days after the procedure and repeated every 3 to 4 days, depending on the bitch's tolerance to amitraz. Metoclopromide (Emequell; Pfizer Animal Health) was dispensed to deal with post-dipping nausea, as the owner had complained that this was a problem with the animal. Wisely, the prednisolone was immediately stopped and the bitch was given meloxicam (Metacam; Boehringer Ingelheim) to treat the inflammation. Antibiotic therapy was continued.

The biopsy report described follicular hyperkeratosis with folliculitis and many *Demodex* spp mites. Yeast infection was also present in the tissue. It was suggested that the bitch may have T-cell suppression and that cure might not be possible.

The culture and sensitivity report showed profuse *Staphylococcus intermedius*, sensitive to lincomycin, erythromycin, co-trimeprothrin, enrofloxacin, cephalexin and amoxicillin clavulanate. *Malassezia pachydermatis* was also identified.

Diagnosis and prognosis

This bitch was suffering from generalised demodicosis with secondary pyoderma, caused by *S. intermedius* and a yeast infection caused by *Malassezia*. T-cell suppression was suggested so the prognosis for cure was guarded.

Treatment

Amitraz dips commenced on a weekly basis. Cephalexin, at a dose rate of 250 mg b.i.d. was prescribed and chlorphenamine 4 mg (Piriton; Stafford-Miller) was added, to be given every 8 hours to control the pruritus and resulting self-trauma. A probiotic supplement was also prescribed to counteract the effects of long-term antibiotic treatment. Baths in Malaseb (Leo Animal Health) were prescribed bi-weekly. The owner was advised that the dips must continue past the clinical cure of the bitch.

Follow-up and outcome

One month after the work-up, the bitch had gained weight and experienced some hair regrowth, although the pinnae still showed some crusting. Another week's worth of cephalexin was prescribed. The pruritus had eased considerably, according to the owner's reports. Skin scrapings showed three small, moribund *Demodex* mites.

Two months post-diagnostic procedures the dog was again quite pruritic and showed slight folliculitis and erythema on the ventrum. The owner had dropped the amitraz dips to one every 10 days so she was asked to maintain the frequency of one dip per week. Skin scrapes showed one live *Demodex* mite. Cephalexin treatment was restarted and the owner was reminded to continue with Malaseb baths at least once weekly.

At the 3rd month post-investigation, there was 90% hair regrowth right up to, but excluding, the paws. The owner had decreased the amitraz to one dip every 3–4 weeks. She was reminded to step up the treatment to once a week, for at least 4 weeks consecutively as we still had not achieved two negative skin scrapings. Skin scrapings on this visit did not show any mites but scrapings cannot be relied on entirely as mites may not always be included in the sample gathered. Antihistamines were again prescribed for 8-hourly intervals and cephalexin was prescribed for a 2-week period.

Three days later the ventrum was exhibiting infection. Amitraz dips were increased to one every 5 days and Malaseb baths were to be performed between dips. Additionally, the owner was advised to give large doses of essential fatty acids – as much as the bitch could tolerate without having diarrhoea, to help decrease the inflammation and pruritus.

The bitch is not cured but is being maintained on a treatment programme of:

- amitraz dips weekly
- chlorphenamine 4 mg tablets three times per day
- pulse antibiotic therapy – her last prescription was for a month of cephalexin
- essential fatty acids to tolerance level.

It is likely that treatment, on some level, will be lifelong.

Discussion

This bitch had a long history of skin problems that may have all along been due to demodicosis. If extensive skin scrapings had been done at the onset of skin disease, perhaps an earlier diagnosis could have been made and prevented initial mismanagement of this case. Due to the nature of the disease, we know that the bitch carried *D. canis* from puppyhood but we do not know when the presence of the mite developed into a full-blown disease. The bitch may have been genetically destined to develop the disease.

At the presentation for generalised dermatitis, skin scrapings and hair pluckings should have been performed, possibly preventing the need for a general anaesthetic later in the investigation. Something as simple as hair pluckings can be quite useful in diagnosing *D. canis* (Grant 1998). Proof of the mite's presence may have inspired the owner to be more compliant and certainly would have contraindicated the use of prednisolone to control the pruritus (Paterson 1998). However, it is not always possible to harvest a mite even when demodicosis is strongly indicated and skin biopsies are a definitive means of diagnosis for this disease. By the time the owner presented the bitch for a second flare up of pyoderma the skin condition had become so severe that the attending veterinary surgeon felt that skin biopsy was a necessary measure.

It needed to be explained to the owner that demodicosis can actually be fatal if aggressive treatment is not given faithfully. Because of the complicating factors the owner also needed to be made aware that treatment could easily last 6 months, if not longer.

As the owner was so worried about the chemical properties of amitraz, other treatment modalities may have been explored. Some good reports have been given of treatment with either ivermectin or milbemycin (Scott et al 2001). These are simple treatments to give orally; however, it can be difficult to convince the owner to continue with treatment well beyond clinical cure. Additionally, milbemycin must be imported under special license. A variety of immune-system stimulants have been suggested as helpful, though not curative. Vitamin E, selenium, levamisole and coenzyme Q (Ackerman 1993) may have appealed to this health-conscious client.

Finally, our treatment protocol may have been changed to advantage. It is considered best to fully clip the animal and bathe it in a sulphur and salicylic acid product to remove scale and crust prior to beginning amitraz treatment (Paterson 1998). This procedure may have improved the efficacy of the dips.

REFERENCES

(for the Case Study)

Ackerman L 1993 Diagnosis and management of parasitic skin disease. In: Ackerman L (ed) Pet skin and hair coat problems. Veterinary Learning Systems, Trenton, NJ, p 47–49

Grant D 1998 Parasitic skin conditions. BVNA Scottish Region Scientific Weekend Lecture Notes, Crieff, p 5–6

Paterson S 1998 Parasitic skin diseases. In: Paterson S (ed) Skin diseases of the dog. Blackwell Science, London, p 91–95

Scott D W, Miller W H, Griffin C E 2001 Parasitic skin disease. In: Scott D W et al (eds) Muller and Kirk's Small animal dermatology, 6th edn. W B Saunders, London, p 427, 430–431, 457–473

Chapter 5

Bacterial and fungal infections of the skin

CHAPTER CONTENTS

Bacterial and fungal infections of the skin are very common cutaneous conditions. Generally, these conditions exist secondarily to some underlying problem such as an ectoparasite burden, allergy or an endocrine disorder. Regardless of the actual cause, cutaneous infections need to be identified in their own right and treated appropriately.

Pyoderma occurs in dogs frequently and often on a recurrent basis. In cats, pyoderma is a relatively rare occurrence. Technically, pyoderma is defined as a cutaneous pyogenic infection, i.e. pus is involved. There are three categories of pyoderma, with each category involving deeper layers of the epidermis and eventually the dermis.

SURFACE PYODERMA

Pyotraumatic dermatitis

Surface pyoderma occurs in the interfollicular epidermis. One example of surface pyoderma is the hot spot, or more correctly termed, pyotraumatic dermatitis. A hot spot looks almost like a wound. The area of skin has been denuded of hair and the spot itself is an erosion of the upper epidermis. The lesion is erythematous, moist, and it weeps exudate. Hot spots occur usually secondarily to a parasite burden or an allergic skin condition. The dog will lick and chew at a particularly pruritic area, and in this process transfer bacteria from the oral mucosa to the site of pruritus. This inoculates the region with *Staphylococcus intermedius* bacteria, which cause an inflammatory response, increasing the pruritus and thus a vicious circle is set up.

When examining a hot spot, one should clip around the lesion looking for satellite lesions. If additional lesions exist, the problem may be more complicated. It is also important to be sure that the hot spot is just a hot spot and not furunculosis, which is a deep infection of the skin. If there is a dark patch within the lesion this is a sign of haemorrhage and indicates a deep rather than surface lesion.

Treating a hot spot is fairly straightforward. The area needs to be clipped and cleaned and then an antibiotic ointment can be prescribed to apply to the lesion twice daily. Usually an ointment which also contains a steroid is chosen in order to help control the pruritus. Some dogs will also need an Elizabethan collar to prevent further self-trauma. The underlying cause must be addressed or the dog will only create another lesion in an alternative site.

Skin fold pyoderma

A second type of surface pyoderma is skin fold pyoderma, also known as intertrigo. Unfortunately, this disease is often a result of anatomy. Dogs and cats with facial skin folds (Persians, Himalayans, Shar peis, Pugs, Bulldogs, etc.) have perfect environments for bacterial or fungal overgrowth. The skin folds are moist and warm, encouraging the commensal organisms to multiply rapidly. Once the population reaches a certain level, the toxins released by the organisms damage the skin. Washing the skin reduces the population of the organisms and limits the toxin damage. Other areas of concern are folds around the tail base in pugs and bulldogs and vulval skin folds in overweight bitches. If the fold is the consequence of obesity, the simple solution is to put the animal on a diet. If the folds are anatomical, in some cases corrective surgery is in order. Generally though, the course of treatment prescribed is frequent cleaning. A swab or cotton bud should be used daily to wipe the folds clean and to dry them. If an infection has been diagnosed via cytology, cleansing can be instituted with dilute chlorhexidine (Hibiscrub, SSL) diluted 1:5 or with a shampoo containing antibacterial or antifungal ingredients. The owner does need to be informed that the maintenance of skin folds is a life-long, daily task.

Bacterial overgrowth and mucocutaneous pyoderma

Two other types of surface pyoderma include bacterial overgrowth and canine mucocutaneous pyoderma. In bacterial overgrowth there is an unusually high population of the normal commensal skin bacteria. Clinical signs include pruritus and a foul odour. Bacterial overgrowth has been linked to allergy and endocrine disorders and is best treated with shampoo therapy. Mucocutaneous pyoderma is most common in the German Shepherd dog where it appears with crusts and erosions on the lips, eyelids, vulva, perineal region and anus. Antibacterial ointments and washes can be used, but with care, due to the location of the lesions. Some clinicians prefer to treat systemically with antibiotic therapy.

SUPERFICIAL PYODERMA

Superficial pyoderma is defined as a skin infection occurring in the hair follicle but not yet jeopardising the hair shaft. Papules and pustules characterise superficial pyoderma. Secondary lesions include crusts, plaques and epidermal collarettes. These secondary lesions are the result of ruptured pustules and the damaging action of the bacteria. Superficial pyoderma usually occurs on the abdomen and medial thighs. Other truncal areas are possible but less likely, and lesions on the face and pinnae are very rare. Superficial pyoderma nearly always has an underlying cause which needs to be ascertained in order to prevent recurrence. While surface pyoderma can be treated topically, superficial pyoderma generally benefits from systemic treatment. Antibiotics should be given for 7–14 days past clinical cure. Usually a 3-week course is anticipated. Topical shampoo therapy can assist with cure, given twice weekly with a contact time of 10–15 minutes.

Impetigo

A specific type of superficial pyoderma is impetigo. This commonly occurs in puppies but can manifest in adult dogs experiencing some form of immunosuppression. Pustules develop between follicles in the areas of the axillae and inguinal regions. In puppies, impetigo resolves spontaneously but topical treatment can be given to alleviate owner's anxiety. In the adult, the immune system will need assistance with antibacterial systemic treatment. Parasite burdens, poor nutrition and dirty kennelling can be underlying agents for puppy impetigo. Recommendations relating to improved standards of husbandry are worthwhile when dealing with the owners of impetigo-affected puppies.

Bacterial folliculitis

Papules, follicular pustules, epidermal collarettes and patchy alopecia characterise bacterial folliculitis. This disease is probably the most common form of superficial pyoderma and is often associated with allergy, parasites or endocrine disease. An idiopathic form can occur in shorthaired breeds of dog.

Superficial spreading pyoderma

This condition manifests with haemorrhagic bullae that turn into epidermal collarettes. There is erythema at the edge of the collarettes, with a slight exudate. Generally, it is only the secondary lesion that is observed. Clipping can be useful to ascertain the extent of the disease. The cause of the spread has not yet been determined. The disease itself leads to intense pruritus. Systemic and topical treatment is advised in the treatment of this disease. Steroids are tempting due to the pruritus but should be avoided

Deep Pyoderma

Deep pyoderma occurs when follicular infection causes the hair follicle to rupture, releasing hair and bacterial debris into the dermis. Lesions consistent with deep pyoderma are nodules, furuncles, ulcers and draining tracts. As the dermis is vascular, haemorrhage can occur and be seen at the epidermal level as black patches. Cellulitis takes place when furunculosis has developed and inflammatory exudate has infiltrated throughout the dermis. Localised furunculosis can occur on the chin, interdigitally, and at the site of pressure sores. German Shepherd dog pyoderma manifests with draining tracts on the lateral thigh, trunk, groin and lips. This usually occurs in dogs older than 5 years of age with a history of skin disease, such as flea-allergic dermatitis. Deep pyoderma is shown in Figure 5.1.

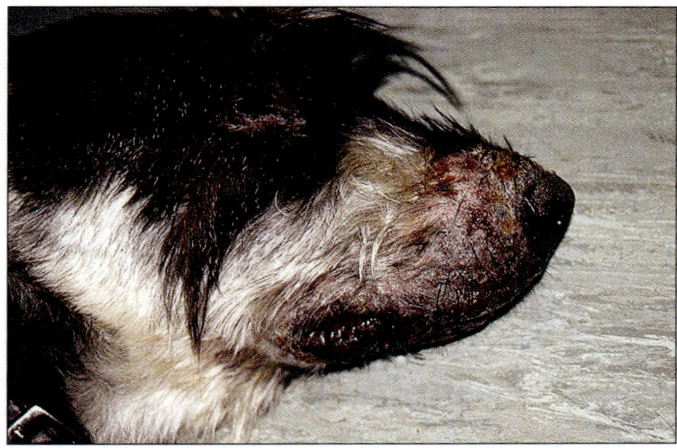

Figure 5.1 This dog is exhibiting a deep pyoderma in which *Streptococcus canis* was identified. Photograph by Annette Loeffler, with permission.

Deep pyoderma always requires systemic antibiotic therapy. Topical treatment can be given for its palliative effect and to help reduce pruritus; however, only systemic treatment will prove curative. In deep pyoderma, systemic antibiotics will need to given 3–4 weeks past clinical cure. A course of 6 months of antibiotic therapy is not at all unusual for the treatment of deep pyoderma, and no deep pyoderma should ever be treated for less than 6 weeks. Deep pyoderma is often the result of superficial pyoderma that was not adequately controlled. Again, a search for an underlying cause is imperative for the condition to be resolved.

The majority of cases of pyoderma (over 90%) are caused by the organism *Staphylococcus intermedius* (Lloyd et al 1996). Streptococcal infections are very rare. *Pseudomonas, Proteus* and *Escherichia coli* (*E. coli*) infections can occur in the right sort of microenvironment – moist, humid, and dirty – but again, these are much less frequently encountered. There are a few recorded cases of MRSA (methicillin-resistant *Staphylococcus aureus*) but these have occurred with pets whose owners have had direct contact with MRSA. Therefore, choosing an antibiotic should be fairly straightforward. In the majority of cases, an antibiotic with proven efficacy against *Staphylococcus intermedius* should be appropriate.

The dog or cat which appears to have pyoderma needs a thorough work-up. While true pyoderma is bacterial, fungal infections can manifest in a similar manner as can sterile pustular disease. Pyoderma is rare in the cat, necessitating a particularly detailed investigation in this species. Pyoderma in cats is often associated with severe systemic disease such as FeLV (feline leukaemia virus), FIV (feline immunodeficiency virus) or diabetes. In addition, clues to the underlying cause must be unearthed and cytological examination of tape strips is probably the best place to start. Several samples should be taken from various lesional sites, being careful to stick the tape to the sample site three times in order to acquire an adequate number of cells. Romanowsky stains (Diff Quik, Dade Behring or Rapi-Diff, Triangle Biomedical Services) can be used and the cells can be examined under high power. Coccal bacteria can be identified as spherical, dark objects between cells, alongside cells and occasionally within keratinocytes. Cocci can be distinguished from melanin granules by the fact that cocci stain lighter (purple versus black or brown), are larger and are more likely to occur outside the cells. Neutrophils may also be seen in abundance in severe infections. Basophils or eosinophils and macrophages may also be visible. However, only the presence of cocci is necessary to make a diagnosis of bacterial infection. If there are rods present rather than cocci, a Gram-negative infection should be suspected. In this case, swabs should be taken for culture and sensitivity. Antibiotic choice will definitely be affected by the presence of rods.

If pustules are present, it can be useful and interesting to pierce the pustule with a needle and make an impression smear by applying a slide to the burst pustule. The slide should be fixed or air-dried and then stained for microscopic observation at high-power magnification. Neutrophils along with bacteria would be expected in a slide taken from a pustule.

The above tests are used to establish pyoderma. Further testing needs to be done to investigate the underlying cause. Skin scrapes and coat brushings should be taken for ectoparasites. Demodectic and sarcoptic mange can easily cause secondary bacterial infections. Any superficial or deep pyoderma, especially a furunculosis, warrants skin scraping for underlying demodicosis. Flea and *Cheyletiella* spp infestations have also been known to lead to bacterial infection. It is wise to put any animal with pyoderma on a strict flea-control programme, selamectin being the treatment of choice because that drug will treat sarcoptic mange as well. Environmental treatment and treatment of in-contact animals should also be advised. A dog suffering from demodicosis is shown in Figure 5.2.

Along with parasites, allergic conditions play a major role in causing secondary pyoderma. If the possibility of ectoparasites has been eliminated and the animal is pruritic, allergic conditions should be investigated. Flea allergy, food sensitivity and atopy can all lead to various degrees of pyoderma. Once good flea control has been established, a food trial may be necessary to eliminate that sensitivity as a possibility. Following the food trial, a work-up for atopy would be the course of investigation.

Hormone imbalances such as hypothyroidism, hyperglucocorticoidisim and growth/sex hormone imbalances should be investigated if ectoparasite and allergy testing proves negative. Hormone investigations require blood sampling. Laboratory fees can be justified by explaining to the owner that identi-

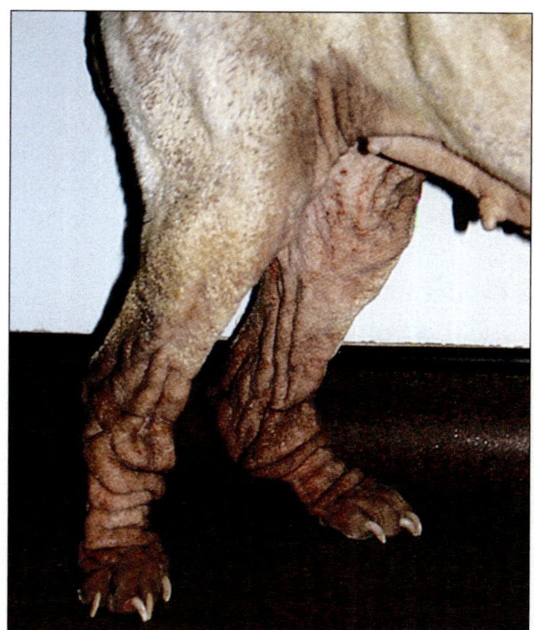

Figure 5.2 This dog is suffering from demodicosis. Infestation, along with the dog's anatomy makes it prone to bacterial and fungal infection. Photograph by Annette Loeffler, with permission.

fying and treating the underlying cause will prevent future incidents of pyoderma, thus eliminating the need for future courses of expensive antibiotics.

Dermatophytosis, and fungal infections in general, can lead to secondary pyoderma. If the history reveals that the problems began with a single lesion, especially in the facial area, a fungal culture is required. Patchy alopecia with scaling is suggestive of dermatophytosis. If you are dealing with a Persian cat, *M canis* should always be a differential diagnosis. Dermatophytosis has been seen to be linked to furunculosis and interdigital pyoderma. Any deep draining tract should make one suspicious of a fungal infection.

Other underlying causes include keratinisation defects, immune-mediated diseases or immunosuppression. Unfortunately, immunosuppression can be iatrogenic by the over-use of corticosteroids. A thorough history will help to identify this problem. Specific diseases, namely, sebaceous adenitis, follicular dystrophy and demodicosis, can cause recurring pyoderma. Rarely, poor nutrition can lead to pyoderma, especially in young or old patients. Finally, neoplasia can be an underlying cause. Figure 5.3 shows a dog with pyoderma.

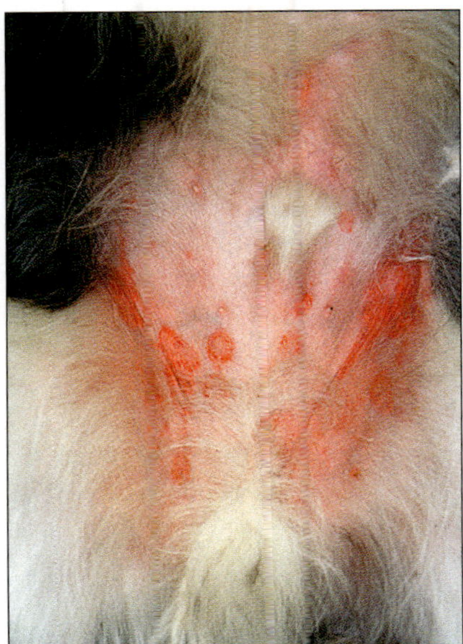

Figure 5.3 In this example of pyoderma, the pustules have ruptured, leaving behind epidermal collarettes. Photograph by Frances Gaudiano.

A summary of pyoderma conditions and examples of common causes

Condition	*Possible cause*
Intertrigo	Obesity, anatomy (skin folds)
Hot spot	Flea allergy
Bacterial overgrowth	Allergy or endocrine disorder
Impetigo	Poor husbandry, parasites
Bacterial folliculitis	Allergy, parasites, endocrine disorders
Superficial spreading pyoderma	Dermatophytosis, drug reaction, epitheliotrophic lymphoma
Chin acne	Demodicosis (pyodemodicosis)
Furunculosis	Demodicosis, dermatophytosis
Clinical sign	***Diagnostic test***
Pruritus	Cytology for yeast, allergy eliminations
Patchy alopecia and scales	Fungal culture
Interdigital lesions	Fungal culture, deep skin scrapings/trichogram for *Demodex*
Surface pyoderma	Coat brushings for fleas/flea-control trial
Any superficial or deep pyoderma	Skin scrapes for mites
Draining tracts	Fungal and bacterial cultures
Furunculosis	Fungal culture, biopsy for demodicosis

Basically, the plan of action when presented with a case of pyoderma is as follows:

- Treat the pyoderma topically twice weekly with an antibacterial shampoo.
- Provide systemic antibiotic therapy for at least 1 week past clinical cure. (Usually a 3-week course for superficial pyoderma and 6 weeks for deep pyoderma.)
- Re-evaluate mid-treatment to assess progress. Adjust treatment as necessary.
- Do not give steroids.
- Identify and treat the underlying condition.

To make sure that you have explored all avenues for underlying causes do the following tests as suggested by the clinical signs and history:

- Tape strippings and impression smears for cytology.

- Skin scrapings and coat brushings for parasitology.
- Establish good flea control.
- Food trial and, if necessary, atopy investigation if allergy is suspected.
- Fungal culture, particularly if patchy alopecia is present, if lesions are interdigital and/or furunculosis has developed.
- Blood testing for hormonal conditions.
- Biopsy for follicular dystrophy, sebaceous adenitis, demodicosis, keratinisation disorder, dermatophytosis.
- If empirical choice of antibiotic is not effective, take swabs for microbiology and culture and sensitivity.

The choice of antibiotic should not be overwhelmingly complicated. Cost and convenience (once daily versus twice daily) do need to be considered for the client's sake, but should not be priorities. The drug chosen needs to be beta-lactamase resistant because *Staphylococcus intermedius* produces this enzyme. The drug should also be readily available to the skin, keeping in mind that the skin receives only 4% of the cardiac output. Distribution to the skin can be slow, a factor which contributes to the need for long courses of treatment. Many treatment failures can be blamed on the fact that the drug wasn't given for long enough or at the correct dose. The animal must be weighed and dosed according to formulary guidelines. If you are dosing correctly, there are a variety of antibiotics that will be bactericidal. Resistances have developed over the years but the percentages of resistance are still fairly low for the average dog or cat seen in first-opinion practice.

Some commonly used antibiotics

Cephalosporin

This is a good choice of antibiotic for deep pyoderma and recurrent cases of pyoderma. Anorexia and vomiting are possible side-effects. Giving the tablet or capsule with a meal tends to reduce side-effects. Resistance rates of 0.6% were measured in 1996 (Lloyd et al 1996).

Clavulanate-potentiated amoxicillin

This drug can be used on recurrent and deep pyodermas. As amoxicillin is a penicillin derivative, hypersensitivity reactions can occur. While *S. intermedius* has developed a resistance rate of nearly 80% to penicillin, clavulanate-potentiated amoxicillin (Synulox, Pfizer) has remained largely effective (Lloyd et al 1996).

Clindamycin

Vomiting and diarrhoea can be side-effects of this drug. Because it comes in capsule form, it can be opened and hidden in food, mixed with water and syringed per os or poured directly into an abscess (a technique used with rabbit abscesses).

Enrofloxacin

This drug is a broad-spectrum antibiotic in the fluoroquinolone group. It cannot be used on animals less than 1 year of age because it can damage cartilage development. Dose rates for cats must be accurate as overdosing is not well tolerated by this species. Enrofloxacin is useful for deep and recurrent pyoderma. Many clinicians prefer to save this drug for use against Gram-negative bacteria.

Erythromycin

The need for this drug to be given every 8 hours reduces owner compliance and heightens the possibility of the animal not receiving the full course of treatment. Gastrointestinal distress is not uncommon. Resistance develops rapidly, limiting the use of erythromycin.

Lincomycin

Vomiting can be a side-effect of this drug. It can be useful on first-time cases of pyoderma but as resistance is reported at 10–40% (Noli 2003) this drug is not helpful for recurrent pyoderma.

Marbofloxacin

This is another wide-spectrum antibiotic in the fluoroquinolone family. Marbofloxacin is used for deep and/or recurrent pyoderma but is often reserved for cases where Gram-negative bacteria have been identified. Vomiting and diarrhoea are possible side-effects, and this drug may lower the seizure threshold in epileptics (Hill 2002).

Oxytetracycline

With *S. intermedius* showing a resistance rate of 40.5% (Lloyd et al 1996), this is not a good choice for the treatment of pyoderma.

Trimethoprim-potentiated sulphonamides

These drugs are a possible choice for first-time pyoderma but not appropriate for recurrent or deep pyoderma. Keratoconjunctivitis sicca (dry eye) can be a side-effect in some cases. It is prudent to perform a Schirmer tear test (diagnostic test for measuring tear production) before prescribing this medication. Polyarthritis has also been recorded as a side-effect with Doberman Pinschers prescribed trimethoprim-sulphonamides. Resistance to this drug is 1–30%, with some countries reporting much higher levels of resistance than others (Noli 2003).

Topical treatment

The use of topical treatment, primarily in the form of shampoo, is a very helpful adjunct to systemic therapy. Topical treatment applies the active molecule directly to the affected area, thus allowing much more rapid access than by systemic therapy. Shampooing has a soothing, anti-pruritic effect, as well as reducing the bacterial population present on the skin surface. Removing debris from the skin surface also removes a food source for the microbes, which is a satisfying concept.

Clients do need to be educated regarding the use of medicinal shampoos. Contact time must be at least 10–15 minutes. Using the shampoo for less time reduces its efficacy, causing a bacteriostatic, rather than bactericidal effect. This can lead to resistance further along in treatment. Practical tips, such as, shampooing the dog and taking it for a walk before rinsing, can be helpful to clients. Rinsing should be thorough as residual shampoo can be an irritant. Eye creams should not be used protectively because they will retain the shampoo ingredients, thus causing increased contact of the ingredient to the eye. Clipping the dog increases the efficacy of shampoo therapy and should be strongly encouraged.

Benzoyl peroxide is the strongest ingredient available in shampoo form for antibacterial treatment. This ingredient is quite good at follicular flushing, making it useful for both superficial and deep pyoderma. A patch test should be done before applying shampoo to the whole dog, because some dogs react adversely to benzoyl peroxide. This shampoo should never be used in cats. As benzoyl peroxide is quite drying, using a conditioning spray afterwards is advisable. This sort of shampoo is a good starting point for topical therapy, but is probably too potent for long-term use.

Chlorhexidine works by disrupting the bacterial cell membrane. It is safe to use on cats and can be found in a variety of formulations. Some clinicians choose to dispense chlorhexidine skin disinfectant and ask the owner to dilute the product in a 1:5 solution. However, the shampoos are more user-friendly. Chlorhexidine is rarely irritating.

Ethyl lactate is useful in mild cases of pyoderma or for long-term maintenance therapy. It has a soothing effect on the skin and is particularly helpful for reducing pruritus. It is mild enough to use on cats.

Piroctine olamine is actually effective against *Pseudomonas* spp infections. As it is not related to the other antimicrobial washes it can be used in cases where resistance has developed to more common ingredients.

Topical ointments, creams and gels are especially helpful when treating surface pyoderma but can be soothing and can accelerate healing with the deeper levels of pyoderma. These types of topical treatment work best with focal areas of infection. Most of the treatments available are polypharmaceuticals, containing antibacterial, antifungal and anti-inflammatory agents. Judicious use must be advised as steroids can be absorbed from topical treatment and can cause side-effects if not used wisely. Owners should be advised to wear gloves when applying topical treatment of any sort.

Autogenous bacterins are another line of treatment that can be used in refractory cases. This formulation is made from the dog's own bacteria and given as a vaccine quite frequently at first, and later on a monthly basis. The preparations vary and adverse reactions can be severe; however, if you are able to obtain a reliable source, this treatment can be effective in as many as 50% of cases. It is especially useful for the treatment of recurrent pyoderma where underlying causes cannot be identified.

If you have followed the treatment protocol for pyoderma (please see below) and find that the case is not resolving a re-examination of procedure must take place. It is possible that you have chosen the wrong antibiotic or that there is a resistance to the antibiotic chosen. If this scenario is assumed, a swab should be taken for culture and sensitivity. Harvesting from a pustule is best but if there are no intact pustules the swab can be rolled along lesional areas and should still collect bacteria. If there is a deep pyoderma, the swab should be inserted deep into the lesion as the bacteria within the lesion may be a different population from those living on the surface. Use a reliable laboratory for your swabs and don't be afraid to ask questions. Laboratories can make mistakes and if the results don't seem to correlate with the clinical picture, ring the laboratory and ask for re-testing.

There may be a simple reason for treatment failure. Perhaps the cat is spitting the tablets under the sofa. Maybe the client is forgetting to give the tablets twice daily and is under-dosing the dog. More embarrassingly, perhaps the dose was not calculated properly for the pet's actual weight.

A main cause of recurring pyoderma is the fact that the underlying cause has not yet been identified. Surface bacteria are commensal. They live happily with the animal without becoming pathogenic, unless there is some reason for microbial overgrowth. Finding the reason may take some time but will save a lot of discomfort on the dog's part and expense on the owner's part. There is the diagnosis of idiopathic pyoderma, especially in German Shepherd dogs, but don't resort to this diagnosis till all else is proven impossible.

Diagnosis of pyoderma

Identify bacterial infection by:

- tape strip cytology
- pustule rupture and impression smear.

Rule out ectoparasites as underlying cause:

- coat brushings
- skin scrapings
- flea-control programme (with product also effective for sarcoptic mange)

Treat pyoderma with systemic and topical therapy. Re-examine within 20 days:

Box

Some improvement but still pruritic

- Carry out food trial (see chapter on allergy)
- Still pruritic after food trial: investigate for atopy (see chapter on allergy)

No improvement

- Check that you are giving an adequate dose rate
- Check owner and pet compliance
- Swab for culture and sensitivity
- Harvest a sample for a fungal culture
- Consider changing treatment

If pyoderma recurs after all of the above, take blood samples to test for endocrinopathy relevant to clinical signs and history:

- hypothyroidism
- hyperadrenocorticism
- reproductive hormone imbalance.

In cats, remember to test for FeLV/FIV

or

biopsy for:

- demodicosis
- dermatophytosis
- follicular dystrophy
- sebaceous adenitis
- other keratinisation disorders.

If none of the above diagnoses is found to be appropriate:

- idiopathic pyoderma.

FUNGAL AND YEAST INFECTIONS

Fungal infections in the form of dermatophytosis (ringworm) are fairly common in cats and somewhat less common in dogs. However, yeast infections, primarily caused by *Malassezia pachydermatitis*, are frequently seen in the dog. Yeast infections often occur concurrently with pyoderma as a secondary phenomenon to allergy or ectoparasites. On the other hand, dermatophytosis can be the underlying problem in a case of pyoderma.

Dermatophytosis is defined as a dermatophyte infection of the hair, nail or stratum corneum. Dermatophytes such as *Microsporum canis* and *Trichophyton* spp digest keratinous debris but not living tissue, thus limiting themselves to the upper layers of the skin and non-viable parts of the hair shaft. An animal becomes infected by having contact with an infected animal or with any object that has been contaminated by fungal spores. Thus, if an infected cat is groomed at a salon, the kennel the cat was in and the grooming table and all grooming equipment can become 'fomites', that is, inanimate objects that can carry a disease. As hairs carrying the spores are swept around the salon, fungal spores are spread throughout the environment. Even ventilation systems and vacuum cleaner bags can harbour fungal spores. Being hardy microorganisms, fungal spores can live in the environment for up to 18 months. One infected cat can wreak havoc.

Luckily, dermatophytosis is a self-limiting disease that generally resolves on its own if the animal has a healthy immune system. The reason we attempt to treat ringworm is not because it is particularly damaging but because of its ability to contaminate an environment, thereby infecting other animals, and because of the zoonotic nature of dermatophytosis.

There are many different species of dermatophytes; however, only a few are relevant to veterinary dermatology and to the UK in particular:

Microsporum canis. Ninety percent of cats with ringworm have the *M. canis* variety. Persian cats are genetically predisposed to *M. canis* infections and can be particularly difficult cases to manage. Of dogs with a ringworm infection, 60% have *M. canis*, which they most likely caught from cats. Probably 99% of the personnel working in rescue catteries have had *M. canis* at one point. The usual source of an *M. canis* infection is a cat. A culture of *M. canis* is shown in Figure 5.4.

Trichophyton mentagrophytes. Wild rodents carry this form of dermatophytosis. It is the type of ringworm most commonly identified in pet guinea pigs. About 30% of dogs with dermatophytosis have *T. mentagrophytes.* Jack Russell terriers figure largely in this group, either due to a breed predisposition or because they frequently attack wild rodents.

Trichophyton erinacei. As you can tell by the name, this is the dermatophyte of choice among hedgehogs. It is found rarely in dogs, because even Jack Russells find hedgehogs difficult to swallow.

A fungal infection caused by *Trichophyton* is shown in Figure 5.5.

Microsporum periscolor. This dermatophyte is found in voles and rarely in dogs.

Microsporum gypseum. This type of ringworm is contracted through contact with contaminated soil. While rare in the dog and cat in the UK, it is a problem in the USA.

Epidermophyton floccosum. This is a dermatophyte found in human beings. It is rare in dogs and cats but they do catch it from their owners from time to time. Nursery schools are a good place to catch *E. floccosum.*

Infection occurs when arthrospores attach to the upper layer of the epidermis, the stratum corneum. The spores germinate and fungal tubes, known as 'hyphae', reach out into the stratum corneum through the aid of keratinases, which are enzymes

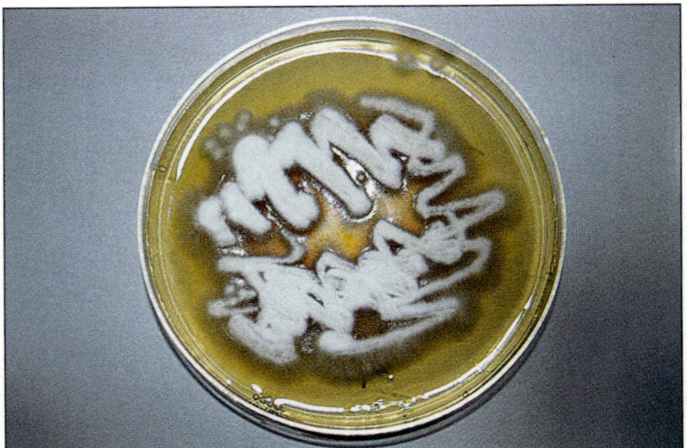

Figure 5.4 *Microsporum canis* is growing on this plate of Sabouraud's dextrose agar. Photograph by Annette Loeffler, with permission.

produced by the fungal spores. As enzymes break down the stratum corneum, they cause an inflammatory reaction. The invasion of the spores continues to the hair shaft, which is penetrated during the anagen phase. Damaged hair falls out easily, leading to the tell-tale patchy alopecia. Eventually, usually within 1–3 months, the immune system is able to overcome the dermatophyte invasion and the disease is resolved. Dermatophytosis becomes chronic if the immune system inadequately suppresses the infection.

The clinical signs of dermatophytosis usually begin focally and can then progress to a more generalised infection. Lesions can be well demarcated or patchy. Typically, there is an inner circle of alopecia surrounded by crust. The lesions tend to heal from the centre outwards, a point to remember when gathering material for samples. The healed area is smooth and shiny. Secondary lesions can include bacterial folliculitis and furunculosis, making it easy to suspect demodicosis instead. Severe dermatophytosis on the face can be similar in appearance to some autoimmune diseases. Generalised dermatophytosis can manifest as seborrhoea sicca with hair loss.

In unusual circumstances, a kerion will be the primary lesion of dermatophytosis. A kerion is a nodule accompanied by a deep, suppurating inflammatory response. This type of lesion is mostly associated with *M. gypseum*, although kerions caused by *M. canis* have been reported.

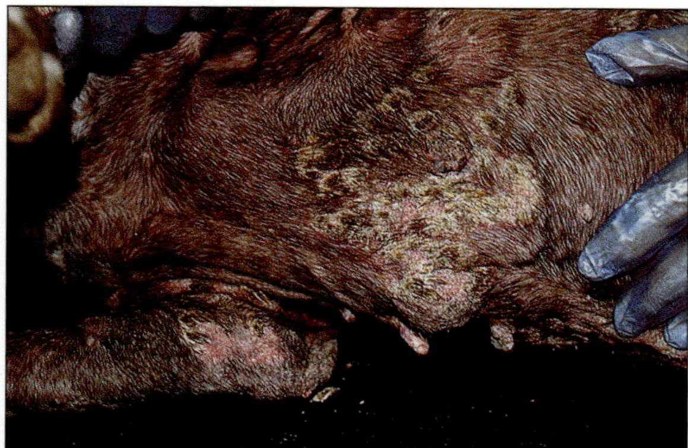

Figure 5.5 This is an example of a fungal infection caused by the organism *Trichophyton*. Photograph by Annette Loeffler, with permission.

Dermatophytosis of the nail is termed 'onychomycosis' and is rare. This type of ringworm is quite difficult to diagnose. Swabs should be inserted as deep as possible into the nail bed to obtain a sample. Nail samples can be gathered by clipping the claw back completely or shaving off bits of nail with a scalpel blade. Yet, these methods may still not be adequate and removal of a claw may be required for a successful biopsy/culture. Amputation of a claw, other than a dewclaw, is a fairly traumatic method of diagnostic testing. If going to these extreme lengths, make sure that the claw is preserved in the correct medium for its transit to the laboratory. A desiccated claw is of no use to the pathologist.

In the cat, any of the above types of lesion is possible for dermatophytosis. Thus, any skin disease in the cat should have dermatophytosis as a differential. Kittens tend to show scale and crust on their face and extremities. Miliary dermatitis can also be a form of dermatophyte lesion, as can recurrent chin acne. Pseudomycetomas – ulcerating nodules with granulomatous perifolliculitis and/or panniculitis – are unusual but can occur in Persian cats with dermatophytosis. Most frustrating is the asymptomatic cat, blithely spreading spores far and wide. These cats are known as 'fomite carriers' and are often Persians carrying *M. canis*. The warm, moist facial folds of Persians serve as anatomical reservoirs of fungi.

When dealing with a suspected case of dermatophytosis it is important to obtain a thorough clinical history, as usual. Because dermatophytosis is a contagious disease, lesions on in-contact animals or humans are good clues. A thorough physical examination of the patient is required, because any systemic problems may lead to the animal's inability to overcome the infection. Any condition that can compromise immune function (e.g. FeLV, FIV) should be noted and any use of steroids is highly relevant. A compromised immune system makes it very difficult to control a dermatophyte infection.

Diagnosis

There are a variety of ways of diagnosing a dermatophyte infection and it is important to remember that dogs can be infected by more than one species of dermatophyte simultaneously.

The Wood's lamp

Probably the most well known method of diagnosis is the use of a Wood's lamp. This is an ultraviolet lamp which, when shone on infected hair, will fluoresce apple green. Unfortunately, this is possible only if the infesting dermatophyte is the species *Microsporum canis* – and even then it is only about 60% accurate. False positives are common as other substances can fluoresce. For example, kitten formula has an interesting glow under a Wood's lamp and medications and even greasy seborrhoea can create false positives. It is important to remember that the lamp needs at least 5 minutes to warm up and that the examination must be done in a very dark room (X-ray processing rooms are often used!). Be sure that the colour appearing is actually apple green. Most dermatologists would agree that the Wood's lamp is not completely diagnostic. Fluorescing hairs should be plucked and examined under the microscope and/or used for a fungal culture. Thus, the Wood's lamp is best used for identifying good sample material. It has been suggested that the Wood's lamp is also useful for locating environmental contamination.

Hair pluckings

Hair pluckings from the edges of lesions or skin scrapes from the same location can be fixed in liquid paraffin or potassium hydroxide (KOH) and examined under a microscope. The low-power lens should be used to locate debris around a hair shaft and then the high-power lens for the identification of fungal hyphae or spores. Spores are alongside and tightly adhered to hair shafts. However, locating and identifying spores and hyphae is difficult and takes much practise to master.

Fungal culture

The same sort of samples, i.e. hair pluckings, can be used for imbedding in Sarbouraud's agar for fungal culture. The area of the lesion can be clipped and lightly cleaned with surgical spirit. Hair shafts should be gently rolled out of the follicles in order to maintain the debris necessary for identification. Scales as well as hair are good to gather for culture. If a generalised disease is suspected, one can use a rubber brush over the entire coat, later pressing the rubber bristles into the agar. This is known as the 'Denman brush technique'. Some clinicians will use a new toothbrush for brushing around likely lesions and then press the toothbrush into the plate.

These cultures must be incubated aerobically – the lid should be loose. The ideal temperature is 26°C for an incubation period of 2–4 weeks. The plate should be kept somewhere free of exposure to ultraviolet light (not on the laboratory windowsill!). The culture should be checked daily as the colour change to red must be identified as soon as it occurs. Dermatophytes metabolise proteins, which liberate alkaline metabolites, causing the pH indicators in the medium to change from yellow to red. However, non-pathogenic fungi can also go through this process. Non-pathogens prefer carbohydrates, and will digest those first, but once all the carbohydrates have been consumed the proteins will be ingested. A late change to red is more indicative of non-pathogenic fungi. With dermatophytes, the colour change will go to red usually within 10 days. Then a white to buff coloured colony will grow on the plate. The colony can be sampled and the exact type of dermatophyte identified. This is useful in terms of locating the source of infection.

Fluorescence microscopy

Fluorescence microscopy utilises skin scales and fluorescent dye. The samples are then examined under an ultraviolet microscope. Naturally, this diagnostic method is not available in general practice but some universities do have this facility.

Biopsy

The most definitive method of diagnosis is biopsy. Fungal invasion of the hair follicle is conclusive proof of dermatophytosis. Depending on your laboratory, biopsy may also be a quicker method of detection than fungal culture; however, it is obviously more traumatic for the patient and more costly for the owner. Special stains can help the pathologist to identify fungi in biopsy specimens.

Treatment

Once ringworm has been identified, one can explain to the owner that it is a self-limiting disease and will go away in a couple of months, or treatment can commence. Treatment is usually preferred due to the contagious nature of dermatophytosis.

Clipping

Firstly, the hair around the lesion, or the entire hair coat if the condition is generalised, must be clipped. The removal of hair reduces environmental contamination. Hair colonised by spores is damaged and is easily shed, spreading spores throughout the environment. Clipping removes this possibility, although it does contaminate the area where the grooming is done. Thorough vacuuming and scrubbing of the area should be undertaken in the area where clipping has taken place. The clippers need to be disinfected, making sure the disinfectant is sporicidal. Even the used vacuum bag should be disposed of.

Shampoo therapy

Clipping encourages new hair growth. Healthy shafts will push out the old diseased hair, helping to speed recovery. Clipping also has the advantage of making shampoo therapy more effective. Miconazole/chlorhexidine shampoo (Malaseb, Leo Laboratories) is licensed as an adjunctive therapy in the treatment of ringworm. While the shampoo cannot cure the infection, it can alleviate the inflammatory response and further reduce environmental contamination and contagion by removing spores from the skin surface. Additionally, keratinous debris, the nutrient source of dermatophytes, is kept to a minimum through the use of shampoo therapy.

Rinses

Enilconazole (Imaverol, Janssen-Cilag) is a topical dip licensed for use on dogs. It should be applied once every 3 days. This dip has also been used with some good effects on guinea pigs, although it is not licensed for this type of pet.

Topical creams

Topical antifungal creams such as clotrimazole (Canesten, Bayer) or miconazole (Daktarin, Janssen-Cilag) can be tried on focal lesions. While ointments have been proved to be effective on humans, they tend to be less successful for pets. The cream or ointment should be applied just before walking the dog or before feeding the cat. This gives the medication some time to be absorbed before it is licked off.

Systemic treatment

Sadly, topical therapy does not penetrate into infected hairs so it can't actually shorten the duration of the disease; it just limits the spread of the disease. For cure, systemic treatment is required. Griseofulvin is the drug usually utilised in the treatment of dermatophytosis if, and only if, a definitive diagnosis has been made. This drug is able to penetrate the hair shafts and treat the fungal invasion. Griseofulvin does have its drawbacks. Treatment is usually extended and the drug is not inexpensive. Griseofulvin should never be given to an animal with impairment of hepatic function, and in doubtful cases a blood sample for the assessment of liver enzymes should be performed before the onset of treatment. Griseofulvin should not be given to any pregnant animal due to the teratogenic effects of the drug. Pregnant owners should have someone else medicate their pets. Cats with FIV do not tolerate griseofulvin very well and can develop neutropaenia. Anorexia, vomiting and diarrhoea are reported with griseofulvin use. Idiosyncratically, there can be bone marrow suppression and neurological signs. Owners should be advised to wear gloves when administering the drug.

Itraconazole, in an oral solution (Itrafungol, Janssen), has recently been introduced to the veterinary market. This drug is licensed for use in cats and is preferable to griseofulvin as it has fewer severe side-effects and does not pose as great a risk to pregnant owners. However, the drug should not be given to cats with impaired kidney function or to pregnant queens, and owners should wear gloves when administering the drug. This medication is given for three alternate periods with treatment given for 7 days in a row, followed by a rest period of 7 days.

Ketoconazole, another antifungal, is rarely used in the treatment of ringworm because it is not licensed for animal use, is very expensive, and is usually less effective than griseofulvin. Again, there are side-effects, and blood tests should be performed before the onset of treatment, with careful monitoring of the patient throughout the treatment regime. All of the antifungal drugs are best given with a fatty meal. A spoonful of fish or safflower oil in the food is adequate. Doses should be divided into two smaller amounts, given twice daily to increase the ease of tolerance.

Lufeneron, as found in Program (Novartis), has been tried in the treatment of ringworm. Doses from two to six times the flea-control dose have been reported to be effective. However, only one controlled study has discussed the use of lufeneron and the rest of the reports have been anecdotal. The concept behind the usage of lufeneron is that it is a chitin inhibitor. Chitin is in fungal walls as well as flea eggs so, in theory, lufeneron should inhibit fungi. The study did show remission in several cases but there is not yet enough evidence to promote this as an effective treatment and it is not licensed at such high dosage.

Antifungal therapy needs to continue until two negative fungal cultures have been obtained. In the meantime, clients should be advised that thorough environmental decontamination is necessary. Obsessive vacuuming is essential and the vacuum bag should be disposed of after use. Full-strength household bleach is needed in order to destroy spores. Chlorine dioxine or enilconazole can be used to disinfect pet utensils and home surfaces. Bedding should be laundered on a very hot wash or even disposed of. Carpets and furnishings should be vacuumed assiduously or replaced. Probably only cat breeders will go to the lengths of replacing their household furnishings, although it is a good excuse for redecorating!

Yeast infections

Both mammals and birds live comfortably with a genus of commensal yeasts called *Malassezia*. For a long period of time, these yeasts were ignored as they were considered part of the normal skin environment. More recently, *Malassezia* has proved to be pathogenic when it multiplies and aggregates in large populations. *Malassezia pachydermatis* is associated with carnivores and, in the pet population, dogs. Cats may have *M. pachydermatis*, but also *Malassezia sympodialis* and *Malassezia globosa*.

M. pachydermatis is a single-celled yeast with a thick wall. Its appearance has been likened to a footprint, a dumbbell, snowman or a peanut. These yeasts stain dark purple and are larger than both melanin granules and cocci. *Malassezia* can be found on pups as young as 3 days of age, presumably transferred by the mother's grooming. Favoured locations for population centres are the ear canal, anal sacs, interdigitally and at mucocutaneous junctions. Animals with facial folds and wrinkles have additional anatomical reservoirs for *Malassezia* populations. Figure 5.6 shows *Malassezia* under the microscope.

Under the right circumstances *Malassezia* will spread from its normal locations and colonise over wider body areas. Increased temperature and humidity promote its growth. An alteration in the lipid barrier of the stratum corneum may also promote growth. If the animal's immune system is compromised it is unable to resist colonisation. Unfortunately, *Malassezia* works synergistically with staphylococci. Thus, if an overgrowth of one microorganism occurs the other one is likely to overgrow as well.

Malassezia secrete proteases, lipases, phospholipases and lipoxygenases, all enzymes that lead to inflammation of the skin and help to breach the

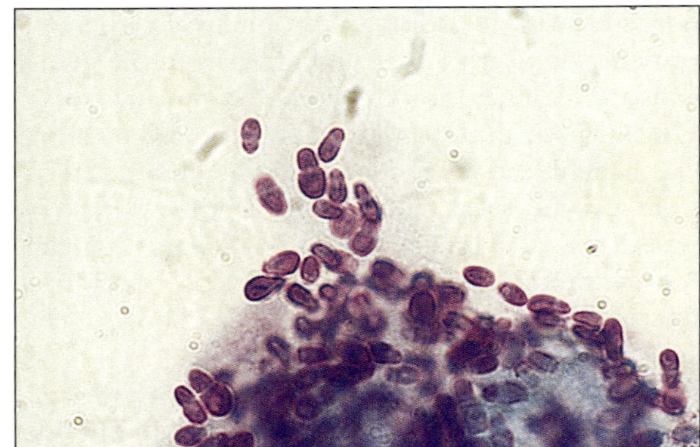

Figure 5.6 *Malassezia* yeast under the microscope. These yeasts are often described as having a 'dumbbell' shape. Reproduced with permission from Medleau L & Hnilica K A Small animal dermatology, W B Saunders, London, 2001.

skin's barriers. The skin becomes pruritic and self-trauma can ensue. Chewing and licking make the skin's environment even more suitable for the yeast.

Certain breeds have a predisposition to yeast infections – Basset Hounds, West Highland White Terriers, Cocker Spaniels, Shih Tzus, Dachshunds, Miniature Poodles, German Shepherds, Silky Terriers and English Setters. Anatomy, as in the Basset Hound's wrinkled and drool-moistened ventral chest, along with an inclination toward allergic disease, make some breeds particularly good candidates for *Malassezia* infections. Allergic disease is often associated with *Malassezia* infection because the pruritus and resultant self-trauma of allergy disrupts the upper skin layers, creating an opportunity for yeast to infect. Other skin diseases also create favourable microenvironments for the development of yeast populations. Keratinisation disorders and endocrine diseases are frequently associated with *Malassezia* dermatitis.

Malassezia is an opportunist and can find favourable conditions for overgrowth in the wake of a variety of maladies. Scabies, demodicosis and even a zinc deficiency can be prequels to *Malassezia* overgrowth. In cats, *Malassezia* dermatitis is much less common but can be secondary to paraneoplastic syndrome, thymoma, FeLV, FIV, feline acne, stress and immunosuppressive therapy. There is no age or sex that most favours yeast infections.

The major clinical signs in dogs include pruritus, which, on the face, can be so severe as to be confused with neurological problems. Erythema is present, along with scale and crust from the greasy exudate. A rancid odour often accompanies infection. Chronic *Malassezia* infection can lead to alopecia, lichenification and hyperpigmentation. Infections can be focal or generalised, with diffuse or well-demarcated lesions. Rarely, *Malassezia* can manifest as interdigital 'cysts', furunculosis, stomatitis, pharyngitis and tonsillitis. Figure 5.7 shows a dog suffering from *Malassezia* dermatitis.

Typical areas of infection are the ears, lips, feet, muzzle, ventral neck, axillae, and ventrum of body, medial limbs, perianal skin and ventral tail. Generally, these are areas of the body with more warmth and moisture.

In the cat, clinical signs of *Malassezia* infection may include otitis externa, erythema, comedones, dark, adherent scales or generalised scale and erythema. There is usually less pruritus than seen with dogs. Waxy, red/brown nails have been noted in paronychia caused by *Malassezia* infections in cats.

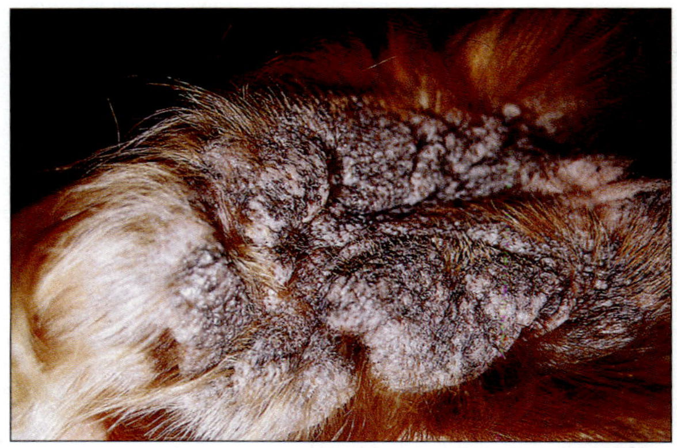

Figure 5.7 This dog is suffering from chronic *Malassezia* dermatitis. The skin has become hyperpigmented due to the yeast infection. Photograph by Annette Loeffler, with permission.

Malassezia dermatitis must be considered whenever an animal presents with any of the following signs:

- erythema
- scale
- greasy exudate
- hyperpigmentation
- lichenification.

Underlying causes can include:

- ectoparasite infestations (fleas, *Sarcoptes scabiei*, *Demodex*, etc.)
- allergies (flea, food, atopy, drug reaction, contact dermatitis)
- dermatophytosis
- staphylococcal infection
- seborrhoea (sicca/dry or oleosa/greasy)
- endocrine disorders (hypothyroidism, hyperglucocorticoidism, reproductive hormone imbalance).

Examination and work-up should include testing for the above underlying conditions. Thus skin scrapings and hair pluckings should be obtained in the first instance. Good flea control should be instituted. A fungal culture should be considered, especially for feline patients. Blood testing may be necessary for endocrine disorders if there are systemic indications of that type of disease. Often an allergy work-up is necessary.

To diagnose *Malassezia* overgrowth, acetate tape strip cytology is an easy and economical method. A strip of tape should be tightly adhered to a likely location three times in order to collect an adequate amount of material. The tape is then looped onto the slide and stained in rapid stains (e.g. Diff-Quik, Dade Bering), using all three stains or just the last two. Some dermatologists choose to skip the fixative as this can 'melt' the greasy sample collected. Stains need to be changed at least weekly as old yeasts floating around in the stain can give false positives. Once staining is finished, the tape can be unlooped and pressed onto the slide. The back of the slide should be rinsed and the slide dried with a paper towel. Wearing gloves is advisable unless you want blue fingers.

Under ×40 magnification, the slide should be scanned for areas of interest. Then a drop of oil can be applied and the oil-immersion lens utilised. *Malassezia* stains blue/purple in Diff-Quik or Rapi-Diff (Triangle Biomedical Services) and will look like a peanut/dumbbell/snowman/footprint. Finding one yeast per high-power field is considered normal but more than one yeast is generally considered significant. If necessary, a sample for a fungal culture can also be submitted, but only if the specific species of *Malassezia* needs to be determined. The plate should be held against the skin for 5–10 seconds and then incubated at 32–37°C for 3–7 days. *M. pachydermatis* produces a creamy-yellow colony.

We are fortunate that there is an effective topical treatment for *Malassezia* in the aptly named Malaseb shampoo (Leo Laboratories) which contains miconazole and chlorhexidine. The client must be reminded that the shampoo needs a 10-minute contact time to be effective. Bathing two or three times weekly is advised. If lesions are focal (for example, the feet) it is acceptable to bathe the affected area only, thus saving the owner time and money.

Other topical treatments for *Malassezia* are enilconazole rinse (Imaverol, Janssen-Cilag) chlorhexidine in a 1–4% solution or 1% selenium sulphide (Seleen, CEVA Animal Health). All of the topical treatments can be drying so prescribing an emollient spray or conditioner may be helpful.

If the *Malassezia* infection is based in the ear, antifungal eardrops should be prescribed. The ear should be cleaned thoroughly on a daily basis in order to change the microenvironment into one less favourable to yeast.

If the animal has a generalised infection, systemic treatment may be required. Griseofulvin, while effective on dermatophytes, is less effective against *Malassezia*. Ketoconazole and itraconazole are preferred. These drugs should be given in split doses with a fatty meal to increase effectiveness. Patients should be closely monitored for side-effects such as anorexia, vomiting and increased liver enzymes. The considerable cost of systemic antifungals needs to be discussed carefully with the client.

While treating the *Malassezia* should reduce symptoms markedly, underlying causes should not be ignored. *Malassezia* and concurrent staphylococcal infections may clear up with only one of the organisms being actively eliminated. A course of antibiotics or treatment with a topical antifungal may actually sort out both infections. Diagnostic testing still needs to be performed to locate the initiating problem and prevent or control recurrence.

FORMULARY

Drugs marked with an asterisk are not licensed for small animal use.

Dose rates given are from the BSAVA Small animal formulary, 4th edition, edited by Bryn Tennant.

Antibacterial shampoos

Allermyl, Virbac – *Pseudomonas* spp. and other bacterial infections (active ingredient: Piroctine olamine)

Etiderm, Virbac – Bacterial infection (active ingredient: ethyl lactate)

Malaseb, Leo Laboratories – bacterial and *Malassezia* infection (active ingredients: chlorhexidine and miconazole)

Nolvoson, Fort Dodge – bacterial infection (active ingredient: chlorhexidine)

Paxcutol, Virbac – bacterial infection (active ingredient: benzoyl peroxide)

NB: Only a few of these shampoos are safe to use on cats. Check label carefully.

Topical treatments for bacterial infection

Benzoyl peroxide 2.5% (PanOxyl Aquafel 2.5, Stiefel)
Fusidic acid and betamethasone (Fuciderm, Leo Laboratories)
Fusidic acid (Fucidin gel, ointment, Leo Laboratories)
Malic, benzoic and salicylic acid (Dermisol, Pfizer)
Povidine-iodine ointment (Betadine, Seton Health Care Group)
Thiostrepton and neomycin (Panalog, Novartis)

Systemic treatment for bacterial infections

Amoxicillin–clavulanate (Synulox, Pfizer)
Cats and dogs: 8.75 mg/kg intramuscular, subcutaneous q 24 hours or 12.5–25 mg/kg PO q 8–12 hours
Cephalexin (Ceporex, Schering-Plough; Rilexine, Virbac)
Cats and dogs: 10–30 mg/kg intramuscular, subcutaneous, PO q 8–12 hours
Clindamyacin (Antirobe, Pharmacia & Upjohn)
Cats and dogs: 5.5–11 mg/kg PO q 12 hours (suggested for initial use in cases of pyoderma, not for recurrent infection)
Enrofloxacin (Baytril, Bayer)
Cats and dogs: 5 mg/kg subcutaneous q 24 hours; 2.5 mg/kg PO q 12 hours, or 5 mg/kg PO q 24 hours
Marbofloxacin (Marbocyl, Vetoquinol)
Cats and dogs: 2 mg/kg PO q 24 hours

Topical treatment for fungal infections

Acetic and boric acids (MalAcetic Wet Wipes, Dermapet UK)
*Clotrimazole (Caneston lotion and cream, Bayer)
Enilconazole (Imaverol dip, Janssen-Cilag). Licensed only for use in dogs and large animals
Miconazole (Malaseb shampoo, Leo Laboratories)
*Miconazole (Daktarin Cream, Janssen-Cilag)
Nystatin with thiostrepton and neomycin (Panalog, Novartis)

Ear treatments for fungal infections

Acetic and boric acids (MalAcetic Otic, Dermapet UK)
Clotrimazole, marbofloxacin dexamethasone (Aurizon, Vetoquinol)
Miconazole, polymyxin B, prednisolone (Surolan, Janssen Animal Health)
Nystatin, fusidate, framycetin sulphate, prednisolone (Canaural, Leo Laboratories)

Systemic treatment for fungal/dermatophyte infections

Griseofulvin (Grisovin, Glaxo)
Cats and dogs: 15–30 mg/kg PO q 24 hours with a fatty meal
Itraconazole (Itrafungol, Janssen) 52 ml oral solution. Licensed for use in cats. 5 mg/kg once daily for 7 days on, followed by 7 days off for three periods of treatment.
*Itraconazole 100 mg capsules (Sporanox, Dowelhurst Ltd)
Cats and dogs: 2.5–5 mg/kg PO q 12–24 hours
*Ketoconazole 200 mg tablets (Nizoral, Janssen-Cilag)
Cats and dogs: 5–10 mg/kg PO q 8–12 hours with fatty meal

References and Further Reading

Hill Peter 2002 Small animal dermatology. Elsevier Science, Oxford, p 245

Lloyd David, Lamport Anne, Feeney Ciara 1996 Sensitivity to antibiotics amongst cutaneous and mucosal isolates of canine pathogenic staphylococci in the UK, 1980–96. Veterinary Dermatology 7:171–175

Noli Chiara 2003 'Dermatophytosis' and 'Staphylococcal pyoderma'. In: Foil C, Foster A (eds) BSAVA Manual of small animal dermatology. BSAVA Publications, Gloucester, p 159–174

Nuttal Tim 2003 Malassezia dermatitis. In: Foil C, Foster A (eds) BSAVA Manual of small animal dermatology. BSAVA Publications, Gloucester, p 175–180

Tennant Bryn (ed) 2002. Small animal formulary, 4th edn. BSAVA, Gloucester

Yair Ben Ziony, Boaz Arzi 2000 The use of lufeneron for the treatment of fungal infection of dogs and cats: 297 cases. JAVMA 217(10)

CASE STUDY 1

Bacterial infection in a young beagle bitch

Signalment

The bitch was a 5½-month-old entire beagle at a weight of 9 kg. She was fully vaccinated and up to date on worming. Pet-shop rather than veterinary flea control was in use. The bitch was being fed a commercial puppy food diet and was in good general health. The animal is shown in Figure 5.8.

Problem

A 2 cm × 2 cm nodule of unknown origin below the left eye. The beagle was very boisterous and lived with three children so the possibility of trauma was high.

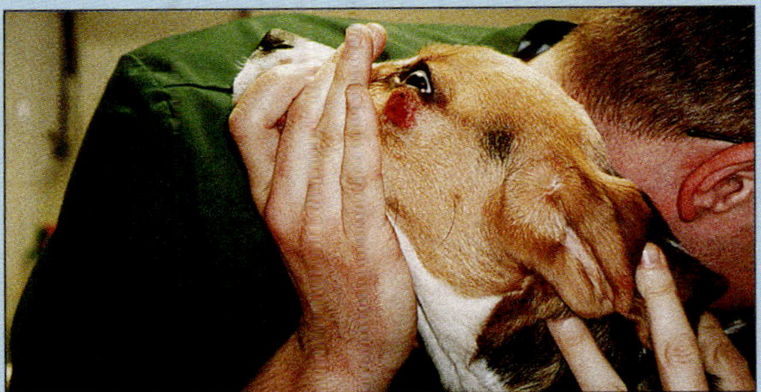

Figure 5.8 Bacterial infection in a beagle. This young dog developed a bacterial infection of unknown origin. Photograph by Frances Gaudiano.

History

The bitch was fully vaccinated and wormed but she was receiving only a pet-shop flea-control product. Treatment for otitis externa had occurred 3 months earlier and continued for some weeks. The ears had been cleaned with a strong cleaner containing anti-inflammatory agents (Epiotic, Virbac). Twice-daily treatment with ear drops (Canaural, Leo Animal Health), continuing for 3 weeks, had also been part of the treatment regime. The bitch had also suffered from colitis at the age of 2½ months. It was felt that the colitis was due to dietary indiscretion but the cause of the otitis had not been identified.

Physical examination

The beagle was a young, healthy dog with an outgoing disposition. The coat was in good condition and there was no sign of external parasites. The owner reported a good appetite and normal elimination patterns. There was no sign of the earlier otitis and the toenails were reasonably short, as they had been clipped at a nurses' clinic a few weeks earlier. The bitch was well exercised and stimulated, living in a family situation. Temperature, pulse and respiration were normal, as was capillary refill type. There was no evidence of lymph node enlargement. The only complaint seemed to be a small lesion below the left eye. It was unknown how the lesion had developed but the bitch seemed irritated by it.

Differential diagnosis

- Surface pyoderma
- Superficial pyoderma
- Dermatophytosis
- Demodectic mange
- Sarcoptic mange
- Flea-allergy dermatitis
- Food sensitivity
- Atopy (unlikely at this age)

Diagnostic procedures

A swab was taken and rolled onto a glass slide. The slide was stained with 'Diff-Quik' stain and examined under an oil-immersion lens. Cocci were present in the sample. It was presumed that the cocci were *Staphylococcus intermedius* as this is the most common of the residential bacteria of the canine skin. Skin scrapings and acetate tape strip examinations were also taken but proved negative. A dermatophyte culture would have been desirable but was not economically feasible in this case. A trichogram did not reveal any fungal hyphae but evidence of self-trauma (broken hair shafts) was noticed.

Treatment and diagnosis

The wound was probably of traumatic origin with a secondary superficial pyoderma caused by opportunistic bacteria.

The area around the wound was carefully clipped clean and the wound was flushed with sterile saline. The owner was given an antibacterial gel (Fuciderm, Leo Laboratories) and told to apply it to the wound twice daily for 1 week. A follow-up appointment was made for a week later.

Three days later the owner returned requesting a buster collar as the beagle had been scratching at the wound. In retrospect, the buster collar should have been given at the initial appointment. Self-trauma to the area was certain to aggravate the condition.

Follow-up and prognosis

At the follow-up appointment, the wound was substantially larger. Erythema, swelling and some erosion were obvious. The bitch's scratching at the area had complicated the problem and the wound could now be described as a deep pyoderma. It was decided to place the bitch on systemic antibiotics, 250 mg of clavulanate-potentiated amoxicillin (Synulox, Pfizer Animal Health) twice daily for 8 days. Ideally, antibiotic for skin cases should be given at least 1 week past clinical cure; however, financial constraints again limited ideal treatment. The owner was also advised to keep the buster collar on his pet at all times.

At a final visit 8 days later the wound had resolved completely. The buster collar was removed and treatment ended. There have been no recurrences of the problem over a 3-month period.

Discussion

Canine skin is more susceptible to pyoderma than is other mammalian skin. This is due to the fact that dogs have fewer squames per layer and poor lipid seal protection (Mason 1995). Therefore, the fact that this beagle developed a deep pyoderma from what began as a small nodule is not an extraordinary event. Pyoderma of varying depth is a daily problem to deal with in small animal practice (Ihrke 1996). The question is: what started the chain of events that led to the bacterial invasion of skin layers? Pyoderma can't develop spontaneously and can recur endlessly if the root cause is not discovered. As the owner was completely unaware of what could have caused the lesion, a process of elimination had to be determined.

Consulting the BSAVA Dermatology manual chapter on 'Facial dermatoses', I found a long list of possible causes (Bond 1993). One must first rule out any parasitical or fungal infestation, hence the skin scrapings and acetate tape strippings. No mites or yeast organisms were found; however, the location of the lesion is typical for *Demodex canis*, but the type of lesion was atypical of that mite. I was worried about the odd flea bite as the dog was not on veterinary flea treatment, but no evidence of external parasites were found.

The face is also a favoured location for atopy, but the dog's age made that diagnosis unlikely. This beagle may in the future develop atopy as otitis has already been experienced. It is possible that scratching at the ear led the dog to inadvertently scratch her face, leading to a wound that was colonised by opportunistic bacteria. Certainly localised deep pyoderma can often be caused by self-trauma (Paterson 1998). Foreign bodies, such as a grass seed, are also well-documented causes of localised deep pyoderma. This was another strong possibility as this beagle was active and frequently exercised outdoors. As a draining sinus was not present, a grass seed as a cause was eliminated, but another foreign body could have been present.

Food sensitivities can occur in canines of this age and certainly this beagle had a history of colitis (and suffered from another attack shortly after her facial lesion cleared up). However, the bitch had been on the same puppy diet for several months with no problems and her earlier colitis attack had been closely linked with bin raiding.

There were many other possibilities, including immune-mediated disorders, but testing for a huge array of possibilities was not reasonable. There had been a good response to systemic treatment and the bitch was a healthy, happy puppy once her facial disfigurement was healed. We concluded that the underlying cause was 'unknown trauma/ foreign body', and advised the owners to get the bitch on veterinary flea treatment.

REFERENCES

(for Case Study 1)

Bond Ross 1993 Facial dermatoses. In: Locke P H, Mason I (eds) Manual of small animal dermatology. BSAVA, Cheltenham, p 121–122

Ihrke Peter J 1996 Overview of canine pyoderma. Bacterial skin disease in the dog. Bayer Corporation, Kansas, p 1

Mason Ian S 1995 Canine pyoderma. Educational video produced by Leo Laboratories, Princes Risborough, UK

Paterson Sue 1998 Skin diseases of the dog. Blackwell Scientific Publications, Oxford, p 34

CASE STUDY 2

Dermatophytosis in a guinea pig

Signalment

A young guinea pig, 6–8 weeks of age, was presented for treatment. The guinea pig was of the 'Tort-White Smooth' breed and weighed 350 grams. The animal was female and was not pregnant.

Problem

The guinea pig had multi-focal lesions that were erythematous and pruritic (see Fig. 5.9).

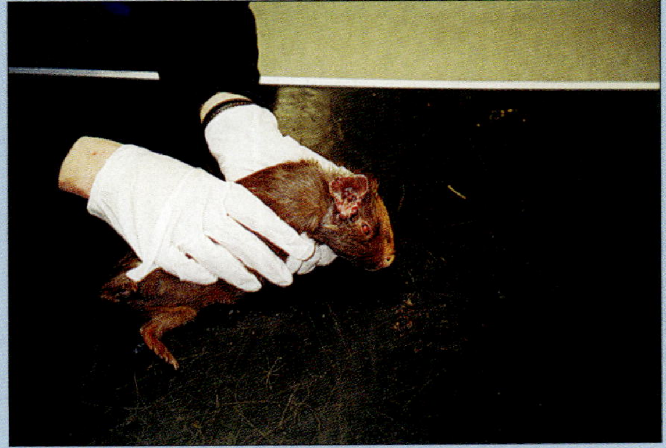

Figure 5.9 Guinea pig with dermatophytosis. Photograph by Frances Gaudiano.

History

The animal had been acquired from a breeding establishment 1 week earlier. The breeder had stated that his entire delivery were at least 6 weeks old but on veterinary examination some of the guinea pigs were as young as 3 weeks of age. The delivery was deposited at a large pet store and the young guinea pigs were placed in communal hutches. This particular animal shared a hutch with two other guinea pigs and a rabbit. The hutches were wooden runs with no ceiling (i.e.

open to the public) with a ramp leading into a covered area at the end of the hutch. The hutches were lined with sawdust. Hay, water and guinea pig and rabbit mixes were provided. Pelleted feeds were not offered. In the mornings, fresh fruit and vegetables were offered. Vitamin C was provided via the mix, although the potency was in doubt as vitamin C has a short shelf life and the age of the mix was unknown. Different store personnel cleaned out the hutch daily. In addition, the small furries were exposed to a fairly steady onslaught of visitors and people passing the hutch with dogs and cats to attend the veterinary surgery in the back of the store. In other words, these animals lived in a very stressful environment!

Physical examination

The guinea pig was slightly underweight, but not knowing her exact age made it difficult to determine exactly how small she was in relation to healthy growth rates. Respiratory rate (RR) and heart rate (HR) were within the normal range (RR 90–150/minute, HR 130–190/minute). The chest sounds were clear. There was no evidence of ocular or nasal discharges. The stools were normal. Appetite was difficult to ascertain due to the communal living arrangements. The feet were clear of pododermatitis and none of the joints appeared swollen. Body temperature was not taken, as this procedure is extremely stressful to conscious guinea pigs.

Dermatological examination

Crusting and erythema were evident with a number of multi-focal lesions. Scabbing was occurring on nasal lesions while less mature lesions appeared on the ventral chest, dorsal shoulder region, on the left and right flanks and on the rump. The lesions were annular in appearance and alopecia existed at the site of each lesion. Hair around the lesions was easily epilated. The guinea pig was exhibiting signs of pruritus but was not frenzied with itchiness as can sometimes occur with a mite infestation.

Differential diagnosis

- *Trixicarus caviae* infestation
- *Glirocola porcelli* infestation
- *Psoroptes cuniculi* infestation
- Demodicosis
- Dermatophytosis (*Trichophyton mentagrophytes* most likely)
- Trauma
- Self-trauma/barbering

Diagnostic tests

Skin scrapings were performed to investigate the possibility of mites. A number 10 blade was used to perform both superficial and deep scrapes. The sample was mounted in liquid paraffin and examined under both low and high magnification. No mites or lice were identified. The possibility of trauma was discussed with the pet store assistants. Housing guinea pigs with rabbits is not generally recommended, as rabbits tend to be much bigger and stronger. However, the evidence of pruritus eliminated the likelihood that the wounds were trauma-related.

Next, a trichogram was performed by plucking hair samples from the edges of several lesions. The hairs were examined at low- and high-power magnification. Again, no mites or lice were identified and no hyphae were obvious either.

Finally, pluckings were taken for a dermatophyte culture. While samples from a sterile toothbrush are often recommended, we chose to pluck samples from the edges of three different lesions. The samples were placed in the medium Sarbouraud's agar. After labelling the sample, it was placed in our laboratory for daily examination. A Wood's lamp investigation was not performed because only *Microsporum canis*, which is not a common fungus of guinea pigs, will fluoresce.

On the fourth day the culture medium had turned red (see Fig. 5.10). It was important to examine the sample daily as protein metabolism can cause the medium to alkalinise (and thus change colour) fairly quickly. It would have been possible to continue to grow a culture and later examine it microscopically for specific species identification; however, that was not deemed necessary.

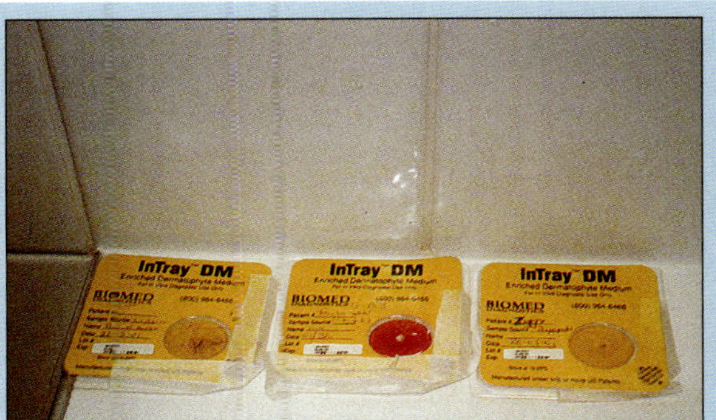

Figure 5.10 Dermatophytosis of guinea pig. The red tray indicates a positive result for fungal infection. Photograph by Frances Gaudiano.

Treatment

Initially, we gave the guinea pig an injection of ivermectin (Panomec, Merial) at a dose rate of 0.4 mg/kg, i.e. 0.14 ml subcutaneously. This was done before we had established a diagnosis of dermatophytosis and also because there had been numerous mite infestations in previous pet-store guinea pigs. False negatives are quite possible on skin scrapings.

Once the culture medium had turned red we made a diagnosis of dermatophytosis, most likely *Trichophyton mentagrophytes*, as that is the most common form of fungal infection in guinea pigs. Several texts were consulted and The Cambridge Cavy Trust was contacted regarding the appropriate treatment of a fungal infection in a young guinea pig. We decided on topical treatment with enilconazole (Imaverol, Janssen Animal Health). A solution was made with one part enilconazole to 50 parts water. This solution was sponged onto the guinea pig's lesions and surrounding skin every third day.

Re-inspection and final outcome

The guinea pig was examined on a weekly basis and progressive improvement was observed. All signs of lesions were gone after 3 weeks; however, treatment was continued for another 3 weeks to eliminate any possibility of contagion to the public as the guinea pig was to be sold. A further fungal culture would have been desirable but was not carried out. Pet-store staff were advised to examine themselves for lesions. The staff were also told to wear aprons and gloves when caring for the infected guinea pig. The original hutch was scrubbed with a bleach solution and the in-contact hutch mates were quarantined for 2 weeks in case of infestation. Ideally, all of the hutch mates should have also been treated for ringworm, but this was considered too labour-intensive by the pet-store staff. Later, a guinea pig purchased from the store was brought to the clinic for a skin condition, which proved to be dermatophytosis. Asymptomatic carriers were also a worry as these animals were destined to be children's pets. The animals in the adjoining hutch were not quarantined, again, a risky choice as infection via fomites and common handling is very likely.

Discussion

There are very few veterinary medicines licensed for use in small mammals. This is probably why we were given such varied treatment modalities for dermatophytosis in guinea pigs. Griseofulvin (Grisovin, Schering Plough) at a dose rate of 0.25 mg/kg daily for 4–6 weeks was recommended, but only with caution in young guinea pigs due to a reportedly high mortality rate (Richardson 2000). Clipping and bathing in enilconazole and miconazole was another treatment proffered (Tilley & Smith 1997). I was curious to see whether anyone had tried treatment with a miconazole/chlorhexidine shampoo (Malaseb, Leo Laboratories) or with lufeneron (Program, Novartis) but no studies with these drugs had yet been performed on guinea pigs. A final suggestion was euthanasia because guinea pigs were usually children's pets and very likely to infect children (Flecknell 1991).

Although we realised that topical treatment would not completely eradicate the dermatophytosis, it would limit the spread of the disease. As the guinea pig lived in a pet store, limiting the disease was of major concern. It was also felt that systemic treatment would have been risky due to the young age of the guinea pig. There was additional concern that the systemic treatment would not be handled with due concern for health and safety. Supportive care, in terms of good nutrition and husbandry, helps the animal's immune system to overcome dermatophytosis. With time, a healthy animal can eliminate a dermatophyte infection without systemic treatment.

Dermatophytosis is a frustrating disease to treat for several reasons. In guinea pigs it can be difficult to diagnose without doing a dermatophyte culture, an expense many people will not go to for a children's pet. Dermatophytosis is often mistaken for a mite infestation (*T. caviae*). However, fungal infections generally appear on the nose and spread backwards. The lesions from dermatophytosis are oval and are not nearly as pruritic as infestation with *T. caviae*. Mite infestation by *T. caviae* also has a different pattern of appearance, as lesions generally start in the neck and trunk region and self-trauma is quite evident. To add to the confusion, very stressed guinea pigs can be harbouring both mites and a fungal infection (Tilley et al 1997).

Asymptomatic carriers of dermatophytosis are common but stress can lead to the development of symptomatic dermatophytosis. Elements such as abrupt change, poor nutrition, crowding and youth can cause the disease to manifest. In this case, the poor animal was suffering from all of these elements. In general, any young guinea pig placed in a pet store situation is a prime candidate for dermatophytosis. The spores are then spread into the bedding and all in-contact animals can become infected. Cross-infection is furthered by handling both from pet store personnel and members of the public who do not wash their hands in between each contact! Secondary bacterial infection can also easily follow in these less than ideal situations (Flecknell 1996). Luckily, dermatophytosis can often resolve on its own, eventually. Unfortunately, chaos can be wrought in the meantime as spores are spread around and live in the environment for up to 18 months.

In retrospect, not nearly enough precautions were taken in this case. Probably the guinea pig should have been clipped prior to topical treatment. Bathing in an antifungal shampoo at least twice would also have been advisable. Neither of the above measures would have led to a more rapid cure; however, they may have decreased environmental contamination markedly. The bedding in the hutch should have been burned and the hutch cleaned with enilconazole on a weekly basis. A thorough vacuuming of the store and the store's air vents should have been undertaken. All in-contact animals, including the animals in nearby hutches, should have been tested and isolated for 3 weeks and then re-tested (Carlotti 1993). These measures may have prevented future outbreaks.

REFERENCES

(for Case Study 2)

Carolotti Didier N 1993 Management of dermatophyte disease. BSAVA Manual of dermatology. BSAVA, Cheltenham, p 257–262

Flecknell Paul 1991 Guinea pigs. In: Beynon P H, Cooper J E (eds) Manual of exotic pets. British Small Animal Association, Gloucestershire, p 56

Flecknell Paul 1996. Diseases of guinea pigs. In: Lewis-Laird K, Swindle M M, Flecknell P (eds) Handbook of rodent and rabbit medicine. Pergamon Press, London, p 121–122

Richardson V C G 2000 Diseases of domestic guinea pigs. Blackwell Science, London, p 1–2, 110.

Tilley Larry P, Smith Francis W K Jr 1997 Dermatophytosis. The five-minute veterinary consult. Williams & Wilkins, Baltimore, p 506–504

Chapter 6

Allergic skin disease in the dog and cat

CHAPTER CONTENTS

Allergic skin disease is caused by the body reacting in an inappropriate way to an ectoparasite or to an element in the diet or environment. With allergy, ordinary substances are interpreted to be a threat to the body, causing an immune response of a hypersensitive nature. There are four different types of hypersensitivity reaction, although only two play a primary role in allergic skin disease.

The *type I hypersensitivity* reaction occurs in the following way: There is cutaneous absorption of a substance, known as the allergen. The allergen can be flea saliva, dust mites, pollens, et cetera. Langerhans cells in the basal areas of the epidermis collect the allergens. The Langerhans cells travel to local lymph nodes to present the foreign substance to lymphocytes. At the initial exposure, helper T-cell lymphocytes become sensitised to the foreign substance.

Cytokines are chemical messengers that are released from cells and cause direct actions within the body. Once the helper T-cells are sensitised by an allergen, they will be stimulated to produce cytokines on subsequent exposure to the allergen. Allergic animals are genetically programmed to send the wrong kind of cytokines to B-lymphocytes and plasma cells, resulting in the production of allergen-specific immunoglobulin E (IgE). IgE is an antibody and acts as part of the immune system's reaction to ward off dangerous elements entering the body and multiplying. Unfortunately, the immune system in allergic animals is stimulated by innocuous substances such as dust mites and pollens.

Immune reaction: hypersensitivity

- Allergen enters percutaneously
- Allergen attaches to Langerhans cells
- Allergen presented to T cells in lymph nodes
- T cells (Th2) release cytokines
- Cytokines stimulate plasma cells and B cells to produce IgE antibodies
- IgE antibodies coat mast cells
- Allergen contacted again and carried to lymph nodes by Langerhans cells
- Sensitised T cells recognise allergen and initiate inflammatory response
- IgE-coated mast cells degranulate
- Histamine, heparin, prostaglandins, leukotrines, proteolytic enzymes released from mast cells
- Heat, erythema, swelling, pruritus, pain, i.e. cardinal signs of inflammation

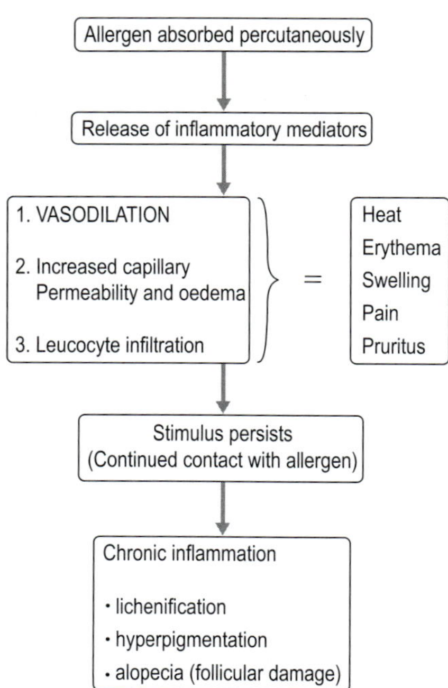

Figure 6.1 Inflammatory cascade.

Once IgE antibodies are produced they bind to mast cells and basophils in the dermis. The helper T cells and specific IgE are primarily sensitised to protein within the allergen, known as the antigen. The next time the dog or cat inhales, ingests, is injected with the allergen, or contacts it percutaneously, there will be an immediate reaction as the antigen is recognised and interacts with the IgE. The interaction will cause the mast cells to degranulate, leading to inflammatory changes in the skin.

Degranulating mast cells can distribute histamine, heparin, proteolytic enzymes, prostoglandins, leukotrenes and other inflammatory mediators. Vasodilation and increased capillary permeability are caused by the chemicals released from mast cells. This reaction is observed as swelling, pain, heat and erythema at the site. Pruritus occurs as neuroreceptors within the skin are stimulated. Leukocyte infiltration follows in the inflammatory cascade. The area of inflammation will be uncomfortable, causing the animal to lick or chew, leading to more inflammation. (See Fig. 6.1.)

If an area of the skin is chronically inflamed the epidermis and dermis themselves will change. The follicles will become damaged and hair growth may become impossible, leading to alopecia. Layers of cornified cells (in the stratum corneum) will increase in response to the insult and the speed of epidermal turnover will increase. This can lead to lichenification and hyperpigmentation (see Fig. 6.2). Left long enough, chronic inflammation can cause irreversible damage to the skin.

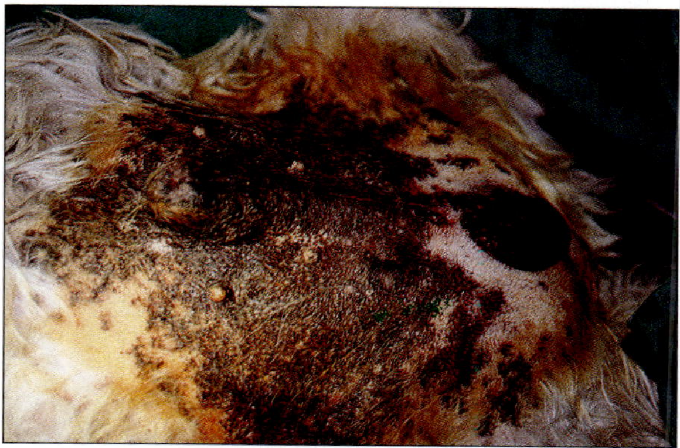

Figure 6.2 Marked post-inflammatory hyperpigmentation is visible in this example. Demodicosis was diagnosed, possibly related to a suspected hormone imbalance caused by a testicular tumour. Photograph by Annette Loeffler, with permission.

There are three other types of hypersensitivity, although type I is most relevant to dermatology. *Type II hypersensitivity* is termed 'cytotoxic hypersensitivity' because in this type of hypersensitivity the target cells are destroyed after being bound by IgG or IgM antibodies. Often the target cell is an erythrocyte. Thus we have nasty conditions such as autoimmune haemolytic anaemia and transfusion reactions. However, autoantibodies can destroy skin cells as well. In the pemphigus group of diseases, the adhesion molecules necessary for holding keratinocytes together, known as desmosomes, are annihilated by autoantibodies.

Hypersensitivity type III involves the formation of immune complexes within tissues. This leads to local inflammation. This is a normal process in most immune responses; however, phagocytosis usually occurs to remove the complexes. With a hypersensitivity reaction, so much complex is created that it cannot be removed by phagocytosis. If the complexes are deposited at a site in the body, there will be an inflammatory response at that site. This is known as an 'Arthus reaction', and an example is the hypersensitivity to *Otodectes cynotis* infestation that occurs in cats. If the excess complex enters the circulation it can deposit in the kidneys, joints, eyes or skin. Conditions such as systemic lupus erythematosus are caused by the hypersensitivity type III reaction.

Hypersensitivity type IV is also known as the 'delayed type' reaction. It is usually a local reaction and will occur 24–72 hours after exposure to the antigen. As with the type I reaction, helper T cells recognise the antigens and release inappropriate cytokines. Cytotoxic destruction of target cells can occur along with changes in the vascular endothelium, leading to more lymphocytes, neutrophils and macrophages congregating at the site. A visible reaction in the form of papules and pustules will become evident. Chronic stimulation can lead to granulomas. Type IV reactions are sometimes seen in flea-allergic dermatitis and, more rarely, in atopic disease.

The most common allergic skin disease, and indeed, the most common skin disease, is flea-allergic dermatitis (referred to as FAD). Any time an itchy dog or cat enters a practice, top of the differential list must be FAD. Some animals are born predisposed to hypersensitivity and will rapidly become flea-allergic upon exposure to flea saliva. However, most dog and cats, if exposed over an extended period of time, will develop a flea allergy. Dogs exposed for 15 minutes per day for 40 weeks become allergic to flea saliva. Once the hypersensitivity has developed, it remains a part of the animal's immune response throughout its life. Flea-allergic-dermatitis is shown in Figure 6.3.

There are three different ways in which the dog or cat will react to flea saliva as an antigen: immediate, delayed and a combined immediate and delayed reaction.

1. An immediate reaction can take place within 15 minutes. This is a hypersensitivity type I reaction, based on IgE antibodies to flea saliva antigen.
2. A late-phase reaction, occurring 4–6 hours after flea bites, which is based on IgE antibodies and basophil infiltration.
3. A cell-mediated type IV hypersensitivity reaction can occur 1–2 days later. About 15–30% of flea-allergic animals display a type IV delayed reaction. This type of reaction cannot be measured by in vitro testing for flea saliva. Thus a very flea-allergic dog can test negative for flea allergy on in vitro testing. If tested by intradermal skin test, the reaction will be seen, but will not appear till 24–48 hours later. This is why owners are asked to observe and report any developments when intradermal skin testing is performed.

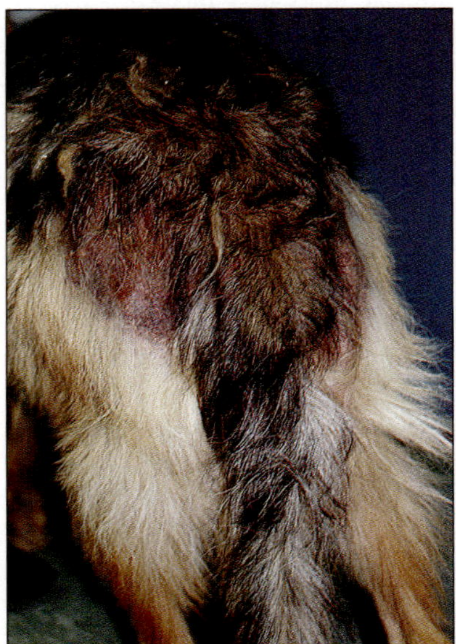

Figure 6.3 The lumbar dorsal spine is the typical area for lesions to develop with flea-allergic dermatitis. Note the erythema and alopecia. Photograph by Annette Loeffler, with permission.

Some very unfortunate animals will display immediate and delayed reactions. Additionally, atopic dogs and cats are predisposed to flea allergy, and flea-allergic animals can also be food sensitive. Therefore, severely allergic animals can suffer from all three – atopy, FAD and food sensitivity. Regardless, the flea situation has to be controlled first.

The average range of onset for a flea allergy is 6 months to 6 years. In dogs, flea allergy will appear as a papular eruption on the caudal dorsum and tail base. Lesions will progress from this primary area to medial to caudal thighs and generalise from there. Cats usually display a miliary dermatitis on their dorsum. These 'millet-like' lesions appear as tiny, crusting papules along the cat's back and can easily be felt when stroking the cat. Some cats do develop other forms of allergic lesion, including linear granulomas and plaques. However, miliary dermatitis is the most common form of allergic reaction in the cat.

In both the dog and cat, the secondary lesions caused by self-trauma can be significant. Secondary pyoderma is also common as the commensal population of bacteria is encouraged by the erosional lesions of scratching and the moist, warm environment created through chewing. Pyotraumatic dermatitis (hot spots) is often the result of incessant chewing and worrying at a focal site of inflammation caused by allergic reaction to flea antigen. Chronically flea-allergic animals will have suffered from long-term inflammation plus extensive self-trauma. In these cases alopecia, hyperpigmentation and lichenification of the skin are expected.

Severe pruritus is always one of the clinical signs of FAD. A flea-allergic animal can be seen suddenly jumping up as if shot, and frantically scratching or chewing with a frenzy. Other allergic animals may prefer to do their grooming in private. Although an owner may never see her cat ripping out its fur, it can still be happening. Taking hair plucks to look for broken hair shafts and chewed ends can identify 'secret' over-groomers. Because FAD animals spend so much time attending to their itchy skin the likelihood of actually finding a flea is remote. This can make it difficult when trying to convince the owner that his or her pet is flea-allergic. Sometimes taking a tape strip from mid-dorsum (an area the animal finds difficult to reach) can help you to obtain flea dirt. This sort of proof may be required with some owners. People do still associate fleas with a dirty home and are deeply offended by the insinuation that their home has fleas. Also, it is a commonly held misbelief that indoor cats do not get fleas. Explaining how hypersensitivity works in that even just a few bites from one flea can cause so much damage may help to alleviate an owner's sense of outrage at being told her pet has fleas.

As fleas complete their life cycle more quickly in warmer weather, FAD is frequently observed in the summer months. However, with modern central heating and fully carpeted homes, fleas can now live and reproduce comfortably all year round so that FAD may be identified during any season. The cat flea, *C. felis*, is the flea most likely to instigate FAD in both dogs and cats. An obligate ectoparasite, *C. felis* lives its entire adult life on the pet, eating, breeding and laying eggs on its host. There is very little travel between hosts and morbidity is caused by grooming or old age. The eggs fall into the environment to develop, evolving through the larval and pupal stages much more quickly in the ideal conditions of 20–30°C with 70% humidity. In less than ideal conditions, the pupae can survive several months, biding their time till weather conditions and an appropriate host are provided. Of all stages in the life cycle, the pupa is the most difficult to eliminate.

The animal with FAD must have its infestation treated in the most thorough manner possible. Topical adulticide treatment is a must. Any of the three veterinary spot-ons are worthwhile treatments (fipronil/fipronil + methoprene, imadicloprid, selamectin). Some households with several animals of varying weights may find the fipronil spray a more economical option. An insect growth regulator may be used concurrently with a spot-on in severe cases. Environmental spray should always be strongly encouraged. The home should be thoroughly vacuumed and the pet's bedding washed at a high temperature. Do remind the owner to dispose of the vacuum bag as the fleas can survive in the bag. The house and car should then be sprayed with a long-acting premise spray containing an adulticide (e.g. permethrin) and an insect growth regulator. Methoprene is sensitive to ultraviolet rays, so in a house with lots of windows and exposure to sunshine pyriproxyfen may be a better choice. If the owner is wary of household sprays, boric acid powders can be effective in environmental control if the powder is applied properly. This can be quite labour intensive so do make sure the owner understands the undertaking of powder application.

There is an argument for using a fast-acting adulticide in cases where the animal needs immediate relief and/or the owner needs visible proof of flea death. Nitenpyram, given in tablet form to dogs or cats, can kill adult fleas within 4–6 hours. This can be given daily and in conjunction with the insect growth regulator lufenuron. Eventually, this combination would eliminate the infestation on the pet and in the home as no viable eggs would survive and the hatching population would be eliminated via the nitenpyram. Some owners may find this combination more acceptable than using a premise spray or powder. You need to work with the individual and devise a plan that will be carried out by the owner and not just given lip service.

In the best of all possible worlds, it will still take a period of time to eliminate the flea population for any particular pet but the animal's pruritus needs to be addressed promptly. Most FAD patients will require corticosteroids for at least a week, to control the pruritus. In dogs, prednisolone at 1–2 mg/kg b.i.d. can be given for 3–5 days and then tapered down till the anti-inflammatory action is no longer needed. In cats, prednisolone at 2 mg/kg b.i.d. for 3–5 days can be given and then tapered off until the pruritus is under control. If the cat is reluctant to take tablets, an injection of depot methylprednisolone acetate can be given as this product is active for approximately 30 days.

A soothing shampoo, with colloidal oatmeal as an ingredient, can be effective in easing the inflammation. Advise that bathing should be performed before applying any sprays or spot-ons in accordance with the manufacturer's instructions, as shampooing and rinsing can reduce the effectiveness of some treatments. Animals with secondary bacterial or yeast infections may need shampoos with ingredients to deal with these infections. Chlorhexidine-based shampoos are good antibacterial agents, and miconazole will act against yeast infections. A shampoo combining both of these ingredients (Malaseb, Leo Laboratories) may be needed.

It is important to address any secondary pyoderma or yeast infection. As part of the diagnostic work-up, tape strippings should be taken for cytological examination. Impression smears can be performed if pustules or hot spots are present. Some surface infections can be treated topically with shampoos. If the lesions are focal, as with hot spots, topical ointments can be utilised. However, superficial or deep pyoderma will need to be treated systemically with oral antibiotics. A broad-spectrum antibiotic appropriate for skin infections should be chosen and given for 1 week past clinical cure. This can be expensive if dealing with a large dog; however, cutting the treatment short may lead to a recurrence of the infection. Controlling the secondary infections will help to control the pruritus and thus decrease the length of time the animal will need anti-inflammatory medication.

If a virulent yeast infection is present, the veterinarian may choose to use systemic anti-yeast medications such as itraconazole or ketoconazole. Unfortunately, these two drugs do have potential side-effects and tend to be very expensive so most anti-yeast treatment is done topically until the necessity for systemic treatment is proven.

Flea allergic dermatitis summarised

- *Clinical signs:* Intense pruritus, papular to crusting lesions, especially in caudal dorsal region in dogs and along dorsum in cats. Chronic cases may show alopecia, hyperpigmentation and lichenification. Secondary pyoderma and yeast infections are not uncommon. Pyotraumatic dermatitis (hot spot) is often related to FAD.
- *Diagnostic tests:* Coat brushings, tape strips, response to flea treatment.
- *Treatment:* Veterinary spot-on or sprays + environmental control. Systemic or topical insect growth regulators in certain cases. Antibacterial and anti-yeast treatment if secondary infection present. Corticosteroid treatment short-term to control pruritus. Soothing and/or anti-microbial shampoos.

FOOD SENSITIVITY

The terms 'food allergy', 'food intolerance' and 'food sensitivity' are often used interchangeably and to describe a wide range of clinical signs. 'Sensitivity' is the most accurate term to use in terms of the disease process that takes place as an allergy process has not yet been verified through research. True food sensitivity is not a common finding. Incidences published in the literature vary from 1% of dermatological patients being affected by food sensitivity to 23% of pets with non-seasonal allergic dermatitis having an underlying cause of food sensitivity (Ackerman & Nesbit 1998). The only way to diagnose a food sensitivity is through a food trial.

The age of the animal must be taken into consideration when considering a food trial. Young animals do not have mature skeletons and an unbalanced diet can cause developmental damage. The manufacturers of an elimination diet should be contacted regarding the diet's suitability for immature dogs and cats. Home-made diets are generally not balanced enough for young animals. There is a further argument espoused by some clinicians that introducing elimination diets at an early age can create additional sensitivities. At any rate, exclusion diets in young animals must be avoided or approached with great caution. However, all itchy animals should be tested for food sensitivities once the possibility of ectoparasite infestation has been eliminated. Coat brushings, pluckings and skin scrapings should be performed to rule out flea or mite infestations. Tape strips for cytology should then be carried out to identify any secondary bacterial or yeast infections. Any positive findings from the above tests would need to be dealt with in order to have an accurate assessment of pruritus at the end of the food trial. However, as a food trial is a lengthy process, it can begin with the first visit.

Dermatological reactions to food substances generally manifest with face, head and neck pruritus via immediate, delayed or immune-complex reactions. Unilateral or bilateral ear involvement frequently occurs. In addition, foot licking and chewing can be observed. There is usually erythema, sometimes with alopecia, hyperpigmentation and lichenification (see Fig. 6.4), secondary to self-trauma and chronic inflammation. Rarely, there can be angioedema and/or urticaria. The age of onset can be as young as 6 weeks (as the animal is weaned) and usually occurs sometime before the dog or cat is 1 year of age. Of patients with dermatological signs, 10–15% will also exhibit gastrointestinal problems such as vomiting and, particularly, diarrhoea.

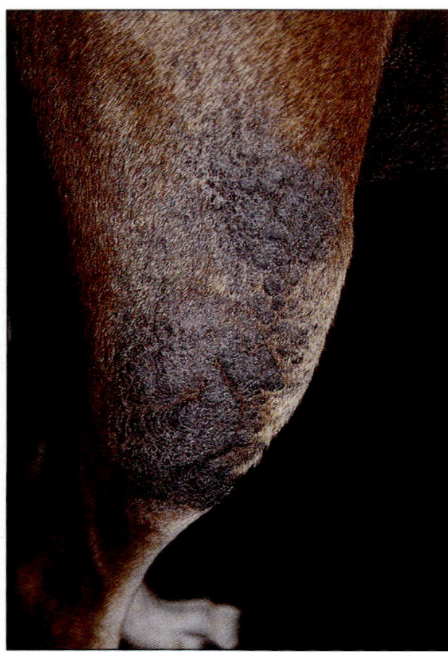

Figure 6.4 Lichenification is a secondary lesion which occurs with chronic inflammation. Dogs with allergic conditions can eventually develop lichenification. Photograph by Annette Loeffler, with permission.

As stated earlier, the only way to test accurately for food sensitivity is a food trial. It would be convenient if blood tests were available for this diagnostic purpose but, currently, enzyme-linked immunosorbent assay (ELISA) testing for food sensitivities is not considered to be reliable. False positives do occur. At present, a food trial with a novel protein and carbohydrate source for 6 weeks is the definitive method of diagnosis. Some clinicians argue that 4 weeks is long enough, while others promote a 12-week trial. The longer trial would render more accurate results; however, owner compliance is very poor for such extended periods. Statistically, 25% of patients with food sensitivity will show improvement in 1–3 weeks, 50% take 4–6 weeks to show improvement, 20% don't show improvement until 7–8 weeks and 5% take 9–10 weeks to improve on a food trial.

Home-made diets consisting of one-third novel protein to two-thirds novel carbohydrate are the gold standard method of assessing food sensitivity. A thorough history of previous diets is necessary to ascertain what the pet has already been exposed to. This is particularly important in the case of wheat exposure. Protein sources can include any one of the following: fish, rabbit, duck or venison for dogs. Kangaroo and ostrich have also been suggested but availability may be difficult. With cats, fish should be avoided. Instead, cats should be offered rabbit, venison or lamb. Some dermatologists recommend the use of lamb and rice baby foods for cats that find the commercial diets unpalatable. Carbohydrate sources for either dogs or cats can be potato, rice, corn (maize) or tapioca. Generally, potato is considered the safest choice in terms of its novelty. Cats can be offered rice or barley. It is important to avoid the protein and carbohydrate sources known to cause the most sensitivity reactions in each species. In dogs the main offenders are dairy products, beef and wheat. Chicken, egg, pork corn and soy have also been reported to cause allergic problems in dogs, but not as frequently as the first three. Food preservatives and dyes can be another source of sensitivity. In cats, reactions to fish, beef, chicken and dairy products are most commonly reported (Roudebush et al 2001).

As a home-made diet is less dense than commercial diets, rather larger quantities need to be served. The 30 kg dog would need 520 grams of protein and 1080 grams of carbohydrate per day. This requires a lot of cooking. Most clients do not have the time or equipment for such large-scale catering. Neither are home-made diets terribly well balanced. As many animals being tested are young, growing pets, it may be unwise to keep them on an imperfectly balanced diet for extended periods of time. Generally, home-made diets are considered too low in calcium, iron and B vitamins, while being too high in protein. Cats should not be on a home-made diet for longer than 4 weeks due to their specific needs for certain amino acids and essential fatty acids.

Luckily, there are many commercial diets to choose from. Several of the major food companies offer sensitivity diets featuring a novel protein and carbohydrate source. Some of these include: Wafcol's salmon and potato, Waltham's capelin and tapioca and Hill's D/D diets. More recently, hydrolysed diets have come on the market. These contain hydrolysed proteins which have been modified so that the molecules are much smaller than normal protein molecules. Making the molecule small, less than 10 000 daltons to be exact, makes the molecule hypoallergenic. Most dermatologists agree that hydrolysed diets are the second best thing to home-made. Hill's Z/D Ultra, Waltham/Royal Canin's Hydrolysed soya hypoallergenic diet and Purina HA are three of the currently available diets on the market.

Pets should be given 2–3 days to change from their normal diet to the diet chosen for a food trial. Cats may take longer to adjust to the change. It is important for cats to accept the new diet, as complete refusal can be dangerous, leading to hepatic lipidosis. Complicating the trial issue for cats is the fact that the cat will need to be confined to the home during the trial period. Otherwise there is no way to control the cat's propensity for hunting snacks or dining out at the neighbour's.

Dog owners will need to be reminded that training treats, table scraps and food dropped from the baby's highchair are strictly taboo while a diet trial is in force. Owners will find this difficult and may need a lot of explanation and encouragement. Explaining how important the trial is as a diagnostic tool and how much difference in the pet's pruritus can be achieved if an actual food sensitivity can be identified may be motivating. It is a good idea to schedule weekly telephone updates to check in with the client and encourage his/her efforts. 'Nothing but the chosen diet and water can pass the lips' must be reiterated over and over. It is surprising how difficult it is for people to really understand what a total elimination diet is. Even vitamins and coloured medications must be avoided. Do ask to see any tablets the animal is currently receiving. Most tablets can be procured in plain white if necessary. Note that pink antibiotics and orange phenobarbitol tablets contain dyes. Uncoloured alternatives are available.

Be prepared to offer ways to make the diet interesting. Mixing the food with warm water can help. Placing the food in interactive toys is a good idea, especially with young dogs. While playing with interactive toys the dog can't chew the furniture or tip over the bin – and it makes the food more interesting. In hot weather, the biscuits can be placed in a rubber toy, moistened with water and then frozen to form a doggy ice lolly. Remind clients that dogs love playing with ice cubes and

Hand-out for food trials

- Take 2 to 3 days to adjust your pet to the new diet.
- If you find after 2 days that your pet will not eat the diet, try adding some fresh cooked source of novel protein (e.g. rabbit, goat, venison) to the diet. Please contact the practice if you need advice at this point!
- Some animals feel less full on hypoallergenic diets. Please keep your bins tightly closed to avoid scavenging.
- Provide interactive toys for your pets to play with. The food can be placed in these toys and will provide your pet with an activity while it is trying to get the food out. Pets find these toys stimulating and it keeps them out of the bin.
- Remind children and visitors not to feed your pet.
- Be vigilant on walks. It may be necessary to keep your dog on a lead to avoid scavenging.
- Cats will need to be curtailed to the home until the trial is finished.
- Always provide plenty of fresh water. Ice cubes can be given as a treat for dogs that enjoy playing with them.
- Contact the practice before giving any medication to your pet. The dyes in medication can spoil the food trial.
- No treats! Don't ruin all your hard work by succumbing to begging!

plain water ice cubes are a legal treat on the food trial. Be creative and be supportive. It can be a long 6 weeks for owners and their pets.

Due to the high cost of hypoallergenic diets (both commercial and home-made) pets don't typically stay on these diets forever. A food trial isn't complete until a challenge has been completed. By challenging the animal with selected proteins and carbohydrates, it is possible to identify the offending allergen and avoid it in the future. Thus, if beef is identified as the food substance which triggers a sensitivity reaction, the pet can eat any diet not containing beef. Surely that is much easier than staying on a pure hypoallergenic diet for life. Yet, you will find clients who have seen so much improvement in their pet that they want to stay on the hypoallergenic diet forever. This should be discouraged, especially in young animals. Most sensitivity reactions occur within 24–72 hours so it is possible to challenge with a variety of ingredients over a fairly short period of time. Many animals will be sensitive to more than one ingredient. A sample challenge chart is shown in Figure 6.5.

It is worth mentioning that a food trial is a diagnostic test; therefore, special diets are covered by some insurance companies. It is certainly worth writing to insurance companies and explaining that the food trial is part of the diagnostic work-up and should be covered by insurance in the same way that X-rays and blood tests are covered by insurance.

At the end of the trial, if the pet is much better, it is a wonderful diagnosis. Avoidance of a food substance is much easier to manage than avoidance of dust mites or pollens. In many cases the pet will be somewhat better but certainly not cured. In this instance you can surmise that food sensitivity plays a part in a whole allergic picture. The animal may also be atopic or the flea control may not be as vigilant as required. It is still worthwhile to treat the animal as food-sensitive and identify which food substances to avoid. If there is no improvement at all, you have at least eliminated food sensitivity as a differential and can go on to investigate other allergic skin diseases, such as atopic dermatitis.

Food sensitivity highlights

- *Clinical signs:* Pruritus and erythema on face, feet, ears. Secondary lesions quite possible.
- *Diagnostic test:* Six-week food trial with hypoallergenic diet. If improves, challenge to identify offending substance.
- *Treatment:* Avoidance of food substance(s) to which the animal is sensitive.

ATOPIC DISEASE

Atopic disease is an allergic reaction to some environmental stimulant. Allergens that commonly trigger atopic reactions include dust and storage mites, grasses and pollens. The primary clinical sign is

Food item \ Day	1	4	7	10	13	16	19	22	25	28	31	34	37	40
Beef														
Dairy (cottage cheese)														
Chicken														
Wheat (wheat germ)														
Egg														
Fish (tuna for cats white fish for dogs)														
Lamb														
Corn (corn meal)														
Rice														

Figure 6.5 Challenge chart.

pruritus, which is often severe. Areas where pruritus occur include the face, feet, ventrum, perineum, axillae and ears, flexor tarsal region and the extensor and flexor carpal region. These areas overlap a great deal with food sensitivity reactions but differ widely from FAD. Erythema is present and there can be secondary bacteria and/or yeast infection. Lesions such as excoriations and erosions due to self-trauma are consistent with the pruritic nature of the disease. Ear infections and conjunctivitis often occur as part of the disease picture. Figure 6.6 shows a dog with alopecia and erythema – conditions that can occur with atopy.

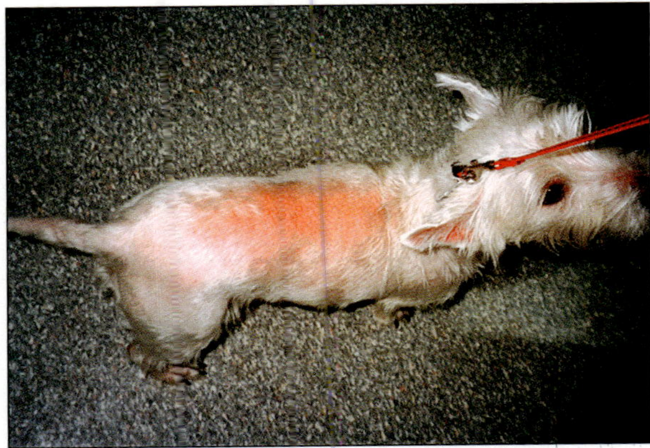

Figure 6.6 West Highland White terriers are frequently afflicted with atopic disease. This dog is displaying alopecia and erythema that can occur with atopy. Photograph by Frances Gaudiano.

Atopy is often seasonal, especially if the animal is sensitive to grasses and/or pollens. In some cases, it can start as a seasonal disease and develop into a year-round problem. The age of onset in the dog is between 1 and 3 years and there is often a family history of the disease as a genetic component is recognised. Some of the dog breeds with a predilection to atopy include Boxers, Bulldogs, Bull terriers, Cairn terriers, Dalmatians, German Shepherd dogs, Golden Retrievers, Labradors, Lhasa Apsos, Jack Russell terriers, Pugs, Scottish terriers, Shar Peis, Shih Tzus, Schnauzers, West Highland White terriers.

Unfortunately, there is no tried and true test for atopic disease. The diagnosis is made via a good clinical history and the process of elimination. There are main and minor criteria which must be fulfilled in order to come to a diagnosis of atopy. Many clinicians use Dr Willemse's list of diagnostic criteria (Willemse 1986; see Table 6.1).

Another method of assessing a patient for atopic lesions is Canine Atopic Dermatitis Extent and Severity Index (CADESI) scoring (Olivry et al 1997). In this method, different sites of the body are examined for erythema, excoriation and lichenification. Each type of lesion is scored on a scale of 0 to 3 (0 = no lesions, 1 = mild lesion, 2 = moderate lesion, 3 = severe lesion). Currently, a modi-

Table 6.1 List of major and minor criteria for atopic dermatitis (Willemse 1986)

Major criteria (at least three must be fulfilled)	Minor criteria (at least three must be fulfilled)
Pruritus	Age of onset less than 3 years
Typical lesions and pattern of distribution	Facial erythema and chelitis (swollen lips)
Facial and/or digital involvement	Bilateral conjunctivitis
Lichenification at caudal tarsal or carpal joints	Superficial pyoderma (staphylococcal)
Chronic or chronically relapsing history	Hyperhidrosis (sweaty skin)
Family history or breed disposition	Skin test reactive to inhalant allergens
	Elevated allergen-specific immunoglobulin G (IgG)
	Elevated allergen-specific immunoglobulin E (IgE)

fied version of the original CADESI template examines 40 different body sites. The maximum score an animal can receive is 360 (a score of 3 for each of the three types of lesion multiplied by 40 sites).

The differential list when looking at an atopic dog should include:

- flea-allergy dermatitis
- sarcoptic mange
- *Cheyletiella* infestation
- pyoderma
- yeast infection
- dermatophytosis
- food sensitivity.

Every element of the differential list must be explored before coming to the conclusion that a dog or cat has atopic disease.

Ectoparasites

After taking a thorough history, one should eliminate the ectoparasite potential. Coat brushings and tape strippings should be performed for fleas and *Cheyletiella*. Skin scrapings should be performed to test for *Sarcoptes scabiei*. Additionally, the animal should be placed on an ectoparasiticidal clinical trial. Environmental spray and selamectin should be used on two occasions, 1 month apart, to help rule out the possibilities of FAD and sarcoptic mange – two other very pruritic disease states.

Bacterial and yeast infections

The initial work-up should also include tape strippings for cytology. With or without an underlying atopic component, bacteria or yeast infestation may be present. Once identified, these infections can be treated and this will greatly reduce the level of pruritus. Treatment can be topical and/or systemic, depending on the severity of the infection.

If there is aural involvement, an ear swab should be taken and tape strippings should be performed on the pinnae. Appropriate otic treatment should be prescribed according to the cytological results. Eye treatment may be needed if there is concurrent conjunctivitis.

Dermatophytosis

Some cases may warrant investigation for dermatophytosis. Generally, 'ringworm' is not a pruritic disease. However, if there is secondary bacterial infection causing pruritus, dermatophytosis is a valid differential. In this case, a dermatophyte culture should be carried out. Hair pluckings or brushing through the coat and then imprinting the agar with the brush, are two methods of gathering samples for culture.

Food sensitivity

After the initial assessment and flea/scabies control measures it is time to move on to a food trial. A hypoallergenic commercial diet or novel protein and carbohydrate source will need to be fed for 6 weeks (see previous section). It may be difficult to explain to the owner that he/she has to wait 6 weeks for a full diagnosis; however, eliminating food sensitivity as a possibility is the only way to come to the diagnosis of atopic disease. In certain circumstances, it may be worthwhile to initiate the food trial at the very first visit. If ectoparasite infestation seems very unlikely and secondary infection is non-existent or minimal, a food trial may be in order from the beginning of treatment.

Once the food trial has been completed and secondary problems have been controlled through shampooing and/or systemic antibiotics/antifungal agents, one can come to the conclusion that the animal is truly atopic (see diagnosis box). It is at this point, only after completing the process of elimination, that you would begin testing for specific allergens. Generally, clinicians will not proceed with allergy testing unless the client has agreed to hyposensitisation therapy because if the owner is not willing to submit their animal to the monthly injections, specific allergy testing is of limited use.

Serum allergy testing is simpler in that it only involves taking a few vials of blood. With serum allergy testing, the animal does not need to be off steroids and antihistamines for as long a period as intradermal skin testing. Unfortunately, serum testing varies greatly in its reliability. False positives can occur. If hyposensitisation vaccines are created on the basis of false positives, the treatment will be deemed a failure and still have cost the owner a considerable sum. This does not lead to good client–practice relations. Serum tests can be useful for identifying IgE and thus convincing clients that there is an allergy problem. Once convinced, clients may be more willing to go for full intradermal testing, which is far more accurate. Simple, in-house tests for IgE antibodies are available and are not too costly. As a client management tool, they are useful tests.

Intradermal testing involves injecting a series of allergens into the skin and monitoring the allergic response. The reason that this test is considered superior for allergy testing is that it not only tests for specific IgE bound to mast cells in the skin, but also tests the tendency for this animal's mast cells to degranulate. Atopic animals can have altered levels of mast cell-derived mediator release. Additionally, the skin's response to the inflammatory mediators released by the mast cells is measured. While serum testing tests only one aspect of an allergic reaction – that is, IgE – intradermal testing tests three different aspects of allergic reaction:

1. the presence of IgE
2. mast cell degranulation
3. cutaneous reaction to inflammatory mediators.

In preparation for intradermal testing, an animal must be off corticosteroid treatment for at least 1 month and off antihistamine treatment for 2 weeks. This can be very difficult in a very pruritic animal. However, these therapies will inhibit reactions and make the test meaningless.

A catheter should be placed in any animal receiving allergen injections. There is the remote possibility of anaphylaxis and intravenous access is a necessary precaution. Also, sedation may be given intravenously. A rectangular area of hair should be clipped on the lateral wall of the chest, large enough to accommodate the number of injections chosen. Rows of dots made with a marker pen should be created in order to regulate the injection sites. Allergens can be purchased from several different companies. Unfortunately, however, it is currently necessary to import these allergens. Due to the hassle of importing the test and the quite steep price of the injectables, only dermatology referral centres are likely to carry out intradermal skin testing. The allergen panel is composed according to the region of the country the animal lives in. Certain grasses and pollens will be specific to each region and would be the allergens the animal is exposed to. Most test kits will also include flea saliva, dust and storage mites and epithelial mixes. Sometimes as many as 50 injections are given. Under the circumstances it is important to number each allergen and create organised rows of injections so that reactions can be correlated to the correct allergen.

Sample test kit

- Negative and positive controls (histamine and saline)
- House dust mites (*D. pteronyssinus*), Farina mite (*D. farinae*), Meal mite (*Acarus siro*), Copra mite (*Tyrophagus putrescentia*), Hay mite (*Lepidogylphus destructor*)
- Flea saliva
- Cat, dog, horse epithelium
- Moulds – *Aspergillus*, *Penicillin*
- Trees – Privet, Sycamore, English oak, White birch, White poplar, European beech, European ash, Hazel, Willow, Elm, Elder, Linden

- Grasses – Oat grass, Timothy grass, Meadow fescue, Rye grass, Sweet vernal, Velvet grass, Bermuda grass
- Weeds – Ragweed, Curly dock, Dandelion, Nettle, Red sorrel, English plantain, Pigweed, Mugwort

Fifteen minutes after injections, the skin test can be read. The positive control wheal is an injection of histamine, while the negative control blep is caused by an injection of saline. The diameter of each wheal is measured and then the mean between the positive and negative controls is calculated. For example, if the histimine wheal measures 10 mm and the saline blep measures 5 mm, the mean is 7.5 mm. Any wheal measuring larger than 7.5 mm is considered a positive reaction. By assessing the wheals, the proper allergens are chosen for mixing into a hyposensitisation treatment. The majority of treatments use about four ingredients. Very sensitive animals may need up to eight ingredients. Some animals will display a delayed hypersensitivity and develop wheals up to 48 hours post-injection. Owners should be asked to assess the wheals and report to the veterinarian if there are any changes.

The hyposensitisation treatments are created by the same companies that distribute the test kits. Each treatment is individualised for that particular animal. Injections are given on a regular basis and eventually a maintenance schedule is reached when animals are typically injected every 3–4 weeks. Hyposensitisation treatments are usually given long term as it can take up to 1 year for improvement to be seen. Improvement is achieved in about 50–80% of cases. The first injection should be given in a veterinary surgery as there is a slight risk of anaphylactic reaction. Subsequently, owners can learn to do the injections at home; however, the animal should always be monitored for at least 30 minutes post-treatment.

While hyposensitization treatments do not 'cure' atopy, the treatments are promoted because they reduce the need for other forms of medical management of atopic disease. By desensitising dogs through continued, controlled exposure, hyposensitisation treatments reduce the level of reactivity to the allergens contained in the treatment.

Generally speaking, it is not possible to avoid the allergen. Dogs allergic to dust mites can be confined to kennels but that is hardly a satisfactory solution. Pollen-allergic dogs can be kept indoors during the pollen season, but again, this can create more problems than it solves. As the allergens cannot be avoided, the animal will continue to suffer allergic reactions in the form of inflamed, pruritic skin.

Essential fatty acids (EFAs) are one innocuous method of helping to reduce the inflammatory response. EFAs alter epidermal lipid barriers and help to shift the type of inflammatory mediators to less potent versions. There are two types of essential fatty acids – Omega 3 and Omega 6 fatty acids. An example of an Omega 3 essential fatty acid is eicosapentaenoic acid (EPA) as found in fish oils. Omega 6 fatty acids are made of gamma-linoleic acid (GLA.) Gamma-linoleic acid can be found in evening primrose oil. Either type of fatty acid can be given singly; however, combining Omega 3 and Omega 6 fatty acids is more effective. A ratio of 5–10:1 is recommended, with the Omega 6 supplement being the greater quantity.

A dose rate of 50 mg/kg of a combined essential fatty acid supplement can help to resolve pruritus in 50–70% of cats. EFAs may be less successful in dogs in eradicating pruritus but are useful as part of an overall programme to control discomfort. Cases with dry skin conditions are particularly responsive to fatty acids. Veterinary EFA supplements can be prescribed or owners can purchase evening primrose capsules and cod liver oil as supplements to the pet's diet. It is safe to dose up to, but not exceeding, the diarrhoea threshold. Higher doses are more effective but the effect on the gastrointestinal tract, as well as the input of extra calories, cannot be ignored. A small risk of pancreatitis must also be acknowledged.

Along with EFAs, antihistamines can be given. Given together, EFAs and antihistamines have a synergistic effect. There are a variety of human preparations available. If one antihistamine doesn't work it is definitely worthwhile to try another. Statistics show that 30% of dogs and 70% of cats improve with antihistamine therapy. Animals will exhibit individual reactions to different preparations. Trial periods should last 10–14 days before abandoning a particular format. Some owners will complain about drowsiness as a side-effect, but this effect should wear off in 3–4 days. It is worth noting that drowsy pets scratch less.

The immunosuppressant drug cyclosporin (Atopica, Novartis) is also used in the treatment of atopic disease. This drug works by inhibiting the release of the cytokine from T-cells which stimulates the production of IgE. Cyclosporin is expensive but doses can be reduced if cyclosporin is given in conjunction with ketoconazole. If the animal has a concurrent yeast infection, this drug regime may be worth utilising. Otherwise, two expensive drugs are being employed and the side-effects possible with ketoconazole must be taken into consideration. Alternate-day doses of cyclosporin can be employed when the animal has been stablised. Some animals are even maintained on twice-weekly doses. There are some side-effects associated with cyclosporin – vomiting and diarrhoea often occur initially. Diabetic animals may become unstable at the onset of cyclosporin treatment and it is advised that cyclosporin be stopped for 2 weeks either side of vaccination.

Recently a herbal therapy has become available to help decrease the skin irritation suffered by atopic dogs. The supplement is provided in sachets that are mixed into the dog's food. The product, Phytopica (Phytopharm), is administered at a dose rate of one sachet per 10 kilograms. Clinical studies have shown that the supplement is well tolerated, safe and, in a majority of dogs, does provide some relief from the clinical signs of atopy.

There is no avoiding the fact that some atopic animals will need corticosteroid therapy. As we all know, steroids have some nasty side-effects. First of all, steroids make animals drink more, urinate more and eat more. Generally, owners find these behavioural changes annoying, to say the least. More serious side-effects include: lethargy, exercise intolerance (coupled with polyphagia = weight gain!), tendency towards secondary infections, poor wound healing, muscle wastage and Cushing's disease. Using hyposensitization vaccines or essential fatty acids and antihistamines will decrease the amount of steroid needed. The lowest possible dose of steroid should be the goal. One might need to begin at an anti-inflammatory dose of 1 mg/kg daily, but hopefully this can be reduced to dosing every second or third day. Cats are more tolerant of corticosteroids, but no animal should be given these drugs needlessly. It is acceptable for the atopic animal to still be a little bit itchy. If pruritus ceases entirely, the anti-inflammatory treatment is excessive.

Secondary infections from yeast or bacteria will arise from time to time in the atopic animal. In the initial stages of management, full courses of antibiotic or antifungal medications will need to be given. Usually this involves at least 3 weeks of treatment with an antibiotic with good efficacy at skin level. Cephalosporins are generally chosen. A full course of treatment may seem expensive at first but it will prevent lingering or recurrent infections, saving money in the long run.

Antibacterial and antifungal shampoos can be used alone or as an adjunct to systemic treatment. Soothing shampoos, which include colloidal oatmeal or ethyl lactate, are excellent for reducing pruritus. Spray-on conditioners can also be comforting to inflamed skin. Most medicated shampoos require 10 minutes contact time and may need to be used two or three times weekly. Expense and hassle can be reduced by instructing the owner to shampoo the affected areas only. Most owners will need instruction on bathing and correct use of shampoo therapy.

Some clinicians have recommended avoidance as a means of reducing flares in the atopic animal. A pet allergic to dust mites cannot completely avoid the allergen but the exposure can be reduced by washing all pet bedding at high temperatures weekly, vacuuming often (preferably with a filter approved for allergy control) and limiting access to rooms with lots of soft furnishings. This is not to say that the pet should be locked in the kitchen all day, but bedrooms can be avoided and rooms with carpeting and sofas could be visited for just a few hours per day. Removing carpeting from the house is helpful but not a step every owner would be willing to take.

Pets allergic to pollens can be restricted from very long romps in fields and woods. Rinsing after a walk can remove some pollen from the coat. Keeping the lawn tidy in the pet's garden can also be helpful. If the animal is allergic to moulds, damp shelter should be a no-go area – these pets should not be locked in garages or sheds. Compost heaps should be off-limits, as should dustbins and houseplants. Unfortunately, while avoidance may make the owner feel more in control of the situation, statistics do not really support it as a means of treatment. Studies done with allergic children only showed mild improvement from severe restriction regimes. Generally speaking, avoidance techniques are a lot of work on the owner's part and do not improve the animal's quality of life. For the minimal amount of relief obtained, avoidance is not really a worthwhile strategy.

Atopy is a disease in which life-long management is required. The owner needs to understand that there is no cure for allergic skin disease and that dedication will be required to keep his or her pet healthy. Adjustments in treatment will be needed from time to time. Some animals have a seasonal component to their disease and may need more supportive therapy during certain times of the year. In many pets, atopy is a progressive disease and these animals will need a gradual increase in treatment over time. Clients with atopic dogs and cats will need a lot of education and guidance on a long-term basis.

Atopy highlights

- *Clinical signs:* Pruritus of face, feet, carpus, tarsus. Chronic relapsing dermatitis, family history, breed predisposition. Onset before 3 years of age, bacterial conjunctivitis, otitis.
- *Diagnostic tests:* Eliminate possibility of ectoparasites through coat brushings and skin scrapes. Do cytology to test for bacterial or yeast infections. Six-week food trial.
- *Treatment:* Strict flea-control programme, treat secondary infections with systemic treatment and/or shampoo therapy, antihistimines, essential fatty acids, corticosteroids if necessary. Hyposensitisation treatment if intradermal testing is done.

Diagnosis of atopic skin disease

- Diagnostic tests for ectoparasites: coat brushings for fleas, lice, *Cheyletiella*
- Skin scrapings for scabies
- Flea and scabies clinical trial: Two doses of selamectin 2–4 weeks apart, plus treat at home with environmental spray
- Cytology for yeast and bacteria, include dermatophyte culture if suspicious
- Treat as needed for infections at least 3weeks or 1 week past clinical cure
- Food trial: 6 weeks on hydrolysed or home-made novel protein and novel carbohydrate diet
- If clinical signs are consistent with atopic disease (for example, pruritus and erythema of face, feet, ventrum, perineum and ears), if the age of onset is 1–3 years, and if the breed has a predilection or family history:

then:

- Diagnosis of atopic disease
- Serum assay or intradermal skin test to identify allergens and compose hyposensitisation therapy. And/or manage with drug therapy, shampoo and supplements

ACUTE CUTANEOUS HYPERSENSITIVITY REACTIONS

A sudden onset of urticaria or angioedema is an acute hypersensitivity reaction to a substance the animal has been exposed to. Urticaria consists of wheals with erythema and localised oedema. The wheals usually subside over a relatively short period of time. Angioedema is a large area of swelling, usually of the face. This can be life threatening if there is obstruction of the airway.

These cutaneous reactions are the result of mast cell degranulation leading to an acute inflammatory response. Vaccines, antibiotics (especially sulphonamides) and non-steroidal anti-inflammatories are notorious agents that can trigger an IgE response. An acute inflammatory cascade follows. If this occurs, make sure the allergy is recorded in an obvious place in the pet's file. Other stimulating agents include food substances or additives, insect stings, vegetation (e.g. nettles) chemicals or intestinal parasites. Even extreme physical factors, such as heat, cold, pressure or exercise, can lead to angioedema/urticaria episodes.

A definitive diagnosis can only be made by challenging the patient with the supposed allergen. This may not be wise though, as a second reaction could be an anaphylactic one.

Drug reactions are usually in a fixed pattern. Severe reactions may lead to erythema multiformae, characterised by annular, erythematous, pruritic lesions. Toxic epidermal necrosis is an even more severe drug reaction that leads to the sloughing of the skin. If the patient has a history of recent or recurrent drug ingestion and a cutaneous reaction develops, take it as a sign not to administer that drug to that patient ever again.

Other allergens tend to cause less severe and less uniform reactions. Avoidance of the substance is best but in case of accidental exposure the client should be given antihistamines to have on hand as needed. Generally urticaria/angioedema is treated with corticosteroid therapy. Severe cases may need adrenaline. Antihistamines are adequate for mild reactions.

Acute allergic reactions: highlights

- *Clinical signs:* Usually sudden onset after exposure to irritant/allergen. Wheals, oedema. Lesions should resolve within 24 hours
- *Diagnosis:* Via history
- *Treatment:* Corticosteroids, adrenalin if needed, antihistamines, avoidance

CONTACT DERMATITIS: ALLERGIC OR IRRITANT

Contact dermatitis is a type IV hypersensitivity disorder if the reaction is an actual allergic reaction with an IgE response. Otherwise, the resultant dermatitis is merely the result of irritation. Reactions often appear on the ventral abdomen or at the neck, underneath collars. The abdomen is an area of skin not protected by hair so it is by nature more sensitive. An animal may lie on vegetation that causes a reaction, a carpet with irritating fibres or a floor just cleaned with potentially irritant chemicals. A maculopapular rash will appear in the areas of exposure. Severe cases may develop vesicles and even ulcers. Diagnosis is made via the clinical history. Re-challenging is not as dangerous in this case. Treatment is generally given in the form of corticosteroids.

Contact dermatitis: highlights

- *Clinical signs:* Papules on area of contact. History of exposure to irritant/allergen
- *Diagnosis:* Rule out ectoparasites, pyoderma, atopic disease. Obtain history
- *Treatment:* Corticosteroids/avoidance

ALLERGIC PATTERNS IN CATS

Miliary dermatitis is one of several allergic patterns that cats uniquely suffer from; it is the most common pattern, exhibited by 85% of allergic cats. This papulocrustaceous dermatitis is highly pruritic and accompanies not only flea-allergic dermatitis but can be seen with atopy, food sensitivity, cheyletiellosis, trombiculosis, pediculosis, dermatophytosis and bacterial folliculitis. Due to the severe itching, alopecia may be a secondary complaint.

Symmetrical alopecia can also occur without miliary dermatitis. Some allergic cats will respond to pruritus by excessive grooming. This behaviour usually begins on the ventral abdomen but will move on to include the flanks, medial forelimbs and, occasionally, the dorsum. Hair pluckings are useful to determine whether this condition is occurring. Over-grooming will lead to traumatised, broken hair shafts. Endocrine disorders would not show this sort of damage and are rare in cats. Showing damaged hair (magnified of course!) to the client may convince the sceptic that his/her cat is indeed over-grooming. Symmetrical alopecia is most commonly seen with FAD.

Indolent/eosinophilic ulcers are unilateral or bilateral, shallow ulcers appearing on the cat's upper lip. While associated with FAD, atopy and food sensitivity, differentials can also include trauma, bacterial infection or neoplasia (especially squamous cell carcinoma). A biopsy is a worthwhile aid in assessing this condition. If the results confirm that the ulcer is a product of superficial and deep dermatitis with a predominant eosinophilic population, then it is an allergic reaction and corticosteroids should help to alleviate the condition.

Linear granulomas are well-demarcated linear lesions of granulomatous pathology. These usually occur on the caudal thighs but can be seen on the chin and in the oral cavity. Linear granulomas will respond to steroid therapy if they are caused by cutaneous allergy. Again, a biopsy should give the definitive diagnosis, eliminating the possibilities of neoplasia or infection. A biopsy report stating that the lesion is granulomatous dermatitis with degenerative collagen would point one towards the conclusion that the lesion is caused by a cutaneous allergy.

Eosinophilic plaques consist of raised, red, well-demarcated, often eroded areas. Plaques can be single or multiple and tend to appear on the ventral abdomen or medial thigh. Again, the differentials should include neoplasia and infection, and a biopsy can be done to ascertain the underlying cause of the lesion. Corticosteroid treatment is usually advised.

Any, or all, of the above lesions can be seen in conjunction with miliary dermatitis!

FORMULARY FOR THE TREATMENT OF ALLERGIC SKIN DISEASE

This is not an exhaustive listing.
Dose rates given are from the BSAVA Formulary, 4th edition, 2002.
Asterisked items are not licensed for small animal use in the UK, but if no comparable veterinary product is available they may be dispensed to animals at the veterinary surgeon's discretion and with informed consent from the owner.

Allergy testing and hyposensitisation treatment

Axiom Veterinary Laboratories – for serum allergy testing
Artu Biologicals (Holland) – intradermal test kits and *hyposensitisation treatment
Fax: 0031 320253030
Biophady (Belgium) – intradermal test kits and *hyposensitisation treatment
Fax: 0032 25227758
Greer Laboratories (USA) – intradermal test kits and *hyposensitisation treatment
Fax: 01 828-7545320
Heska – serum allergy testing and hyposensitisation treatment
Tel: 01626 778844/Fax: 01626 779570
Leo Laboratories, Allercept E-Screen – for the presence of IgE
(order through veterinary wholesalers)
ST Allergens (France) – intradermal test kit and *hyposensitisation treatment
Fax: 0033 155592002
(There are numerous other UK companies that offer serum allergy testing and treatment. However, referral dermatologists have traditionally used continental European and American companies.)

Antihistamines

*Chlorpheniramine 4 mg tablets (Piriton, Stafford-Miller)
Small dogs to medium dogs: 2–4 mg PO q 8–12 hours
Medium to large dogs: 4–8 mg PO q 8–12 hours
Cats: 2 mg PO q 12 hours
*Chlorpheniramine maleate, 10 mg/ml injectable (Chlorpheniramine, Link)
Small dogs to medium dogs: 2.5–5 mg IM q 12 hours
Medium to large dogs: 5–10 mg IM q 12 hours
*Cyproheptadine hydrochloride 4 mg tablets (Periactin, Merck)
Cats and dogs: 0.1–0.5 mg/kg PO q 8–12 hours
*Hydroxyzine 10 mg or 25 mg tablets (Atarax, Pfizer)
2.2 mg/kg q.8 hours, for both dogs and cats

Corticosteroid treatments

Betamethasone (Betsolan, Schering-Plough) 0.25 mg tablets; 0.12 betamethasone is equivalent to 1 mg prednisolone but betamethasone has a much longer duration of activity
Dexamethasone (*Decadron, Merck) 0.5 mg tablets
Cats and dogs: 0.07–0.16 mg/kg IM, subcutaneous, PO q 24 hours for 3–5 days maxiumum
Methylprednisolone (Depo-Medrone V, Pharmacia) 40 mg/ml
Cats: 5 mg/kg subcutaneous every 2 months
Methylprednisolone (Medrone V, Pharmacia) 2 mg and 4 mg tablets
Cats: 1 mg/kg PO q 24 hours, reducing to 2–5 mg/cat PO q 48 hours
Dogs: 0.2–0.5 mg/kg PO q 12 hours

Prednisolone – various pharmaceutical companies (1 mg, 5 mg and 25 mg tablets)

Cats: 1.1 mg/kg PO q 12 hours, taper to 1.1–2.2 mg/kg q 48 hours

Dogs: 0.5–1 mg/kg PO q 12 hours, taper to 0.5–1 mg/kg q 48 hours

Essential fatty acids

Dose rates vary – see the manufacturer's instructions. Some clinicians will give higher doses. The contents of each ml or capsule is shown below.

Coatex (Vet Plus) capsules or liquid form
- Docosahexaenoic acid (DHA) 10.7 mg
- Eicosapentaenoic acid (EPA) 15.4 mg
- Gamma Linolenic acid (GLA) 110 mg
- Linoleic acid (LA) 190 mg
- Vitamin E 10 iu
- Vitamin A 100 iu
- Vitamin D3 30 iu

Complederm (Virbac) liquid form
- DHA 150 mg
- EPA 224 mg
- LA 1824 mg
- GLA 38 mg
- Vitamin E 19 iu
- Vitamin A 574 iu
- B6 0.5 mg
- Biotin 9184 mg
- Zinc 10.1mg

Efavet (Schering-Plough) capsules:
- Efavet Regular
  - DHA 11 mg
  - EPA 17 mg
  - GLA 34 mg
  - LA 276 mg
- Efavet 560
  - DHA 6.5 mg
  - EPA 9.8 mg
  - GLA 31 mg
  - LA 247 mg
- Efavet 330
  - DHA 3.3 mg
  - Epa 4.9 mg
  - GLA 31 mg
  - LA 247 mg
- Efavet High Strength
  - DHA 22 mg
  - EPA 34 mg
  - GLA 68 mg
  - LA 552 mg

Viacutan (Boehringer Ingelheim) capsules and liquid form
- DHA 9.9 mg
- GLA 105 mg
- LA 190 mg
- Vitamin E 10 iu

Immunomodulatory drugs

Cyclosporin (Atopica, Novartis) capsules 10 mg, 25 mg, 50 mg, 100 mg

Dogs: 5 mg/kg PO q 24 hours for 4 weeks, then q 48 hours or two times per week

Not licensed for use in cats

Supplements

Phytopica (Phytopharm) 30 sachets per box

Dogs: one sachet/10 kg

Ordered via email: phytopica@phytopharm.com

Topical treatments and shampoos

Shampoos

Allermyl, Virbac – Pruritus (main ingredient = linoleic acid, vitamin E, Chitosanide)
Dermocanis, Boehringer Ingelheim – pruritus (main ingredient = Borage oil)
Epi-soothe, Virbac – pruritus (main ingredient = colloidal oatmeal)
Etiderm, Virbac – bacterial infection (main ingredient = ethyl lactate)
Malaseb, Leo Laboratories – secondary bacterial and *Malassezia* infection (main ingredients = chlorhexidine and miconazole)
Nolvosan, Fort Dodge – bacterial infection (main ingredient = chlorohexidine)
Paxcutol, Virbac – bacterial infection (main ingredient = benzoyl peroxide)

N.B. Only a few of these shampoos are safe to use on cats. Check label carefully.

Topical steroids

Betsolan cream, Schering-Plough – betamethasone and neomycin
Dermobion ointment, Fort Dodge – neomycin, nitrofurazone, prednisolone as main ingredients
Fuciderm ointment, Leo Laboratories – fusidic acid and betamethasone
*Hydrocortisone cream – various human products are available over the counter
Panalog ointment, Novartis – triamcinolone, neomycin, thiostrepton, nystatin

Food trials

Eukanuba Dermatosis FP – fish and potato with EFAs
  Dogs – 800 g, 5 kg, 10 kg and tins
Hill's Z/D Ultra for Dogs, 3 kg and 7.5 kg
Hill's Feline Z/D Low Allergen 2 kg dry diet
Hill's Canine Z/D Low Allergen, 2 kg and 7.5 kg bags

Z/D diets are hydrolysed protein

Leo Laboratories Specific Diets – Canine Dermatosis Diet, 15 kg bag

Purina Veterinary Diets 'HA', Canine diets in 3 kg and 10 kg

Royal Canine Waltham Hypoallergenic Programme (made with hydrolysed protein)
  Dogs – 2 kg and 14 kg
  Cats – 0.5 kg and 2 kg

Wafcol dog foods
  Fish and corn – 3 kg, 7.5 kg and 15 kg bags
  Salmon and potato – 3 kg, 7.5 kg and 15 kg size bags

Waltham Sensitivity Control
  Catfish and rice or chicken and rice – canine 3 kg, 8 kg and tinned (chicken and rice only)
  Feline format – sachet diet of duck or chicken and rice

References and Further Reading

Ackerman L, Nesbit G 1998 Canine allergic disorders. Canine and feline dermatology. Veterinary Learning Systems, Trenton, NJ, p 109–139

Ackerman L, Nesbit G 1998 Feline allergic disorders. Canine and feline dermatology. Veterinary Learning Systems, Trenton, NJ, p 355–374

Colombini Sarah 2003 Instructing pet owners on the use of a food trial. North American Veterinary Conference Proceedings, Orlando, Florida, 2003.

Day Michael J 1999 Clinical immunology of the dog and cat. Manson Publishing, London, p 48–56, 90–124

Hall E J 2001 Dietary sensitivity. Canine and feline food allergy. Hills Pet Nutrition, p 13–18

Hill Peter B 2002 Small animal dermatology. Elsevier Science, London, p 187–198

Kunkle G, Halliwell R 2003 Flea allergy and flea control. In: Locke P H (ed) BSAVA Manual of small animal dermatology, BSAVA, Gloucestershire, p 137–145

Mueller RS, Jackson H. 2003 Atopy and adverse food reaction. In: Foil C, Foster A (eds) BSAVA Manual of small animal dermatology. BSAVA, Gloucestershire, p 125–136

Olivry T, Guaguere E, Heripret D 1997 Treatment of canine atopic dermatitis with the prostaglandin E1 analog misoprostol: an open study. Journal of Dermatological Treatment 8:243–247

Roudebush P, Guildford W, Shanley K 200_ Adverse reactions to food. Canine and feline food allergy. Hills Pet Nutrition, p 5–11

Tennant Bryn (ed) 2002 Small animal formulary, 4th edn. BSAVA, Gloucestershire

Willemse A 1986 Atopic skin disease: a review and a reconsideration of diagnostic criteria. Journal of Small Animal Practice 27:771–778

CASE STUDY 1

Food sensitivity

Signalment

Large Munsterlander, 6 months old, recently neutered male. The dog weighed 25 kg. (Low normal for the breed average of 25–30 kg.)

Problem

The owner reported frequent episodes in which the dog scratched and chewed to the point of self-trauma. The chewing reaction was focused primarily on the feet. Face rubbing was not evident but scratching at the ears did occur. The pruritus did not have a seasonal component. Diarrhoea occurred in the consultation room and was apparently an intermittent sign.

History

The dog had been acquired at 8 weeks from a breeding kennel. At 9 weeks the pup began showing signs of pruritus and rapidly developed erythema with pustules on the ventral abdomen and medial thighs. The pup had been taken to another veterinarian and antibiotics had been prescribed. An antibacterial wash has also been given to the owner to administer to the dog for several days.

Three weeks later, the owner returned to her first veterinary surgeon for further investigations. The pup's skin had become scaly and the pruritus was continuing. Deep and superficial skin scrapings were taken at this time. The scrapings were sent to Grange Laboratories and blood tests were taken for possible food allergies. A sample for IgG and IgE antibodies to the 'Food Panel' was sent to 'Sensitest Allergy Testing', Animal Care. The dog was prescribed selamectin (Stronghold, Pfizer).

Results for the skin microscopy were negative for both surface and burrowing mites. However, the food panel identified IgE antibodies to various items. An egg and rice exclusion diet was recommended (Hill's D/D, Appendix One).

One month later the pup was treated for an ear infection, the treatment used being an antibacterial/antifungal agent with an anti-inflammatory component (Otomax, Schering-Plough).

The owner did report that she was trying the egg and rice diet, but with added vegetables, jacket potatoes and occasional venison. Also, due to the cost of the prescription diet, the owner had been experimenting with other dog foods. Thus an elimination diet had not been adhered to.

The only other household pet was a cat, which was given selamectin (Stronghold, Pfizer) monthly. The dog slept on the bed with its owner. Neither the owner nor the cat suffered any dermatological lesions.

Physical examination

Pulse, respiration and temperature were normal. No abnormal cardiac sounds were auscultated. The hair coat seemed of good quality but the skin did exhibit a moderate level of generalised scaling.

Differential diagnoses

- *Cheyletiella yasguri* infestation
- *Sarcoptes scabiei* infestation
- *Demodex canis* infestation
- Pediculosis
- *Malassezia pachydermatitis* infection
- Pyoderma
- Flea-allergic dermatitis
- Atopy
- Food sensitivity

Diagnostic procedures

Skin scrapings, coat brushings and tape strippings were performed. Microscopy was unremarkable. Blood samples taken for haematology and biochemistry revealed no abnormalities except for a low urea level: 1.49 mmol/l (normal range 2.5–9.64 mmol/l), which the veterinarian felt was merely a juvenile anomaly. A further blood sample was taken for serological screening for IgE levels (Top Screen, Axiom). All results were negative.

Treatment

Our proposed diagnosis was allergic disease caused by food sensitivity. Atopy had not been ruled out as IgE levels only identify allergens a dog may be sensitive to and do not diagnose atopic disease. However, the early onset of pruritus and the distribution pattern did point towards food sensitivity. In order to confirm this diagnosis it was necessary to place the dog on a complete elimination diet for 6–12 weeks. Waltham Sensitivity diet, Capelin and Tapioca, was chosen for the trial as both the protein and carbohydrate source were novel to this dog. Unfortunately, within 4 days, the dog was violently pruritic. The next diet tried was Wafcol's Salmon and Potato; however, there was a flare within 24 hours. It was deemed best to return to Hill's D/D Egg and Rice as the dog had been partially managed on that diet formerly. Ideally, a home-made elimination diet should have been used but the size of the dog made a home-made diet difficult. Chlorphenamine (Piriton, Stafford-Miller) at a dose rate of 4 mg twice daily was prescribed. Prednisolone (Prednidale, Arnolds) at a dose rate of 5 mg twice daily was prescribed for use only if the dog was exhibiting pruritus. After 1 week, the owner complained that the Piriton was making her dog too sleepy, so she was advised to use it only when needed. An antibacterial/antifungal shampoo (Malaseb, Leo Laboratories) was prescribed on a prophylactic basis. The owner was advised to continue treating both the dog and cat with selamectin monthly.

Evening Primrose oil, in capsule form, was prescribed as a supplement to aid with the skin scaling. Due to cost, only one capsule per day was used, although higher doses would probably have been more effective.

Follow-up

The dog was seen 6 weeks later, following numerous telephone calls regarding the progress with the food trial. No incidents of diarrhoea had occurred over the period and the pruritus had been maintained at a bearable level. We were concerned that the pruritus had not been eliminated completely but it was revealed that the dog had shown flares of clinical signs when it had scavenged food dropped by a visiting grandchild. It was felt that enough improvement had been made to warrant continued treatment with the prescription diet.

Another 3 weeks followed and the dog was seen again. He was lively and his coat showed lustre. There was very little evidence of skin scaling. We decided that a challenge would be appropriate at this point. The owner wanted to try the dog on a lamb/rice diet. Therefore, she was instructed to feed lamb for 3 days and report back with any reactions. It appeared that the dog tolerated a small quantity the first day but when given a larger portion on the second day pruritus developed. Instructions were given to challenge with chicken, then beef, then fish, then eggs, then cottage cheese. Flares occurred with all substances except eggs. Carbohydrate challenges were done later with wheat germ, rice, corn meal and potato. Flares occurred with wheat germ and cornmeal. A maintenance diet of egg and rice was chosen. The owner was told she could supplement with potato, venison and rabbit if the dog lost enthusiasm for the prescription diet. The owner kept a supply of antihistamines and corticosteroids on hand in case of flares due to dietary indiscretions.

Prognosis

In the real world, complete elimination diets are very difficult to put into practice. From the trial we ran, we felt it was safe to conclude that this dog did have an allergic disease in which food was a major contributing factor. Although the prognosis is generally good, sensitivity diets can be expensive and some animals find them unpalatable.

Discussion

Food sensitivity still only makes up 1–2% of the skin disease seen in practice (Paterson 1998). However, this dog did show the classic signs of non-seasonal pruritus with focal spots on the feet, ears and perineum. Pyoderma of the ventral abdomen, which this dog exhibited in puppyhood, can also be seen with food sensitivities. Concurrent diarrhoea can point towards a food sensitivity, with 10–15% of sufferers showing both sets of symptoms (Paterson 2001).

Some authors state that food sensitivities show no age, sex, or breed predilection (Paterson 1998). However, other researchers state that 32–53% of dogs with food sensitivities present before 1 year of age. The theory is that immature gastrointestinal tracts are more sensitive and will see all food as antigenic. Also, the stress of vaccination, moving to a new home, diet changes, and all the other traumas of puppyhood put the gastrointestinal tract in a vulnerable state, predisposing it to hypersensitive responses (Olson 2001).

Defining the problem as sensitivity leads one to question the validity of serum analysis for diagnosis. We were no longer looking for an IgE response but an IgG response. The other complication is the fact that one cannot test for all the antigens in any one type of food (Bond 2001). In fact, one study has shown a serology test to have a 0% success rate in diagnosing food sensitivities (Muller & Tsohalis 2001). Although the test first used on our patient also measured IgG levels, this too can be misleading. Food is full of antigens and the gut has the job of breaking down the glycoproteins into digestible molecules. Even the non-sensitive dog will show some non-immunological responses to an antigenic food load (Hall 2001a).

This brings us back to the elimination diet. The best elimination diet is a home-made diet as there can be false negatives with commercial sensitivity diets (Bond 2001). Home-made diets should utilise a novel protein (e.g. venison, rabbit, capelin) and a novel carbohydrate free of gluten. Adding vegetable oil, dicalcium phosphate, potassium chloride and a multivitamin/mineral complex will help to balance the diet (Hill 1999). For a relatively large dog, as this Munsterlander was, a lot of cooking was involved. Large pots, along with fairly costly chunks of meat needed to be purchased. While the owner was prepared to put in the time needed for preparation, she could not afford the meat and cooking equipment and did not have the refrigeration space.

The new hydrolysed diets are a very good second choice as the altered proteins reduce the potential to cause a hypersensitive reaction (Hall 2001b). The stumbling block is the price.

The owner wanted to know how her dog ended up being so sensitive. There could be a genetic component, especially with gluten sensitivities. Also, the immature gut of the puppy does not yet have a tight enterocyte barrier and large molecules can slip by, leading to later sensitivities (Olson 2001). As a prophylactic measure, we asked the owner to be particularly strict about the diet when the dog is undergoing vaccination, worming or any stressful events. Introducing an antigenic item at this time could create another sensitivity (Olson 2001).

REFERENCES

(for Case Study 1)

Bond R 2001 Food allergy and intolerance: mechanisms and diagnosis. Canine and feline food allergy. Lecture notes. Hills Pet Nutrition, Birmingham, p 13–16

Hall E 2001a Difficulties in diagnosing and treating gastrointestinal food allergy. Canine and feline food allergy. Lecture notes. Hills Pet Nutrition, Birmingham, p 4–8

Hall E 2001b Is it really a food allergy? Veterinary Times December 10th:10

Hill P 1999 Diagnosing cutaneous food allergies in dogs and cats – some practical considerations. In Practice June:287–294

Muller R, Tsohalis J 2001 Evaluation of serum allergen-specific IgE for the diagnosis of food adverse reactions in the dog. Canine and feline food allergy. Hills Pet Nutrition, p 19–21

Olson M 2001 Food allergies in dogs. Insights into pathogenesis, prevention and treatment. Canine and feline food allergy. Hills Pet Nutrition, p 23–26

Paterson S. 1998 Skin diseases of the dog. Blackwell Publishing, London, p 160–162

Paterson S 2001 Paying attention to dietary detail. Veterinary Times March 10th:15

CASE STUDY 2

Management of allergic skin disease

Signalment

The dog presented was a 15-month-old, liver-and-white German Short-haired Pointer. The dog was male, had been castrated, and was slightly underweight.

Problem

The dog was very pruritic and showed evidence of self-trauma, especially to the feet.

History

The dog had been seen at a previous vet where, as a puppy (<6 months), it had experienced several episodes of severe gastritis that had eventually required endoscopic examination. Neither foreign bodies nor gastric ulceration was discovered. The dog was then placed on a low-allergy diet based on fish and potato base (Dermatosis FP Response Formula for Dogs, Eukanuba Veterinary Diets). This seemed to alleviate the gastritis, so the dog remained on the diet long term.

At 6 months of age that dog had been castrated and it was noted that it had been cryptorchid. There was apparently extensive self-trauma at the incision site.

A pinpoint corneal ulcer was identified shortly after the dog had been castrated. The condition was treated with a fusidic acid and genticin ointment (Fucithalmic, Leo Laboratories). As the dog reached 1 year in age it was seen for dry, scaly skin. Skin scrapings were performed and proved negative. A variety of treatments were tried, including a chlorhexidine and miconazole shampoo (Malaseb, Leo Laboratories). One month later the dog was prescribed essential fatty acids and a conditioner/humidifying skin spray (Humilac, Virbac). Otitis externa was also identified at this time and the dog was treated with a fusidic acid, framycetin, nystatin and a prednisolone ear preparation (Canaural, Leo Laboratories).

Finally, a family history of systemic lupus erythematosus (SLE) was recorded, with one litter mate affected and other dogs from the same kennels being positively diagnosed with SLE.

Physical examination

The dog appeared slightly underweight at 27 kg. (The range for a male German Short haired Pointer is 28–32 kg.) Temperature, pulse and respiration were within the normal ranges. There was marked erythema with some erosion on the dorsal aspect of the right forepaw and the caudal tarsi. The left axilla was severely erythematous. The owner reported foot chewing but had not noticed the dog scratching at the axillae. Alopecia appeared around the left eye and on the left flank. The left ear pinna and vertical canal manifested erythema and a dark, purulent exudate. The tympanic membrane was difficult to visualise due to the accumulation of debris. The overall demeanour of the dog was subdued.

Differential diagnoses

- Demodicosis
- *Sarcoptes scabiei* infestation
- Flea infestation
- *Cheyletiella* spp infestation
- Pediculosis
- Pyoderma
- *Malassezia* dermatitis
- Flea-allergy dermatitis
- Food intolerance
- Atopy

Diagnostic tests

As the differential list was extensive, it was necessary to begin with a process of elimination. A trichogram was performed first and this showed a great deal of shaft damage. It was assumed that this was due to self-trauma. The hair was not easily epilated.

Secondly, several skin scrapings, both deep and superficial, were taken and examined with a ×4 and a ×10 objective lens. All of the skin scrapings were negative, which could help to eliminate the ectoparasitic diseases.

A tape-strip test was then performed. The slide was stained with Diff-Quik (Baxter Scientific Products) and examined microscopically under the ×100 oil-immersion objective. *Malassezia* was not identified but some coccal bacteria were present.

An ear swab was taken and also stained as above and examined under the ×10 and ×100 objectives. *Malassezia* was not obvious but bacteria were well evident in the coccal form. They were assumed to be *Staphylococcus intermedius* as this is the most common commensal canine bacterium.

Due to the family history of systemic lupus erythematosus, it was felt that a skin biopsy was in order, although biopsies are not generally used for the diagnosis of atopic disease. A pre-operative blood screen was taken which showed a mild eosinophilia – this can be indicative of either parasitic infestation or allergic reaction. The rest of the haematology and biochemistry results were within normal ranges.

The dog was premedicated with buprenorphine (Vetergesic, Animalcare Ltd.) acepromazine (ACP, Vericore) and carprofen (Rimadyl, Pfizer Ltd.). Amoxicillin (Clamoxyl L.A., Pfizer) was given for antibiotic cover. The dog was induced 45 minutes later by an intravenous injection of propofol (Rapinovet, Schering-Plough) and then maintained on 1.5 % isoflurane (IsoFlo, Schering-Plough) and 2% oxygen. Three biopsies were taken from various sites. The samples were preserved in 10% formalin solution and sent to an outside laboratory for histopathology. Chronic folliculitis/furunculosis was recorded in the histology report. This finding could be indicative of self-trauma due to an underlying allergic condition and certainly justified antibiotic therapy.

At the initial consultation the dog was placed on a food trial. This was carried out for 6 weeks, utilising a novel protein and carbohydrate food (Capelin and tapioca, Waltham). Subsequent dietary challenges did not correlate with significant flares of clinical signs. As pruritus had remained a problem throughout the trial it was assumed that food sensitivity could not be the primary component of this animal's disease.

Through the process of excluding other factors, a diagnosis of allergic skin disease was the veterinarian's ultimate conclusion. Figure 6.7 shows atopic dermatitis.

Treatment

Selamectin (Stronghold, Pfizer Ltd.) at a dose rate of 240 mg was prescribed to use monthly (keeping the ectoparasite burden at bay increases the pruritic threshold). A mild ear cleaner (Leo Ear Cleaner for Dogs, Leo Laboratories) and a medicated otic preparation (Canaural, Leo Laboratories) were dispensed to deal with the secondary ear infection. The skin lesions were treated with a daily chlorhexidine scrub. Chlorhexidine has antibacterial activity and this topical treatment was felt to be sufficient to deal with the secondary surface bacterial infection. Additionally, a low-allergy diet had been introduced. All of these measures were instituted before the biopsy results had been obtained. A full 6-week diet trial was conducted without proving food to be a major factor in the dog's dermatological clinical signs, but the owner chose to stay with a low-allergy diet on a long term-basis due to the dog's gastrointestinal sensitivities. The low-allergy diet may have been helpful in raising the pruritic threshold.

Upon receiving the biopsy results, it was decided to treat the pruritus conservatively at first to see if the problem could be controlled without the use

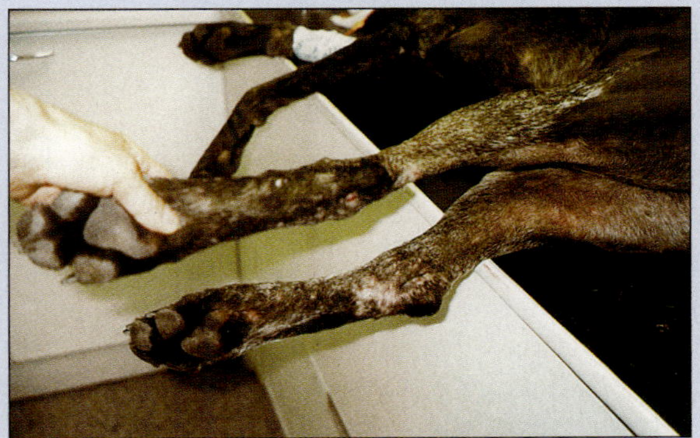

Figure 6.7 Atopic dermatitis. Notice the erythema and alopecia of the hocks – signs of atopic disease. Photograph by Frances Gaudiano.

of corticosteroids. The dog's diet was supplemented with essential fatty acids in the form of Evening Primrose Tablets and Cod Liver Oil. Antihistamines were also employed to decrease the pruritus (Chlorpheniramine, Piriton) at a dose rate of 4mg twice daily. The report of chronic folliculitis/furunculosis indicated that the bacterial infection was more serious than had been assumed on initial examination. Therefore, a course of antibiotics in the form of cephalexin (Ceporex, Schering-Plough) at 20 mg/kg was prescribed for 3 weeks.

Re-inspection and final outcome

Follow-up 3 weeks later showed a much happier, less pruritic dog. The surface lesions had cleared and the ear infection was nearly under control. A further 10 days of antibiotics were prescribed in order to give antibiotic cover beyond clinical cure. The owner was relieved and accepted the fact that treatment might have to be life-long. She was supplied with a practice treatment guideline for allergic dogs and seemed able to comply with the suggestions. As the dog is still quite young, it is likely that the treatment protocol will need to be adjusted because atopy tends to be a progressive disease. At this point, the dog is comfortable with the use of regular flea treatment, a low-allergy diet, essential fatty acid supplementation and antihistamines. Perhaps, in the future, corticosteroid therapy or hyposensitisation treatment may need to be instituted but, fortunately, it was not necessary at this point.

Discussion

Atopic disease is the second most common skin ailment after flea-allergic dermatitis and perhaps should have been suspected earlier. However, the family history of systemic lupus erythematosus was misleading in this case. The mild eosinophilia was indicative of an allergic response; however, it can also indicate a parasitic infestation. In 1986 Plechner suggested that eosinophilia is indicative of food intolerance. Certainly this dog had exhibited gastrointestinal signs earlier and did seem more comfortable on a hypoallergenic diet. Ideally, the dog should have been placed on a food trial for 6 weeks, with later challenges, to determine exactly what part food sensitivity played in his disease process.

The first skin complaint for this dog occurred at about 1 year of age, which is within the average range of onset for atopic disease. Most atopic dogs do start with seasonal problems. This dog presented to its first vet in the summer months, an appropriate time of the year to be responding to environmental and ectoparasitic allergens.

The dog in question exhibited many of the cardinal signs of both atopy and food sensitivity. The face, feet, and ears are considered the focal areas for atopy and food sensitivity. Some 50% of atopic dogs suffer from otitis and conjunctivitis (Craig 2001). It is not known whether the dog's corneal ulcer was secondary to conjunctivitis but the alopecia around the eyes would certainly indicate a pruritic condition in that area. At 15 months, the dog had already experienced two cases of otitis externa. A strong indicator of atopy is a tendency to lick and chew at the flexor and extensor metacarpal and metatarsal regions. Again, this dog exhibited that symptom dramatically.

Enzyme-linked immunosorbent assay (ELISA) or intradermal allergy testing is often performed on atopic dogs. With results from these tests a system of avoidance and possibly hyposensitisation can be carried out. However, this owner was not yet interested in using hyposensitization treatment so identifying specific allergens was not necessary. In the future, referral to a specialist centre for intradermal testing may be required. A treatment could be developed for the dog if it showed hypersensitivity to the antigens in the test. The use of hyposensitization treatment would limit the need for corticosteroid therapy if the disease progresses to that point.

At this early stage, it was decided to manage the case through medications and supplements. The advantages of antihistamines, i.e. a reduction in self-trauma due to the slight sedation, plus the stabilisation of mast cells and the decrease in mediator release, were explained and appreciated. It was noted that 10–40% of dogs can be stabilised on antihistamines alone (Griffin, 1993) but the use of essential fatty acids would have a synergistic effect towards treatment. One Evening Primrose Oil capsule per day can decrease the signs of atopy. In addition, fish oil at a dose of 1 ml/ 4.5 kg. can produce improvement within 4–16 weeks (Bond 2001).

Focal areas of discomfort are best treated with topicals (Griffin 1993) and in this case we chose chlorhexidine scrub as even topical steroids can create undesirable side-effects. The dog will not be completely itch-free – if it were, that would indicate an overdose of treatments (Scarff 2001). If the disease does progress, the use of all of the above treatments should keep corticosteroid usage to a minimum.

REFERENCES

(for Case Study 2)

Bond R 2001 Essential fatty acids in dermatology. BSAVA Congress 2001 – Scientific Proceedings, Cheltenham, p. 159–161

Craig M 2001 Canine atopy. UK Vet 6:50–52

Griffin C 1993 Management of atopy. In: Locke PH (ed) BSAVA Management of atopy. BSAVA, Cheltenham, p 263–268

Plechner A J 1986 Pet allergies. Very Healthy Enterprises, Inglewood, p 34, 64–65

Scarff D 2001 Rational use of steroids in the management of skin. UK Vet 6:54–59

Chapter 7

Endocrine, metabolic and paraneoplastic disorders

CHAPTER CONTENTS

ENDOCRINE DISORDERS

Typically, endocrine disorders manifest dermatologically with non-pruritic, bilateral, symmetrical alopecia. If a skin pattern is symmetrical, that usually indicates that the causative factor is internal, rather than external. Not all cases of endocrine disease have a clear-cut pattern of non-inflammatory symmetrical alopecia. However, if one notes hair loss without pruritus, endocrinopathies should be investigated. Pruritus can occur in endocrine disease, but only as a symptom of a secondary infection, not as a primary clinical sign. The age of onset is another important indicator of endocrine disease. Most endocrinopathies are mid-life disorders. If a young animal appears with non-inflammatory alopecia it could be a congenital endocrinopathy, but these are very rare. More likely, a young animal would be suffering from some other form of follicular disorder.

Hypothyroidism is the most common of the endocrinopathies, but unfortunately it is very frequently misdiagnosed. If thyroxine levels are measured without the utilisation of dynamic hormone tests, false-positive diagnoses are possible. The primary form of hypothyroidism in the dog is caused by lymphocytic thyroiditis or idiopathic thyroid necrosis. Secondary hypothyroidism (only about 10% of cases) is due to lesions at the level of the adenohypophysis, and the rare, tertiary form is due to lesions in the hypothalamus. In cats, a primary form of hypothyroidism is due to a congenital thyroid deformity, leading to an early onset of the disease, but this is a rare disorder. Iatrogenic hypothyroidism, due to bilateral thyroidectomy, or damage to the remaining thyroid during unilateral thyroidectomy, also occurs in cats.

The classic case of hypothyroidism walks in with bilateral, symmetrical alopecia in the truncal area. Alopecia on the dorsal nose and on the tail ('rat tail') are also apparent. The skin has become thickened and hyperpigmented, feeling cool to the touch. What hair that is left is dull and easily epilated. The dog's face has a tragic expression due to myxoedema (thickening of the skin due to mucin accumulation). Bradycardia would be evident on cardiac auscultation. The owner would complain of the animal gaining weight and 'heat-seeking' behaviours. When you take a blood sample, the dog bruises markedly and takes overlong to heal. An animal with these signs makes diagnosis easier; however, one would hope not to see that many dogs this advanced. More likely, you will see a middle-aged dog that has begun to slow down a bit, maybe put on a bit of weight. The coat will look dull and perhaps a bit thin. There might be a secondary pyoderma or, less commonly, a *Demodex* infestation. It would be necessary to investigate further to realise that the dog actually was hypothyroid. It would be terribly easy to treat the pyoderma and not hunt for an underlying cause. Hopefully, if you found *Demodex* in an adult dog you would immediately suspect that something was wrong and start investigating. The initial sites of alopecia with hypothyroidism are shown in Figure 7.1.

The first thing you can do easily is to take some hair plucks. Check whether the hair comes out readily. When examining the hair under a microscope compare the number of telogen hairs to anagen hairs. Telogen hairs have a club-like root and barbed or frayed ends; anagen hairs have a pronounced bulb at the end and look sleek and healthy. If there are significantly more telogen hairs, this would point towards an endocrinopathy. Thyroxine (T4) is essential for new hair growth. A decreased thyroxine level will increase the length of time that the haircoat will stay in the telogen phase. While examining your hair pluck samples you can also look for *Demodex* mites. *Demodex* can be a differential with hypothyroidism because demodicosis also causes alopecia. At the same time, hypothyroidism slows down natural immunity and allows commensal *Demodex* to multiply and create a concurrent state of demodicosis in a hypothyroid animal. With this in mind, deep skin scrapes should also be performed. Of course, in any dermatology case, parasitic infection must be ruled out before proceeding with any other sort of investigation. Do make sure the dog doesn't have fleas first.

Once parasites have been ruled out and it has been determined that the dog is definitely not pruritic, look for the clinical signs listed in Box 7.1.

In the cat you would look for: seborrhoea, dull coat, easily epilated hair, poor hair re-growth after clipping and symmetrical alopecia. A kitten with

Box 7.1 Hypothyroidism: common and less common clinical signs

Common clinical signs with hypothyroidism

Thin, dry hair
Seborrhoea
Pyoderma
Alopecia
Poor hair re-growth post clipping
Weight gain
Lethargy
Weakness
Hyperpigmentation (especially the bridge of the nose)
Hair easily epilated

Less common clinical signs with hypothyroidism

Myxoedema (tragic face)
Ceruminous otitis externa
Ocular and genital discharge
Facial nerve paralysis
Bradycardia
Hypothermia

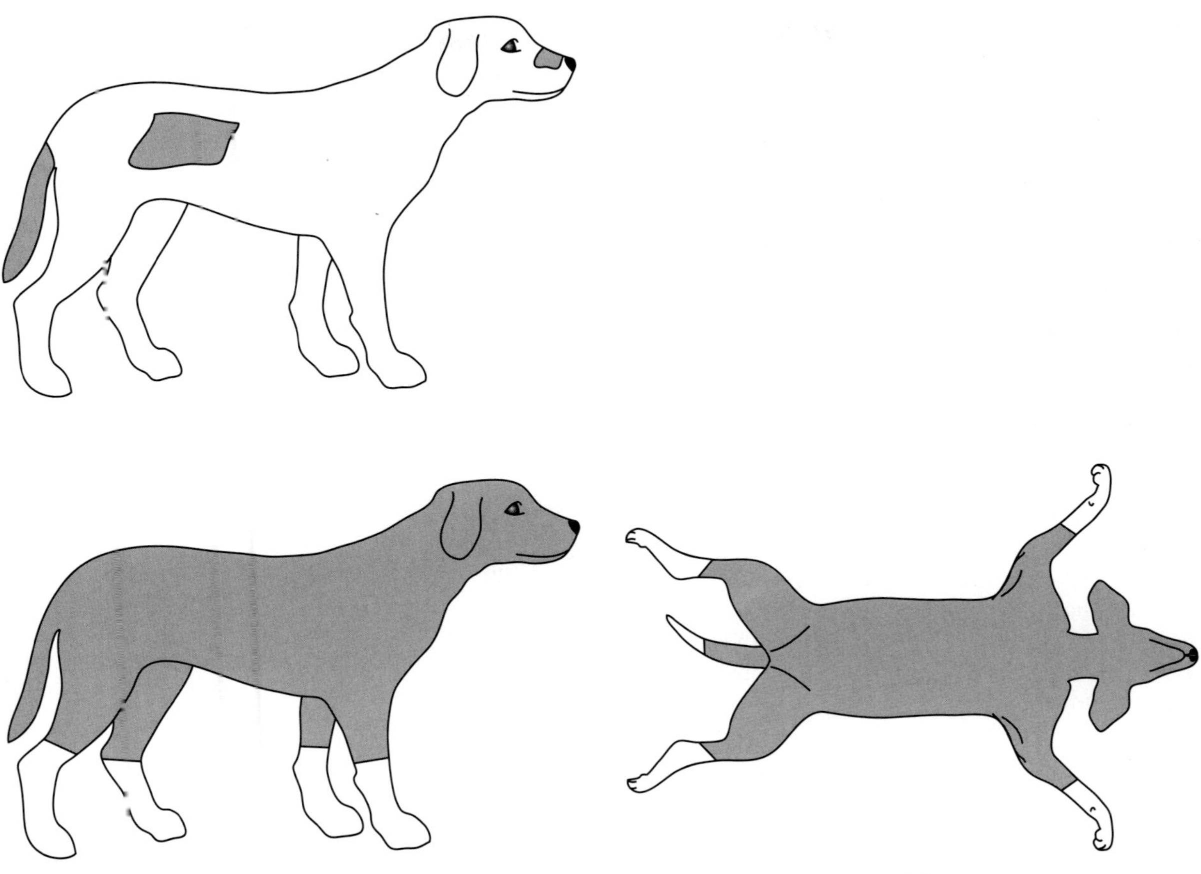

Figure 7.1 A: Initial sites of alopecia with hypothyroidism (proximal tail, bridge of nose, flanks); this leads to the situation shown in B. B: Pattern of distribution of well advanced alopecia with hypothyroidism; a similar pattern is shown in hyperadrenocorticism, although the head isn't typically involved.

congenital hypothyroidism would have secondary hairs but no primary, guard hairs in his/her coat.

Regardless of age, blood testing would be called for at this stage. A young dog or cat could have very rare congenital hypothyroidism (often associated with pituitary dwarfism) but the more commonly presented middle aged dog (3–8 years) would be a prime candidate for acquired hypothyroidism. Mid-sized to larger dogs tend to be more susceptible to hypothyroidism than small dogs. Breeds particularly prone are: Airedales, Beagles, Borzois, Doberman Pinschers, Golden Retrievers, Great Danes, Irish Setters and Old English Sheepdogs.

Routine biochemistry and haematology are performed to rule out other systemic causes. Hypercholesterolaemia is noted in a large majority (33–75%) of hypothyroid cases, while 5–32% of cases may show mild, normocytic, normochromic anaemia. Plasma lipids are usually increased and there can be a mild to marked increase in the liver enzymes alanine amino transferase and alkaline phosphatase in about 25% of cases. Creatine phosphokinase is raised in 10–18%

of afflicted animals. Endocrine assays tests are then needed to come closer to a diagnosis of hypothyroidism. The standard free T4 level is often used; however, on its own it is not diagnostic. Many factors can affect thyroxine levels and cause below-normal results. Systemic illness often lowers total T4. This is known as the 'euthyroid sick syndrome'. The thyroid gland itself is functioning adequately but the illness is slowing down the entire body. Several drugs can also lead to low T4 levels. Among these are: amoxicillin, cephalexin, barbiturates and steroids. If the dog is being seen for a dermatological problem it is quite likely that it has been treated with systemic antibiotics and/or steriods. A wash-out period of a few weeks may be necessary before taking blood samples for thyroxine evaluation.

Along with thryoxine levels, a TSH (thyroid-stimulating hormone) assay should be performed. A high thyroid-stimulating hormone level would indicate that the endocrine system is working very hard to get the thyroid going. If the TSH is high and the T4 is low, then you probably do have hypothroidism. However, if the T4 is low and the TSH is normal, then it is likely that you are only dealing with euthyroid sick syndrome.

There are two more tests used to diagnose hypothyroidism that are generally considered more definitive. The TSH and TRH (thyrotropin-releasing hormone) stimulation tests are both accurate means of measuring thyroid function. Formerly, there were occasionally severe side-effects with these tests and the bovine hormones used also created a concern about communicating unwanted bovine disease. However, TSH tests can now be done with reconstituted recombinant human TSH. The agent can be ordered on a named patient basis from IDEXX laboratories (labhelp@idexx.com). Thyrotropin-releasing hormone (Sigma Chemical Company) is still only available in the bovine form so is rarely used. Briefly, the protocol for these tests is as follows:

TSH stimulation test

1. Collect 1–2 ml as a basal blood sample in a plain or gel tube. Be sure to label the sample as 'pre-injection' and record the time on the sample tube.
2. Inject the contents of the vial of the reconstituted recombinant human TSH intravenously, following aseptic technique.
3. Collect a second sample 4–6 hours later into a second plain or gel tube. Be sure to label the tube 'post-injection' and record the time on the sample tube.
4. Thirty to 120 minutes past collection, centrifuge both samples and separate plasma before sending to an outside laboratory.
5. Submit both samples to IDEXX laboratories, requesting 'TSH stimulation test' on the submission form.

Normal dogs would have total T4 levels one and half times higher in the second sample while hypothyroid dogs would not show a significant difference between pre- and post-injection samples.

TRH stimulation test

1. Collect first sample into gel tube or heparin.
2. Inject 0.02 mg/kg TRH by very slow intravenous injection.
3. Collect second sample 4 hours later into gel tube or heparin. Be sure to label sample 'post-injection'.
4. Have both samples analysed for total T4 levels.

Normal dogs have T4 levels 1.2 times higher in the second sample and the level should be higher than 30 nmol/l. Hypothyroid dogs would have levels lower than 30 nmol/l with less difference between the two samples.

Once the diagnosis of hypothyroidism has been determined based on age, clinical signs and hormone testing, a treatment needs to be given. This is a progressive disease and, if left untreated, the animal's condition may ultimately be fatal. Levothyroxine (Soloxine, Arnolds) is the thyroid supplement licensed for canine use. A loading dose of 20 micrograms/kg twice daily should be given initially. However, animals with cardiac disease should be started at a lower dose. Once the animal is stable, dosage can be adjusted accordingly. T4 levels should be repeated 3 months into treatment. The blood should be taken 6 hours after a dose of levothyroxine is given. Generally speaking, the dog or cat will be brighter in a few weeks time and begin to lose weight. Hair regrowth may take 2 to 3 months. If maintained on an appropriate dose of treatment for the rest of its life, the prognosis is excellent. Of course, the animal should never be bred for fear of passing on the disease genetically to its offspring.

A summation of the procedures to follow when working up an alopecia case is shown in Box 7.2.

Hyperadrenocorticism (HAC), also known as Cushing's disease, is another endocrine disorder of middle-aged dogs. The disease has been reported in the cat but is much less common in that species. There are two versions of HAC: spontaeous and iatrogenic. Spontaneous hyperadrenocorticism can be caused by adrenal neoplasia in 10–15% of the cases and by pituitary malfunction in 85–90% of cases. A microadenoma of the pituitary gland can motivate the gland to produce more ACTH than is needed, thus stimulating the adrenals to produce too much cortisol for the body's needs. Adrenal adenomas/adrenocarcinomas secrete excessive levels of cortisone. The iatrogenic form is caused by the injudicious use of corticosteroids. Through over-supplementation with steroids, the animal's endocrine system becomes deranged and loses the ability to regulate cortisol levels in the body. Regardless of how it happens, too much cortisol is circulating throughout the bloodstream, causing marked clinical signs. Using 'The Five Ps' as a memory device you can recall the most common clinical signs:

- polyuria
- polydypsia
- polyphagia
- pendulous abdomen
- panting

which will often appear in the pet afflicted with hyperadrenocorticism. Dermatological signs include the typical endocrine pattern of bilateral, symmetrical alopecia. Additionally you will find thin skin, causing blood vessels to become more prominent, and loss of elasticity of the skin. There will also be hyperpigmentation and comedones visible. Hair will be easily epilated. Unless there is a secondary pyoderma or dermatophytosis, pruritus will be absent. The dermatological sign most strongly suggestive of hyperadrenocorticism is calcinosis cutis. This is a deposit of calcium in the skin, which can be seen as whitish areas which are gritty to the touch. Radiographically, these deposits will be radio-opaque. However, calcinosis cutis is seen in only about 10% of cases, and usually these cases are quite severe. This is a slowly progressive disease so the dog will have been ill for some time before calcinosis cutis appears.

The cat will show similar systemic and dermatological signs to the dog. Note that thin cat skin is easily torn and one must clip for blood testing with extreme caution. An interesting symptom of iatrogenic HAC in cats is the medial curling of the ear tips. Nearly 90% of cats with hyperadrenocorticism will also be suffering from diabetes mellitus.

If the systemic and dermatological signs are consistent with hyperadrenocorticism, and differential diagnoses have been ruled out, diagnostic testing must begin.

A urine sample can be a non-intrusive test to commence with. If the cortisol:creatinine ratio is normal, then hyperadrenocorticism can be ruled out. If the urine cortisol:creatinine ratio is elevated,

Box 7.2 Alopecia flow chart

Pruritus/inflammation
Scrapings
Cytology
Fungal culture
Biopsy
Treat as diagnosed
If recurrence, investigate further for underlying condition

No pruritus/inflammation
Young animal with systemic signs relating to endocrine function: test for congenital endocrine dysfunction
Treat as diagnosed
Young animal without systemic signs: biopsy for follicular dysplasia, colour dilution alopecia
Treat as diagnosed

No pruritis/inflammation
Middle-aged to mature animal with systemic signs relating to endocrine function: perform haematology, biochemistry, endocrine function tests
Treat as diagnosed
If no systemic signs relating to endocrine function: biopsy and investigate further

further testing should ensue. Cat owners should be sent home with non-absorbing cat litter and the urine sample should be collected at home. Most cats are stressed in a hospital environment and this will result in abnormally high levels of cortisol. Similarly, any animal that has been on steroid treatment for more than a few weeks will present with skewed results. Especially for blood testing, there needs to be a wash-out period before accurate testing can take place. The length of de-toxification depends on how long the pet was on corticosteroid therapy.

If the urine sample is abnormal, the next test can be routine haematology and biochemistry. With Cushing's disease one can expect to see:

- eosinopaenia in 82% of cases (<0.2 ×10 to the 9th/litre)
- lymphopaenia (<1.5 ×10 to the 9th /litre)
- neutrophilia and monocytosis
- raised alkaline phosphatase (ALKP) – in some canine cases it can be very high, although only one-third of affected cats will show raised ALKP
- mild to moderately raised alanine aminotransferase
- raised bile acids
- increased cholesterol levels and lipaemia
- high normal to high fasting glucose – concurrent diabetes mellitus is common
- urea level often low-normal.

These levels, particularly the raised liver enzymes and hyperglycaemia, are strong pointers towards a diagnosis of HAC. However, to definitively diagnose the disease, dyanamic endocrine function tests are necessary. The low-dose dexamethasone suppression test can identify the majority of pituitary-based disease and is even more specific for the identification of adrenal-based Cushing's disease. If the healthy dog is given dexamethasone its endocrine system will respond by producing less ACTH and thus less cortisol, as the body already has sufficient steroids via the injection. Affected dogs will lack the ability to suppress production of cortisol and the levels will rise. The LDD test is practised as follows:

1. Take a baseline blood sample into a serum gel tube or a heparinised tube and label sample.
2. Inject 0.01 mg/kg of dexamethasone intravenously.
3. Collect further blood samples at 4 and 8 hours post-injection. Label samples accordingly.
4. Samples should be centrifuged and sent to a laboratory for analysis.

Normal dogs will be able to suppress cortisol levels to < 40 nmol/l (depending on the laboratory's cut off point) at 4 and 8 hours post-injection. Affected dogs will be unable to suppress effectively and will show levels greater than 40 nmol/l with the 8-hour sample. If the results are borderline and the clinical signs are strongly suggestive, it is worthwhile re-testing 1 month later.

While the low-dose dexamethasone test can diagnose Cushing's, further tests are needed to identify which type of Cushing's the animal is suffering from. The high-dose dexamethasone suppression test (HDDST) is utilised to differentiate between adrenal- or pituitary-based hyperadrenocorticism. The test proceeds as follows:

1. Collect a baseline blood sample in a serum gel or heparin tube.
2. Inject 0.1 mg/kg dexamethasone.
3. Take further blood samples at 4 and 8 hours. Label samples with time taken.

In pituitary-dependent disease, at the 4- or 8-hour test, 55–85% of patients will show suppression of cortisol to <40 nmol/l. Adrenal-dependent cases will typically be unable to suppress cortisol levels. This is the best test to use for identifying hyperadrenocorticism in cats, but the dexamethasone should be given at a dose rate of 0.15–0.2 mg/kg. Unfortunately, none of these tests are 100% accurate. Ultrasound can be used as an additional diagnostic aid to examine the adrenals for lesions; however, very small tumours can be difficult to identify. Magnetic resonance imaging (MRI) has been used to look for macroadenomas of the pituitary, but microadenomas are not always visible on MRI.

One further test can be done to determine whether or not the disease is spontaneous or iatrogenic: the adrenocorticotrophic hormone (ACTH) stimulation test. Stimulation with ACTH will lead to raised cortisol levels in spontaneous HAC, but iatrogenic HAC cases will not respond to ACTH stimulation. The test is performed as follows:

1. Collect baseline blood sample in serum gel tube.
2. Inject intravenously 0.5 ml of tetracosactrin

acetate (synthetic ACTH, known as Synacthen, Alliance pharmaceuticals) into dogs less than 15 kg. Dogs greater than 15 kg should receive 1 ml Synacthen (alternatively this can be dosed as 125 mg or 250 mg).

3. Collect a second blood sample 1 hour later. Samples must be labelled pre and post injection.

If the cortisol level rises to >660 nmol/l (as an example of one laboratory reference range) the patient is suffering from spontaneous HAC. If there is no rise in cortisol, iatrogenic HAC may be the cause of the symptoms. ACTH stimulation is often used as a first test for Cushing's disease, instead of the LDD test, if there is no history of steroid treatment. ACTH stimulation is not terribly accurate in cats as cats show a hyperreaction when stressed. If the ACTH stimulation is used in a cat, the dose should be 125 mg of Synacthen, and post-injection samples should be taken at 30 minutes and 1 hour after the injection. Some 15–30% of cats will display false negatives with the ACTH stimulation test.

A breakdown of when to follow which test procedure is given in Box 7.3.

Operating on the adrenal or the pituitary glands to remove the tumour can be curative if it is a benign tumour. However, tumours can be extremely small and difficult to identify and surgical procedures on the pituitary glands are fraught with risks. Referral to a specialist centre for surgery is advised. For the dog, medical management is usually chosen. Trilostane (Vetoryl, Arnolds) is given at 4–16 mg/kg/day. If side-effects occur, the dose should be adjusted. Mitotane (Lysodren, Bristol-Myers, Squibb) was used prior to Trilostane; however, it tends to cause more side-effects and is a risk to the person handling the medication. Gloves and a mask must be worn when handling mitotane. Ketoconazole has also been used to lower cortisol levels, at doses of 5–10 mg/kg per day, increasing to 10–15 mg/kg/day. Side-effects include vomiting, diarrhoea and liver toxicity. For a small percentage of patients, selegiline (Selgian, CEVA) has been successful. The mainstay of treatment at this point is trilostane. ACTH stimulation testing should be carried out 7–10 days after treatment commences and then every 3–6 months to evaluate the efficacy of treatment. Overdosing can lead to vomiting, diarrhoea and weakness. Prednisolone can be given to stabilise the patient if cortisol levels have been driven too low.

In the cat, bilateral adrenalectomy along with lifelong medication to maintain cortisol levels is one form of treatment. The prognosis is guarded, however, as there tend to be post-operative complications. Medical management with mitotane or ketoconazole is not terribly successful either. The use of trilostane in cats is not licensed but has been discussed in the literature, stating that moderate improvement in clinical signs has been observed in a limited number of cases (Skelly et al. 2003, Neiger et al 2004).

Reproductive hormone imbalances

Reproductive hormone imbalances are a group of conditions that have dermatological signs due to

Box 7.3 ACTH STIM, LDDST, UCCR, HDDST

Borderline cortiso suppression after LDD test or insufficient cortisol rise in ACTH stimulation
+
Urine cortisol:creatinine ratio elevated
+
Clinical signs:
Re-test in 1 month

Raised cortisol after LDD test or ACTH stimulation
+
Urine cortisol:creatinine elevated
+
Clinical signs
HDDST
If cortisol suppressed = pituitary-dependent HAC
If cortisol not suppressed = adrenal-dependent HAC

abnormal levels of sex hormones. These conditions are fairly rare and, aside from hyperoestrogenism, generally less serious systemically than hypothyroidism or hyperadrenocorticism. Reproductive hormone-induced alopecia usually begins at the caudal, ventral abdomen and at the genitalia. There is hyperpigmentation and there can be increased scale. The alopecia can spread to the limbs, flanks and neck areas. Abnormal reproductive hormone levels, discovered through blood tests, can be useful in pursuing a diagnosis; however, the range between normal and abnormal levels is quite large. If adrenal sex hormones are believed to be at fault, an ACTH stimulation test may result in abnormally increased levels of serum progesterone and androgens. One must rely heavily on the clinical signs and the exclusion of differentials in order to make an accurate diagnosis.

Hyperoestrogenism. Older, intact bitches will shows signs of oestrus, such as vulval enlargement, even when not on oestrus. Clinical signs can wax and wane with the oestrus cycle. Polycystic ovaries or ovarian neoplasia may prompt the imbalance but the condition can also be iatrogenic. Uncontrolled cases can develop non-regenerative anaemia, thrombocytopaenia and myeloid hypo or hyperplasia. If left unchecked, in rare cases, the condition can prove fatal. A hormone assay will show a raised basal oestradiol level. Treatment is ovariohysterectomy.

Hypo-oestrogenism. This is an uncommon condition that can be caused by early neutering and thus is usually seen in young bitches. The bitch shows signs of an infantile vulva. Urinary incontinence is a significant side-effect of this condition. Diagnosis is achieved via clinical signs, history and exclusion of differentials. Oestrogen can be given via injection for 3–4 weeks but test for bone marrow suppression, a possible side-effect of stilboestrol. Treatment is not justified unless the urinary incontinence is making life unbearable for the owner or leading to urine scald on the bitch.

Hormone imbalances in the male

Most hormone imbalances in male dogs are caused by testicular tumours – sertoli, interstitial and seminoma. **Sertoli cell tumours** are the most common of these tumours. Cryptorchid dogs are more susceptible to these tumours which cause increased oestrogen levels, a pendulous prepuce, bone marrow suppression and attraction of other male dogs. A visible difference in size between the two testes can be an obvious clinical sign of the neoplasia. Dermatologically, the alopecia will be bilateral, beginning around the perineum and advancing forward from there. Hyperpigmentation occurs along with macular melanosis of the inguinal and perineal skin. The hair coat will be dry and frizzy. Haematology can show thrombocytopaenia, due to the raised oestragen levels. Hormonal assays will show raised oestradiol. Treatment is achieved via bilateral castration. Tumours will be found in both testes in 20% of affected dogs. **Seminoma tumours** present, and are treated the same as sertoli cell tumours. **Interstitial cell tumours** cause perianal and tail gland hyperplasia and can also lead to greasy seborrhoea. Hyperadrogenism can be discovered on the hormone level assays. Diagnosis and treatment is as for sertoli cell tumours.

Male dogs without testicular neoplasia may show similar dermatological signs as with sertoli cell tumours; however, hormonal assays will show increases or decreases of testosterone and oestrogen. Castration can sometimes resolve the alopecia, but not in all cases.

Growth hormone deficiency can be congenital or acquired as an adult, although identification of the adult form is controversial. The congenital form is also known as pituitary dwarfism and is caused by lesions in the pituitary gland. German Shepherd dogs are more prone to this disease than other breeds. Unfortunately, the congenital damage can also cause hypothyroidism and hyperadrenocorticism, so the dog can be plagued with all three conditions. Clinical signs include stunted growth, retention of puppy coat and also bilateral symmetrical alopecia with hyperpigmentation. Dynamic endocrine tests need to be run to diagnose this disease. Treatment is with growth hormone which is difficult to obtain and can cause diabetes mellitus. Generally speaking, the prognosis is quite poor.

The adult onset form of the disease used to be referred to as adult growth hormone responsive dermatitis. However, it is now believed that the adult form of the disease may be caused by an imbalance of reproductive hormones. Known now as alopecia X (and many other names), this disease tends to affect Pomeranians, Chow Chows, Keeshounds and Minature Poodles more than other breeds. There is alopecia at the perineum which extends to the neck, caudal thighs and tail. Hyperpigmentation can be intense and the coat is dry and frizzy. Diagnosis is achieved by ruling out differentials, especially Cushing's disease and hypothyroidism. An ACTH stimulation test may show abnormally high levels of progesterone and androgen, indicating an imbalance in the production of these hormones via the adrenal glands. To check whether a true growth hormone imbalance is present a xylazine stimulation test can be performed as follows:

1. Collect baseline sample in EDTA.
2. Centrifuge and freeze baseline sample.
3. Inject 0.1 mg/kg of xylazine (Rompun, Bayer) i/v.
4. Collect blood 20 minutes later in a gel tube.
5. Centrifuge and freeze second sample.
6. Send samples frozen via special courier to the laboratory. (The laboratory doing this test is in Utrecht.)

Normal dogs will show an increase in growth hormone but affected animals will not. Alternatively, a single sample in a gel tube can be submitted for somatomedin C (also known as IGF-I, insulin growth like factor). This is a protein secreted by the liver in response to growth hormone. Certain laboratories in the UK will perform this test.

Skin biopsy can also be performed to rule out follicular disorders. Once a diagnosis of alopecia X has been accepted, treatment options can include mitotane, growth hormone supplementation and castration. Castration may work only temporarily and the other two options have potentially serious side-effects, so they may not be really justified in what is only a cosmetic problem.

Cyclical flank alopecia, or seasonal flank alopecia, causes hair loss in late winter or spring, with regrowth in the summer or autumn. The seasonal aspect of the disease suggests some link with melatonin but exactly what the link is has not been identified. Some dermatologists classify this disease as a keratinisation disorder. Bilateral symmetrical alopecia of the flanks begins in adolescence with loss of some primary hairs. With each cycle, more hair is lost and the hyperpigmentation increases. The alopecia will spread from the flanks to the whole body, except for the head and limbs. Boxers, Bulldogs, Airedales and Dobermans are the more afflicted breeds. Diagnosis is achieved by ruling out other endocrine and follicular disorders, which involves hormonal assays and skin biopsy. An ACTH stimulation test may show a 17-hydroxyprogesterone imbalance. Treatments tried include melatonin and trilostane. Both are questionable to use for a disease that does not have any systemic signs.

A few other non-endocrine-based alopecias are as follows:

Telogen effluvium and **anagen defluxion**. These incidences of alopecia are caused by systemic insults but are not related to hormone imbalances. These diseases may be part of a differential diagnoses list in the process of examining a case of endocrinopathy. Telogen effluvium occurs when the hair enters its resting phase, telogen, and stays there overlong. Conditions such as pregnancy, lactation and systemic illness can cause this arrest in development. Hair loss is seen later when the hair begins to grow anew and the anagen phase pushes the old telogen hairs out of place. Treatment is not needed as long as the dog has recovered from the earlier stress.

Anagen defluxion is caused by a severe insult such as pyrexia, septicaemia, toxaemia or a major drug reaction, such as can happen with chemotherapy. The hair growth cycle is abruptly interruped during the anagen phase, leading to weak, easily fractured hair. Hair loss is generalised and re-growth may take some time. Treatment of the underlying cause should resolve the problem.

METABOLIC DISORDERS

There is one significant metabolic disorder that affects the skin. **Superficial necrolytic dermatitis** (SND) has a hepatic and a pancreatic form. The cutaneous clinical signs are similar in both syndromes, but the aetiology differs. Both diseases have the dermatological manifestation of surface crusts and hyperkeratosis. Self-trauma is prevalent and causes secondary infection, erosions and ulcers. All cases suffer from hyperkeratotic pads and digits, which are pathological enough to cause lameness. Other lesions occur at the mucocutaneous junctions: oral, ocular, anal, vulva, scrotum and prepuce. The more common syndrome is the **hepatocutaneous syndrome.** In the affected animal, decreased plasma amino acids may be recorded. This may be caused by an inability to metabolise protein efficiently. In humans, there is a recognised abnormality in glucagon metabolism which has a knock-on effect on protein metabolism. We do not yet know whether this is happening in dogs. Abnormal zinc and essential fatty-acid metabolism have also been discussed as part of the disease process. Whether or not an underlying hepatic pathology leads to superficial necrolytic dermatitis or is coincidental has not been firmly established. Figure 7.2 shows a dog displaying lesions that can accompany hepatocutaneous syndrome.

Superficial necrolytic dermatitis usually affects dogs of 5 years or older, with more males suffering than females. Cats can also suffer from SND, but much less often than dogs do. Clinical signs include: lameness, lethargy, anorexia, weight loss and polyuria with polydypsia, if diabetes mellitus has developed concurrently. The history-taking should be thorough to detect any incidence of hepatotoxicity, for example, exposure to toxins, drug overdose, et cetera. The differentials for hyperkeratotic pads should be explored. Conditions such as pemphigus foliaceus, zinc-responsive dermatitis, contact dermatitis and drug eruptions should be included in the differential list. If there are also lesions in haired areas of the body, folliculitis should be considered as a possible differential. Initial dermatological examination should include skin scrapes and hair plucks for demodicosis and dermatophytosis. Cytology should be performed to ascertain whether there is a secondary infection, and whether it is bacterial or fungal. Following these tests, blood tests for haematology and biochemistry analysis should follow. With SND there will typically be marked abnormalities in the blood results:

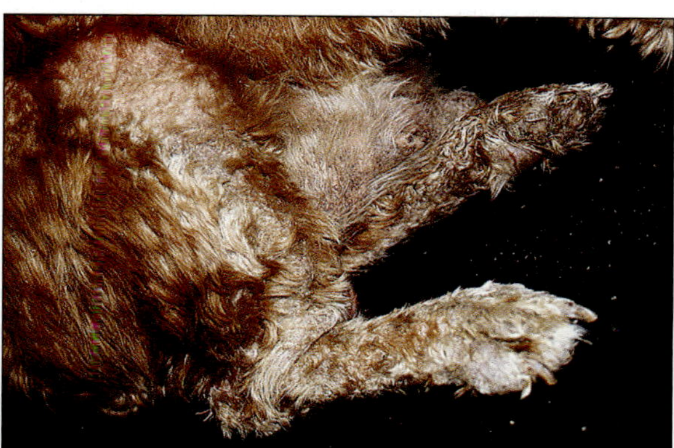

Figure 7.2 This dog is displaying skin lesions that can accompany hepatocutaneous syndrome. Photograph by Annette Loeffler, with permission.

- Alkaline phosphatase (ALKP) will be raised in nearly all cases.
- Alanine transferase (ALT) and aspartamine transferase (AST) will be raised.
- Pre-prandial and post-prandial bile acids will be abnormally elevated.
- Glycaemia levels will be elevated and diabetes mellitus will be diagnosed in some cases.
- Albumin results will be below normal.
- A mild to moderate non-regenerative anaemia and stress leukogram will be recorded on haematology.

Blood results consistent with SND prompt the need for a skin biopsy. Punch or wedge biopsies can be harvested. It is kinder to collect a sample from a non-weight-bearing footpad, e.g. digit one, and if at all possible, the overlaying crusts should be kept intact and submitted with the biopsy sample. Ulcers should not be sampled. Multiple biopsy sites are preferred for accurate analysis. A biopsy report consistent with SND would describe parakeratotic and hyperkeratosis of the stratum corneum and areas of pallor or necrolysis in the superficial epidermis. Hyperplasia of the deep and mid-epidermis along with exocytosis of leucocytes into the epidermis may also be recorded.

To achieve a definitive diagnosis, pre- and post-prandial bile acid tests should be arranged. This involves collecting a basal sample in a serum gel tube. Then the dog must be fed something it will eat promptly, such as a tinned dog food, and a post-prandial sample is taken 2 hours later. It is essential that the dog actually eats the proferred meal or the test is pointless. At this juncture, an ultrasound of the liver is most helpful and, if at all possible, a liver biopsy. However, a definitive diagnosis won't change the fact that the prognosis is guarded at best. The worse the dermatological presentation is, the less likelihood there is of survival. Utilisation of a dermatological and nutritional programme will buy the dog time, maybe a year at best.

The diet must be changed gradually over a period of 3–4 days. Anorexia must be prevented at all costs as it worsens the condition. A gradual increase of the amount of protein must be added to the diet to compensate for the poor metabolism of protein. Along with increasing protein content, zinc and essential fatty acids should be increased. Vitamin E should also be added to the diet. A simple method of adding protein is to feed the normal diet and add three to six boiled egg yolks to the feed. The other three elements, zinc, EFAs and vitamin E can be added in supplement form. Casein supplementation has been used but as it is not very palatable it can increase the risk of anorexia. Intravenous amino acids in an 8.5–10% solution can be given at 25 ml/kg via a jugular catheter over a period of 6–8 hours. This dose should be repeated every 7–10 days. After three doses, the treatment should be evaluated for efficacy. Amino acid supplementation should not be given in cases where hepatoencephalopathy is a component of the presentation.

Dermatological treatment requires clipping around the lesions and shampooing away the crust and exudate. Emollients can be used on the horny projections due to hyperkeratosis of the footpads. The shampoo should be appropriate to treat the type of secondary infection present. Benzoyl peroxide or chlorhexidine-based shampoos should be chosen for a bacterial infection and miconazole or clotrimazole used if a fungal infection has been identified. Systemic antibiotics are necessary for the treatment of any secondary bacterial infection that may exist. The use of systemic antifungals is probably not wise owing to their potential for hepatotoxicity. A culture and sensitivity test may be necessary for the choice of the correct antibiotic. With any medication, keep in mind that any hepatotoxic side-effects will not be tolerated.

PARANEOPLASTIC DISEASE

Paraneoplastic skin conditions are rare skin conditions of the cat, dog and human, related to internal neoplastic disease. The skin conditions are often striking and can be used as a marker or early warning sign, raising the suspicion of an internal neoplasia.

Glucagonoma syndrome is a paraneoplastic syndrome that causes superficial necrolytic dermatitis. This disorder is caused by a malignant tumour of the islet cells of the pancreas. The tumour can be very small and difficult to find on ultrasound. The same dermatological signs will be present as with SND. Blood tests will definitely show hyperglycaemia but raised ALP and ALT will not occur in every case. Pre- and post-prandial bile acids will be within the normal range, indicating a non-hepatic cause. Unfortunately, a serum glucagon assay is not readily available for dogs and as the tumours are difficult to find via ultrasound, the only method of definitive diagnosis is through exploratory laparotomy. However, ex-lap will make excision of the tumour possible and this can be curative if the animal survives the post-operative period. Sadly, many do not. If surgery is not chosen as a treatment, medicating with isotretinoin (Roaccutane, Roche) is another option as this drug inhibits glucagon secretion. However, isotretinoin is an expensive drug and poses some risk to the handler. If the tumour has already metastasised, medical treatment will offer only temporary relief. Dietary and dermatological programmes, as used for SND, may help in some cases but are not usually of great benefit.

Two paraneoplastic syndromes have been recorded in the cat:

1. exfoliative dermatitis, secondary to thymoma
2. paraneoplastic alopecia with pancreatic tumour.

In the first condition, thymomas can lead to exfoliative dermatitis with secondary *Malassezia* dermatitis. Upon removal of the thymus, the dermatological pathology resolves completely. In condition number two, cats present with shiny, glistening skin, revealed by a progressive, symmetrical alopecia of the ventrum, limbs, ears and head. Initially a crust will appear at the margins of the alopecia. Hair is easily epilated. Often, there is a secondary infection with *Malassezia*, leading to pruritus. Systemically the cat will appear depressed and anorexic, with concurrent weight loss. There will be a distended, painful abdomen. A mass may be palpable and ultrasonagraphy may show hepatic nodules and/or a pancreatic mass. The prognosis is poor as usually the mass is inoperable.

As these are very rare conditions, a full dermatological work-up should be performed to eliminate all the more common problems that might lead to alopecia and pruritus. Skin scrapes and hair plucks will rule out demodicosis. Dermatophytosis should also be eliminated via fungal cultures. Allergic conditions can be explored. Complete blood counts and a serum biochemistry should help to point towards an underlying systemic cause.

FORMULARY

Drugs marked with an asterisk are not licensed for veterinary use.

Levothyroxine (Soloxine, Arnolds)
*Isotretinoin (Roaccutane, Roche)
*Mitotane (Lysodren, Bristol-Myers, Squibb)
Trilostane (Vetoryl, Arnolds)

References and Further Reading

Bond Ross 1998 The dog with symmetrical alopecia. In: Torrance AG, Mooney CT (eds) BSAVA Manual of small animal endocrinology. BSAVA Publications, Gluoucester, p 17–24

Byrne Kevin P 2002 Metabolic dermatosis. In: Foster A, Foil C (eds) BSAVA Manual of small animal dermatology. BSAVA Publications, Gloucester, p 206–210

Cerundolo Rosario, Paradis Manon 2002 An approach to symmetrical alopecia in the dog. In: Foster A, Foil C (eds) BSAVA Manual of small animal dermatology. BSAVA Publications, Gloucester, p 83–93

Hill Peter B 2002 Performing and interpreting diagnostic tests. Small animal dermatology. Elsevier Science, Oxford, p 212–230

Neiger R, Witt A L Noble A, German A J 2004 Trilostane therapy for treatment of pituitary-dependent hyperadrenocorticism in 5 cats. Journal of Veterinary Internal Medicine 18(2):160–164

Skelly B J, Petrus D, Nicholls P K 2003 Use of trilostane for treatment of pituitary-dependent hyperadrenocorticism in a cat. Journal of Small Animal Practice 44:269–272

CASE STUDY

Hypothyroidism in a Golden Retriever

Signalment

The dog was an 11-year-old neutered male Golden Retriever weighing 38 kg.

Owner's complaint

The dog was lethargic and was exhibiting hair loss at the flanks. The owner reported a temperament change, with the dog showing signs of fractious behaviour.

History

Although the dog was 11 years old, there was scant history from a previous vet because the dog had not had regular veterinary care. Vaccinations and worming were not up to date and the dog had not been treated with a veterinary flea treatment. The animal lived with another, younger dog, which did not exhibit any dermatological clinical signs. The owner reported that the Golden Retriever was drinking more water and urinating more frequently.

Physical and dermatological examination

Temperature was in the normal range and the owner did not report any heat-seeking behaviour. The heart rate was slightly low at 65 beats per minute. The respiratory rate was within the normal range of 10–30 breaths per minute. The dog was overweight at 38 kg (top range of normal weight for a male Golden Retriever is 34 kg). There were no gross abnormalities felt on examination and no obvious infestation of ectoparasites. Throughout the examination the dog lay flat on the floor with a depressed demeanour.

Symmetrical, bilateral alopecia was evident on the flanks. The coat was slightly dry and thin but not markedly so. There were no signs of pruritus, erythema or seborrhoea.

Differential diagnosis

- Dermatophytosis
- Demodectic mange
- Hyperadrenocorticism
- Hypothyroidism

- Reproductive hormone imbalance
- Growth-hormone-responsive dermatosis
- Cyclic flank alopecia
- Diabetes mellitus

Diagnostic tests

A dermatophyte culture and a skin scraping were done first. Both proved negative. A fasting blood sample was collected for haematological, biochemical and endocrinological analysis. The EDTA sample for haematology showed a low white blood cell count at 2.7 × 10/l (normal range 6–16.9 × 10/l) and a low granulocyte count at 2.7 × 10/l (51%) out of a normal range of 3.3–12.0 × 10/l. Decreased production of granulocytes was suspected.

A heparinised sample and a spun gel serum sample were sent for extensive screening to an outside laboratory (Idexx Laboratories) as a thorough analysis was not possible in our in-house laboratory. Results showed raised levels of bile acids (19.9 μmol/l; range 0.1–5.0 μmol/l), cholesterol (9.9 mmol/l; range 3.2–6.2 mmol/l), triglycerides (1.24 mmol/l; range 0.30–1.20 mmol/l), a decreased sodium:potassium ratio of 26.54 (range 28.8–40.0) and a raised basal cortisol of 154.0 nmol/l (range 25–125 nmol/l).

The raised cortisol levels along with the polydipsia seemed to point towards hyperadrenocorticism (HAC). At this point, a urine creatinine: cortisol ratio should have been performed but in the interests of limiting costs it was omitted and a low-dose dexamethasone test was performed. A fasted sample was taken at 9.00 a.m. The dog was then injected intravenously with dexamethasone at a dose rate of 0.01mg/kg (0.38 ml). Samples were then taken at 12 00 p.m. and 5.00 p.m. The results were within normal ranges.

Three days after the LDD test, the dog was re-examined as it had extensive bruising along both cephalic veins where venepuncture had taken place. One foreleg had been licked repeatedly and a lick granuloma was forming. We bandaged the area to prevent further self-trauma.

As a hypercholesterolaemia was also noted on biochemistry, it was decided that investigation for hypothyroidism was warranted. Blood serum samples were collected for thyroxine levels (T4) and for a thyroid-stimulating hormone (TSH) assay. The T4 level was low at 11.4 nmol/l (normal 17.0–54.0). The TSH was elevated at 0.5 (normal <0.41).

Treatment

The dog was started on one tablet of 0.8 mg L-thyroxine (Soloxine, Arnolds) twice daily. The recommended dose rate is 0.22–0.44 micrograms/kg – dogs needing a much higher dose rate than humans due to a marked difference in metabolism. An antibiotic/anti-inflammatory ointment (Fuciderm, Leo Laboratories) was prescribed for the lick granuloma on the foreleg, to be used twice daily till the lesion resolved.

Re-inspection

One week later the dog was seen and the owner reported a marked improvement in the dog's general demeanour. The foreleg lesion was resolving. One month after initiating treatment, the foreleg lesion had resolved and the alopecic patterns were fast diminishing. The telogen hairs were moulting heavily and new hair re-growth was evident. The dog had lost one kilogram.

Final outcome

Two months after the initiation of treatment the dog was seen again and was doing well. The hair coat was healthy and the heart rate and all other vital signs were normal. The dog had lost another kilogram as well. T4 and TSH assay were monitored 6 hours after the morning tablet had been given. Both levels were within the normal ranges.

Discussion

Hypothyroidism, while the commonest of endocrine disorders in dogs, is also one of the most difficult to diagnose, being known as the 'great impersonator'. A thorough and careful history is essential in the diagnosis of this disease (Grant 1991). The owner's reports of PUPD (polyuria and polydipsia), along with mild flank alopecia and slightly raised cortisol levels, led us to suspect another endocrinopathy, HAC. The clinical signs of lethargy, depression and personality change could be consistent with either HAC or hypothyroidism. The dermatological signs were not specifically typical of hypothyroidism. There was no hyperpigmention or scaling and the alopecia did not begin at the tail. Poor wound healing was obvious only after blood testing had begun and the face did not show myxoedema.

On the other hand, Golden Retrievers have a predilection towards hypothyroidism and the hair coat was easily epilated. It would have been helpful to do a trichogram as many hairs in the telogen phase would have been a good indicator of the disease state (Ferguson 1993). The dog was slightly older than the average age of onset but due to lack of consistent veterinary care it may have been exhibiting clinical signs for some time prior to examination.

In terms of initial laboratory analysis this patient did show a raised cholesterol level, which is seen in 50–75% of hypothyroid cases. Increased triglycerides were another indicative blood measure. Finally, use of T4 and TSH assay tests enabled us to reach an appropriate diagnosis for this case.

Dunn (2001) states that there must be a marked improvement with the use of L-thyroxine or improvement could merely be related to euthyroid syndrome. Because we saw a dramatic improvement in the patient's demeanour within 7 days and dermatological signs resolved within 2 months, we felt confident of our diagnosis. It was noted that the use of steroids, in the form of the skin ointment we were using, could affect the need for L-thyroxine. However, further examinations did not seem to require a dose change. Neither did any cardiac liabilities require dose adjustment. Side-effects, such as panting, PUPD, anxiety and diarrhoea were not reported.

REFERENCES

(for the Case Study)

Dunn K 2001 Hypothyroidism. Veterinary Nursing Times July 1st:6–7

Ferguson Ewan A 1993 Symmetrical alopecia. In: Locke P H, Mason I BSAVA Manual of dermatology. BSAVA, Cheltenham, p 101–113

Grant D I 1991 Skin diseases in the dog and cat. Blackwell Scientific Publications, Oxford, p 67–71

Chapter 8

Keratinisation and pigmentation disorders

CHAPTER CONTENTS

KERATINISATION DISORDERS

Keratinisation disorders are disorders of the skin maturation process. In normal canine skin the process of maturing from basal cells to shed squames at the stratum corneum takes 22 days. If the process is disordered, cells can move from the basal layer to desquamation in as little as 8 days. Additionally, the sebaceous glands and adnexae can become involved, producing increased sebum and other skin secretions. The actual composition of epidermal secretions can change. The end result is excess scale at the surface level, plus or minus greasy exudate.

Historically, keratinisation disorders have been divided into three types of disorder. Seborrhoea oleosa was the scaly, greasy and foul-smelling version of the disease. Seborrhoea sicca was a dry, scaly form of disorder and seborrhoeic dermatitis referred to a scaly, greasy condition with inflammation. Many texts still use these terms; however, it is more appropriate to speak in terms of the degree of scale and grease present rather than dividing into three separate problems. Keratinisation disorders are a disorder of proliferation at the basal cell level, which causes increased loss of cells at the cornified layer. The amount of proliferation is what determines the severity of the disease.

Causes of keratinisation disorders

There are a number of factors that can affect the process of epidermopoiesis. A warm environment with decreased humidity is not especially healthy for skin development – something we experience ourselves when we visit hot climates. What we put into the body, for example, steroids and cytotoxic agents, as well as what we put on it, such as drying shampoos, play a part in the process of epidermal cell turnover. Dietary imbalances, primarily deficiencies of zinc, vitamin A and essential fatty acids also contribute to poor skin health.

Any sort of trauma or infection is seen as an invasion by the skin and cell turnover will increase to rid the body of the foreign invader. Injury to the skin causes water loss, which will affect proliferation. Pruritus, whether from parasites, allergy or infection, can lead to inflammation and hyperplastic change and create trauma, thus stimulating proliferation as well. Hormone levels, particularly thyroxin, affect cell turnover.

Keratinisation disorders are an extremely common skin condition in the dog, although less common in the cat. Of all keratinisation disorders, 80% are secondary to an underlying cause, while only 20% of keratinisation disorders are primary. When examining a patient with a scaling disorder it is essential to work through the vast array of underlying causes in order to come to a satisfactory diagnosis. Treatment of the fundamental cause can control the scaling disorder completely. However, if the disorder is primary, treatment will most often not be curative, only palliative, and must continue throughout that animal's life. Excessive scale is shown in Figure 8.1.

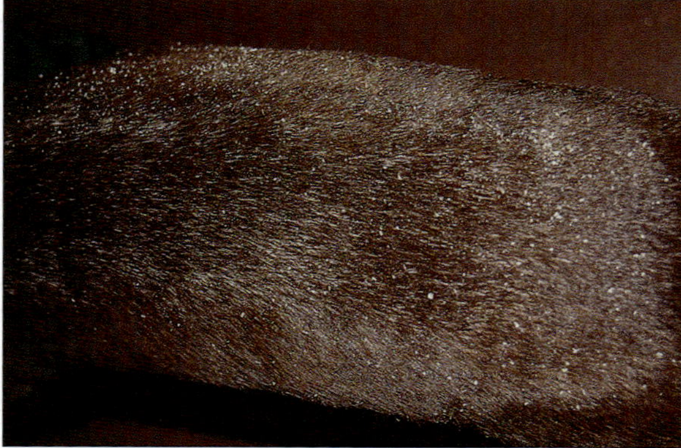

Figure 8.1 Excessive scale can be found with many dermatological conditions, including keratinisation disorders, pyoderma, cheyletiellosis and hypothyroidism. Photograph by Annette Loeffler, with permission.

Breed disposition can be helpful in determining the root cause. Breeds prone to atopy, such as the West Highland White Terrier, Golden Retriever, Labrador, Dalmatian, Wire Fox Terrier and the Shar pei, should obviously be investigated for an allergic condition when they present with a scaling disorder. On the other hand, there are several breeds prone to primary keratinisation disorders. Proper diagnostic protocol requires one to investigate all possible underlying causes before concluding on a diagnosis of a primary keratinisation disorder.

A seasonal component to the disease might point towards allergy or a flea problem, while the presence of pruritus would also suggest a parasite or allergic problem. If the owner reports weight gain and heat-seeking behaviour, thyroid dysfunction should be considered. Polyuria, polydipsia and weakness should make one suspicious of hyperadrenocorticism. Quizzing the owner on diet is important as well. An unbalanced diet or even poorly stored, or out-of-date, food can lead to deficiencies that would manifest as keratinisation disorders. Causes of secondary keratinisation disorders are listed below.

Allergy
- Food
- Atopy
- Contact

Ectoparasites
- Fleas
- *Sarcoptes scabiei*
- *Demodex*
- Lice
- *Cheyletiella*

Endocrine
- Hypothyroidism
- Hyperglucocorticoidism
- Reproductive hormone imbalance

Deficiencies
- Vitamin A
- Zinc
- Essential fatty acids

Infection
- *Malassezia*
- Staphylococcal
- Dermatophytosis

Neoplastic
- Paraneoplastic alopecia
- Thymoma
- Cutaneous lymphoma
- Mycosis fungoides

Metabolic
- Diabetes mellitus
- Superficial necrolytic dermatosis

Immune-mediated
- Pemphigus foliaceus
- FeLV
- FIV

Therefore, every patient with a scaling disorder should be examined firstly, for parasites. This would involve coat brushings, hair plucks and skin scrapes to rule out fleas, mites and lice. Good parasite control should be put in place as a clinical trial for parasites, and for the animal's wellbeing. Reducing pruritus can only be helpful. Cytology should be done to identify any possible *Malassezia* or staphylococcal infections. Samples for a fungal culture may also be deemed necessary.

While taking the history, a discussion of the type of food fed, any supplements given, how the food is stored and even how old the food is, is important. A deficiency could be the root of the problem. Be inquisitive regarding any seasonal aspect to the disease and the level of pruritus the animal feels. A food trial may be in order, followed by a diagnostic plan to eliminate the possibility of atopy.

There should be a full physical examination of the animal, enquiring as to drinking and urinating habits, any recent weight loss or gain and any temperament changes. Endocrine function tests as well as haematology and biochemistry evaluation can be ordered if there are signs of systemic disease. The age of onset and the progression of the disease should be noted.

An early age of onset, generally younger than 2 years of age, is common with primary keratinisation disorders. In fact, some keratinisation diseases can manifest at birth. Breed predilection also plays a major part in identifying a keratinisation disorder as primary, rather than secondary. There are several keratinisation disorders which can be readily identified as hereditary. This information is not only helpful in diagnosis but should definitely be communicated to the owner who may be considering breeding from an affected animal.

The primary keratinisation disorders are listed below:

- acne
- ear-margin alopecia
- epidermal dysplasia
- follicular dysplasia/dystrophy
- icthyosis
- large-plaque parapsoriasis
- lichenoid-psoriasiform dermatosis
- nasodigital hyperkeratosis
- primary idiopathic seborrhoea
- sebaceous adenitis
- Schnauzer comedo syndrome.

A discussion of these diseases will facilitate recognition.

Acne

Acne tends to affect shorthaired breeds of dog such as the Bulldog, Boxer, Doberman and Great Dane, pointing towards a hereditary component. Cats can also be affected. Most animals show clinical signs as they reach sexual maturity.

Acne is a disorder of the follicular keratinisation process leading to papulonodular lesions on the chin, lip and muzzle. Usually, the disease process starts at the chin. There is minimal pruritus but comedones are a common pattern due to the follicular nature of the disease. Papules and pustules are possible in the moist form of acne. Secondary infection can occur, which increases the likelihood of pruritus and pustules of a non-sterile nature.

The differential list with this disease, as with many keratinisation disorders, is demodicosis, dermatophytosis and bacterial folliculitis. Plucks and scrapes must be done to rule out *Demodex*, a fungal culture for dermatophytosis and cytology for folliculitis. Piercing a pustule for a smear impression, as well as tape-strip cytology, is advised. Once underlying causes have been ruled out, idiopathic acne can be diagnosed.

If there is secondary bacterial involvement, at least 7 days of systemic antibiotic therapy should be prescribed, along with hot compresses if deep folliculitis is present. Oedema and inflammation can be managed with prednisolone, if there is no complicating bacterial infection. Antibacterial gels or shampoos are used to treat the acne itself.

Ear-margin dermatosis

Dachshunds are predisposed to ear-margin dermatosis, with lesions usually appearing bilaterally on the pinnal margins. Follicular casts are tightly adhered to the edge of the pinnae, forming soft, greasy plugs over the follicles. There is alopecia, thickening of the skin and ulceration. The resultant head shaking can lead to fissures. The disease can spread and cover the whole pinna.

This is not an easy disease to diagnose as the differential list includes some of the more rare dermatological conditions. *Demodex* can be ruled out with scrapings and pluckings and possibly biopsy if necessary. However, lupus, cutaneous vasculitis and cold agglutination disease cannot really be dismissed via in-house testing. Frostbite is also on the differential list but a good history can rule out that diagnosis. If vasculitis is suspected, biochemistry, haematology and a biopsy are called for. Generally speaking, a biopsy is needed to rule out other causes and to identify the actual disease. The breed should be a useful indicator in diagnosis.

Ear-margin dermatosis is managed through warm water soaks used to loosen the adhered casts. After soaking, an antiseborrhoeic shampoo should be used. Creams containing steroids are used if inflammation is present, or systemic prednisolone can be prescribed. The prognosis is guarded with this disease, and in severe cases the only solution is an ear crop.

Epidermal dysplasia

This is the disease of West Highland White Terriers that causes 'armadillo syndrome'. There is hyperpigmentation, lichenification, scale and alopecia with an age of onset of 6–12 months. Clinical signs affect the ventrum, extremities and face. Pruritus and inflammation can be severe. A ceruminous otic discharge often accompanies the disease picture.

The cause is disorder and disorientation of the basal cell layer. It is currently believed that epidermal dysplasia is a hypersensitivity reaction to *Malassezia*. The condition is caused by self-trauma secondary to allergy. It is a spectacularly severe reaction which appears primarily in Westies.

Secondary infection must be identified and treated in order to make any headway in either diagnosis or treatment. Antibacterial/antifungal shampoos two to three times weekly with 10 minutes contact time will help to alleviate the topical infections. Elimination of dermatophytosis and parasite involvement should be carried out in the usual way. A keratoplastic/keratolytic shampoo will be helpful alongside the topical treatment for infection. Systemic treatment of *Malassezia* or staphylococcal infections may also be required. Searching for an allergic component is always indicated with this breed. Food trials and atopy investigation should be part of the diagnostic work-up.

Follicular dysplasia/dystrophy

Follicular dysplasias and dystrophies present as hyperpigmentation at areas of alopecia. There are four varieties of these disorders:

1. black-hair follicular dysplasia
2. colour-dilution alopecia
3. cyclic alopecia
4. idiopathic follicular dysplasia.

Black-hair alopecia manifests with alopecia and hyperpigmentation at the sites of black hair growth only. This pattern can be found with American Cocker Spaniels, Basset Hounds, Beagles, Bearded Collies, Dachshunds, Gordon Setters, Papillions, Pointers, Salukis and Schipperkes. If the dog is completely black coated, alopecia will occur in a generalised manner.

Colour-dilution alopecia affects the keratinisation of the follicles and hair cuticle. The coat can appear as moth eaten or with generalised alopecia. Scale can also occur with variable degrees of severity. Affected breeds include the blue and fawn variations of Chihuahuas, Chow Chows, Doberman Pinschers, Great Danes, Italian Greyhounds, Minature Schnauzers, Newfoundlands, Poodles, Salukis, Whippets and Yorkshire Terriers.

Even with treatment, affected dogs generally fail to re-grow their coats completely.

With cyclic alopecia, the hair loss waxes and wanes. The areas of loss differ with breed predilections. Airedales, Boxers, English Bull Terriers and Staffordshire Bull Terriers tend to display flank alopecia. Doberman Pinschers can have flank and lumbosacral alopecia along with hyperpigmentation. Irish Water Spaniels and Portuguese Water Dogs will begin with caudal alopecia that progresses forwards. Endocrinopathies should be considered whenever cyclical alopecia is observed.

Siberian Huskies, Alaskan Malamutes and Curly Coated Retrievers are known to suffer from idiopathic follicular dysplasia, which manifests as alopecia without any definite pattern of loss.

Pattern baldness is characterised by miniaturised hair follicles. This occurs primarily in the Yorkshire terrier on the ears, nose and trunk; the Dachshund on the ears and ventrum, and on the Greyhound's caudal thighs.

These follicular disorders can commence as early as 4 weeks of age when the puppy's coat becomes dull, with variable levels of scale and eventually alopecia. Secondary bacterial folliculitis is not uncommon. Most affected pups will show clinical signs by 6–9 months of age.

Any follicular dysplasia or dystrophy must be assessed for the possible underlying causes of demodicosis, dermatophytosis and bacterial folliculitis. Thus, skin scrapings, hair pluckings, a fungal culture and possibly a biopsy would need to be part of the diagnostic work-up. Trichography can be particularly useful in identifying colour-dilution alopecia as dilute hairs tend to have large melanin granules clumped in bunches along the hair shaft. The accumulated granules weaken the hair at these points and cause shaft fracture.

Treatment of these diseases requires a follicular flushing agent such as benzoyl peroxide, sulphur or salicylic acid. Moisturisers in the form of coat conditioners or lotions should follow shampoo therapy in order to counteract the extreme drying effects of these agents. Antibiotic therapy may be necessary in the face of secondary bacterial folliculitis. In the case of pattern baldness, shampoo therapy is not helpful but the use of melatonin has been used with some positive effect.

Icthyosis

This is a hereditary disease that can be accompanied by clinical signs even at birth. Most affected dogs show signs by 1–2 months of age. There are large, thick, tightly adhered yellow to grey scales generalised over the animal. Hyperkeratosis at the footpads and nasal planum can also occur. Malodour and secondary infection, usually with *Malassezia* or staphylococci, is quite common.

Breeds predisposed to icthyosis include: West Highland White Terriers, Cavalier King Charles Spaniels, Jack Russell Terriers, Yorkshire Terriers, Staffordshire Bull Terriers, Bull Terriers, Irish Setters, Labradors, English Springer Spaniels, Rottweilers, Collies and Doberman Pinschers.

A diagnosis is obtained via biopsy. Samples will show mitosis in the basal region, hypergranulosis and microvesicles in the stratum corneum along with hyperkeratosis. Treatment is long term and includes emollient rinses. Systemic treatment is with retinoids, for example isotretinoin (Roaccutane, Roche) daily for 8–12 weeks and then every other day as a maintenance dose. Isotretinoin is a difficult drug to obtain and expensive to dispense. It is a drug that must be given out with clear warnings to the owner as the drug is dangerous if not handled wisely. It is teratogenic so should not be given to breeding dogs and should not be handled by women of child-bearing years. A mild case of icthyosis has a good prognosis but severe cases have a poor outcome.

Large-plaque parapsoriasis

This is a very rare disease which appears as generalised erythematous, scaly plaques on the trunk. There is patchy alopecia. Staphylococcal infection often occurs with this disease and can take the form of expansive, flaccid pustules. These later form significant epidermal collarettes. Erosions can occur as additional secondary lesions.

After excluding other possibilities, a biopsy is needed to make a diagnosis of large-plaque parapsoriasis. Once identified, the disease can be treated with corticosteroid therapy, first at a loading dose, and then decreased to a maintenance dose to prevent relapses. Antibiotics should also be prescribed if a bacterial infection is present. The actual cause of this disease is, as of yet, unknown.

Lichenoid psoriasis

This is a rare disease, which mostly affects English Springer Spaniels with an age of onset between 4 and 18 months. It is believed that the disease is caused by an exaggerated reaction to a staphylococcal infection. Lichenoid psoriasis is non-pruritic, erythematous, with lichenoid papules and plaques in the pinnal, external ear canal, peri-orbital, peri-anal and inguinal regions. There is a generalised greasy scale that may wax and wane.

Diagnosis is based on age of onset, breed and clinical signs. Biopsy is necessary for a definitive diagnosis. Ruling out demodicosis and dermatophytosis hastens diagnosis.

Anti-seborrhoeic shampoos treat the disease topically but systemic treatment is usually required. Oddly, some cases respond to corticosteroid treatment while other cases improve with antibiotic therapy.

Nasodigital hyperkeratosis

Unlike most other keratinisation disorders, nasodigital hyperkeratosis usually appears in the older dog. Cocker Spaniels and English Springer Spaniels have a predilection towards this disease with Labradors having a definite hereditary link (Peters et al 2003). Irish Terriers and Dogue de Bordeaux are also predisposed but only with footpad hyperkeratosis.

Generally, this disease presents as an accumulation of tightly adhered keratin on the nasal planum and/or the footpads. There are usually no other clinical signs, other than that the dog can be lame if the feet are severely affected. Erosions and ulcers will occur in both the pads and nasal region if the keratin becomes thick and dry enough.

The differential diagnosis can include: distemper, cutaneous lymphoma, dermatophytosis, hypothyroidism, lupus erythematosus, nasal solar dermatitis, papillomavirus, pemphigus foliaceus and pemphigus erythematosus, superficial necrolytic dermatitis and zinc-responsive dermatitis. A fungal culture should be taken initially to rule out dermatophytosis. If there are other suggestive symptoms a blood sample should be taken for hypothyroidism. Systemic signs would be significant if considering distemper. Otherwise, diagnosis will rely heavily on biopsy to rule out the many and varied diseases on the differential list. A full physical is most important to rule out any concurrent clinical signs. A diagnosis of nasodigital hyperkeratosis is reliant on the fact that there are no other signs than the isolated skin lesions.

Treatment requires softening of the keratin via warm water soaks or wet dressings. A keratolytic shampoo (salicylic, or tar for example) needs to be applied to the hyperkeratinised areas and left in contact for 12 hours. If fissures are present, topical steroids can be used to decrease inflammation. As long-term management, frequent application of hydrating agents – such as petroleum jelly – is necessary.

Nutritional keratinisation disorders

Essential fatty acid deficiency causes a dull, dry coat with increased scale. If the deficiency has been chronic, the condition will develop into a greasy, scaly coat, especially at the ears and at intertriginous areas. Alopecia is possible – as is pruritus and secondary infections. *Malassezia* and bacteria can both multiply opportunistically.

The deficiency can be caused by a gut absorption problem or an actual feeding problem. Dogs on long-term weight-loss diets may suffer from the effects of their low fat content. Poorly stored food, or food that has gone out of date, can also be low in essential fatty acids and lead to deficiencies.

Diagnosis is based on a dietary history and the elimination of all other possibilities, including: hypothyroidism, sex hormone imbalances, demodicosis, sebaceous adenitis and mycosis fungoides. Skin scrapings and pluckings should be carried out, and blood testing if clinical signs point in that direction. A clinical trial in which essential fatty acids are added to the diet can be both a diagnostic test and cure. The owner should be advised to feed a well-balanced complete diet of good quality. Anti-seborrhoeic shampoo and moisturisers can help to resolve the disease.

Primary idiopathic seborrhoea

This is a disease that affects the spaniel breeds particularly, although other breeds are affected. The primary dysfunction is an increased rate of differentiation at the basal cell layer, causing proliferation and increased scale. The normal keratinisation period of 22 days can be shortened to as little as 8 days. Ceruminous otic discharge accompanies the prolific scale. If there is a simultaneous problem with allergy or secondary infection, inflammation will also be present.

The lesion pattern with this disease can be multi-focal to generalised. Lesions usually start in the skin folds (intertriginous areas) and around the nipples. There can be involvement of the ear margins, chin and nasodigital regions. Follicular hyperkeratinisation takes place, plugging the follicle to form comedones. A ceruminous otic disease often occurs concurrently. The skin may be dry, greasy or inflamed, or may show a combination of these signs.

The age of onset is typically less than 2 years of age, with some animals being affected from birth. Dog and cat breeds most likely to develop primary idiopathic seborrhoea are:

- Cocker Spaniels
- English Springer Spaniels
- Basset Hounds
- West Highland White Terriers
- Doberman Pinschers
- Labradors
- Irish Setters
- Shar Peis
- German Shepherd dogs
- Dachshunds
- Persian cats
- Himalayan cats

Doberman Pinschers, Dachshunds, German Shepherds and Irish Setters are more likely to develop dry, white to grey scale. The scale can appear focally or multi-focally or may be diffuse. The hair coat is dull and dry.

Basset Hounds, Cocker Spaniels, English Springer Spaniels, Labradors, Shar Peis and West Highland White Terriers are prone to malodorous, brown to yellow greasy scale. The neck, feet and intertriginous areas are most commonly affected. Follicular casts will be prevalent as will ceruminous otitis with hyperplasia of the ear canal.

Seborrhoeic dermatitis is the greasy, inflamed form of the disease and tends to affect the above dogs prone to greasy scale. With dermatitis the most damaged areas include the pinnae, ventral neck, chest, perineum and intertriginous regions. There can be hyperkeratotic plaques, bacterial folliculitis and *Malassezia* infection, as an opportunistic invader.

Diagnosis is achieved by noting the breed and age of onset. Tests for ruling out underlying causes should include parasite assessment, especially for *Demodex*, and cytology to ascertain possible infectious causes, especially *Malassezia*. Additionally, deficiencies should be explored by getting a thorough history of the animal's eating habits. Endocrine function tests, particularly hypothyroidism, would be indicated if the animal presented middle aged or older. Immune condition should be considered, particularly FeLV/FIV status in the cat.

Treatment will be life long if the animal is diagnosed as having this primary disorder. The mainstay of management should be shampoo therapy. The particular shampoo chosen needs to correlate with the level of greasiness found in the skin. A particularly greasy animal may require a shampoo with tar or benzoyl peroxide – although neither of these ingredients are safe for cats. A less greasy animal will require a milder shampoo, possibly something with the ingredient ammonium lactate. Shampooing should take place every 4–7 days, depending on the severity of the disease. Medicated shampoos require a minimum of 10 minutes contact time on the animal.

Moisturisers are helpful in counteracting the drying effects of the shampoos. Sprays or rinses are available for the veterinary market. Moisturising ingredients include glycerine, propylene glycol and lactic acid. Essential fatty acids (EFAs), given systemically, will also improve skin health by helping to reduce the inflammation and normalising the natural skin oils. EFAs are available in capsule and liquid form.

Secondary infections should not be overlooked in management of the primary disease. Many affected animals will also have a secondary staphylococcal or *Malassezia* infection. Both of these conditions can be treated topically via shampoo therapy with antibacterial and antifungal agents, for example chlorhexidine and miconazole. In some cases, systemic treatment of the secondary infection may be required.

Severe inflammation may require short-term corticosteroid therapy. Some cases may respond to isotretinoin. A clinical trial of 2 months should be given. If there is no response within that period, treatment with isotretinoin should be withdrawn.

Schnauzer comedo syndrome

As hinted at in the name, this disease affects young, adult Miniature Schnauzers. Crusted papules can appear on the dorsum and spread from the shoulders to the tail. There is often an element of bacterial folliculitis.

Ruling out demodicosis, dermatophytosis and superficial bacterial folliculitis can help to identify the disease, and biopsy will confirm it. If the animal is middle-aged or older on presentation, hypothyroidism can be considered.

Treatment consists of antiseborrhoeic shampoo and systemic antibacterials, if needed. Bathing should take place every 3–5 days in a shampoo containing benzoyl peroxide, sulphur, tar or salicylic acid. Moisturisers can be added to the treatment regime if the shampoos become too drying. Maintenance therapy requires bathing every 1 to 2 weeks.

Sebaceous adenitis

Sebaceous adenitis is a disease of progressive alopecia and scaling. The average age of onset is between 1 and 5 years. Breeds prone to this disease are: the Standard Poodle, the Akita, the Samoyed and the Vizsla.

The poodle displays a pattern of hair loss typical of affected long-coated dogs. There is symmetrical alopecia at the dorsal trunk, neck, head and pinnae. The alopecia can appear in a cyclical manner. The remaining coat is dull and brittle. Follicular casts can be observed on shed and plucked hair. There is mild to heavy scale, depending on the severity of the disease. Secondary bacterial folliculitis is common. Cases with complicating pyoderma are often malodorous. Of affected dogs within this breed, 25% may be subclinical carriers.

Akitas affected with sebaceous adenitis get the worst version of this disease. There is generalised erythema and multiple papules and pustules, in addition to heavy scale. The alopecia can be partial to general. Greasy debris complicates the picture. Systemically, there is pyrexia and weight loss.

Vizslas are affected by the shorthaired version of sebaceous adenitis. In this version, there is multifocal alopecia on the trunk, head and ears, with intermittent swelling of the muzzle, lips and eyelids. Scale accompanies the multifocal alopecia but the disease is usually non-pruritic in this form and folliculitis is rare.

Samoyeds suffer with moderate to severe truncal alopecia and scale. The remaining coat is dull and brittle with profuse follicular casts.

When underlying diseases such as demodicosis, dermatophytosis and bacterial folliculitis have been ruled out, a biopsy should be performed. With sebaceous adenitis, the biopsy will show inflammation of the sebaceous glands or a granulomatous dermal reaction with destruction of the sebaceous glands. It is helpful for the pathologist if multiple samples are harvested both of lesional and non-lesional skin.

Mild cases of sebaceous adenitis can be managed with anti-seborrhoeic shampoos, which contain sulphur, tar or salicylic acid. Emollient rinses would be required post-bathing. If there is secondary bacterial infection, utilising a shampoo with an antibacterial agent such as chlorhexidine, benzoyl peroxide or ethyl lactate will be necessary. Essential fatty acid supplementation has proved to be helpful as well.

Severe cases of sebaceous adenitis are much more difficult to manage. There will be destruction of the sebaceous glands and dermal fibrosis to deal with. Any secondary bacterial infection should be handled with systemic antibiotics. For the treatment of the actual disease, isotretinoin and cyclosporin have both been used as treatment options. However, isotretinoin is extremely teratogenic to both the animal and the handler. Female owners of childbearing age cannot handle this drug and all others should wear gloves and treat isotretinoin with respect. Cyclosporin is a licensed drug but still needs to be handled carefully. There are significant possible side-effects with cyclosporin, including vomiting, diarrhoea, liver and kidney toxicity, papillomatous skin lesions and gingival hyperplasia.

Vitamin A-responsive dermatosis

This is a rare, chronic disease with an age of onset of between 2 and 3 years of age. Cocker spaniels are affected more than other breeds but Labradors, Miniature Schnauzers and Shar Peis can contract the disease. The disease is not caused by a deficiency in vitamin A but clinical signs abate with supplementation of vitamin A. It has been proposed that the disease is caused by faulty vitamin A uptake in the epidermis, but this theory is not proven.

Clinical signs include generalised scale and follicular plugs with a dull, dry hair coat. Hyperkeratotic plaques can appear on the ventral and lateral thorax and abdomen. There are focal areas of papules, crust and alopecia. Ceruminous otitis accompanies the cutaneous features.

Primary idiopathic seborrhoea is a major differential diagnosis, especially in Cocker Spaniels. A complete diagnostic work-up should be done to eliminate parasites, dermatophytosis and other possible underlying factors. Cytology should be performed to identify concurrent bacterial or fungal infections.

A biopsy can be harvested to help obtain a diagnosis of vitamin A-responsive disease. Response to therapy is another method of diagnosis, utilising retinol (vitamin A). Retinol is measured in international units and is given once daily. The condition should be closely monitored for 3–6 weeks. Remission can occur within 10 weeks but treatment will need to continue for life. There are no adverse side-effects from vitamin A given at the correct dose. 10 000 IU once daily is recommended (Kwochka & Shanley 2003).

Retinoids are a synthetic form of vitamin A which are more potent but can cause side-effects such as dry eye, vomiting, diarrhoea, joint stiffness, pruritus and skeletal abnormalities if used long term. Blood tests reveal that retinoids can raise cholesterol, triglyceride levels and liver enzymes. Retinoids also cause risk to the female owner as the drug is dangerous to handle due to its teratogenic effects.

Topical treatment with antiseborrhoeic shampoos containing tar, sulphur or benzoyl peroxide will help to clear the follicular plugs. Moisturising conditioners counteract the drying aspects of the shampoo and decrease scaling. Bathing should commence on a two to three times per week schedule and decrease as the condition improves.

Zinc-responsive dermatosis

This is another disease that is not caused by a true deficiency but responds to treatment with a supplement. There are two forms, both rare, of zinc-responsive dermatosis. Syndrome I affects primarily Siberian Huskies and Alaskan Malamutes, while syndrome II is predominant in Dobermans, Great Danes, Beagles, German Shepherd dogs, German Short-haired Pointers, Labradors, Rhodesian Ridgebacks and Standard Poodles.

Syndrome I is caused by poor absorption of zinc. The dogs may be on a very good quality diet, but a genetic defect in the intestinal absorption blocks zinc from being utilised. Stress, oestrus and other digestive disorders can affect the absorption of zinc as can high levels of calcium and phytates (plant proteins) in the diet. In affected breeds, extraneous factors that affect zinc absorption in any dog will be aggravated by the genetic component of the disease. Young adults usually show clinical signs at 1–3 years of age.

Erythema, alopecia, tightly adhered scales and crust are the typical lesions which affect the periorbital region, chin, ears and prepuce. Heavy crust can appear on pressure points, such as the elbow and hock. The footpads may develop hyperkeratinisation. Chronic lesions will become hyperpigmented. The remaining hair coat is dull and dry. Secondary bacterial and fungal infection is common.

The differential diagnosis list for these clinical signs includes demodicosis, dermatophytosis, *Malassezia* dermatitis and pemphigus foliaceus. Skin scrapings, cytology and fungal cultures should be performed before proceeding to biopsy. If zinc-responsive dermatosis is suggested by biopsy, the report will describe severe, diffuse, surface and follicular parakeratotic hyperkeratosis with hyperplastic superficial dermatitis.

The definitive diagnosis is achieved via a treatment trial of zinc sulphate once daily or zinc methionine twice daily for 4–8 weeks. If there is a good response, then zinc will need to be given for life. Supplements should be given with food and the dose can be divided to increase tolerance; occasionally vomiting can occur. The BSAVA formulary (Tennant 2002) gives a dose rate of 2–10 mg zinc sulphate/kg PO q 24 hours. Intravenous injections of zinc sulphate can be given once every 4 weeks as an alternative to tablets. Maintenance injections may only need to be given once every 6 months, depending on the severity of the disease.

Warm water soaks are used to remove the tight scale and then anti-seborrhoeic shampoos should be used. Any secondary bacterial or fungal infections must be treated.

Syndrome II of zinc-responsive dermatosis affects fast-growing puppies with an unbalanced, excessive level of calcium and/or phytates in their feed. The clinical signs are the same as in syndrome I; however, there can be more plaques present on the pressure points. Systemic signs usually accompany the dermatological disease, with puppies suffering from stunted growth, depression, anorexia, lymphadenopathy and secondary infection. As demodicosis and dermatophytosis are much more likely to occur in young animals, diagnostic testing for both of these problems should occur at the onset of the investigation.

Usually, placing the pup on a well balanced diet leads to resolution of clinical signs. However, supplementing with zinc can hasten recovery. Zinc supplementation need only be given until the disease is eradicated. Relapse will not occur as long as the diet remains balanced. Anti-seborrhoeic shampoos can be helpful, as can essential fatty acid supplementation; however, dogs should be monitored for signs of pancreatitis when receiving essential fatty acid supplementation. The response to zinc supplementation tends to improve with the use of essential fatty acids.

Feline keratinisation disorders

In cats, dry scaling disorders are more common than alterations in the glandular secretions. Follicular casts and comedones, with inflammation, crust and alopecia can and do occur, but scaling is more common.

Feline acne

Acne can strike at any age in the feline, although it usually first appears at about 1 year of age and then re-appears cyclically through life. Predisposing factors include poor grooming habits, abnormal sebum production, stress, viral disease and immunosuppression.

The disease process occurs as telogen hairs fail to escape the follicle and form a keratinosebaceous plug. Comedones appear on the lower lip and chin. Papules, mild erythema and pastules may also develop. The chin and lip can swell. If secondary infection occurs, the papules will become pustules and there will be pain and pruritus. Self-trauma will complicate the disease, leading to furunculosis and ulcers. Nodules may form with erythema, alopecia and finally, scarring.

Impression smears taken from ruptured pustules may show a bacterial infection of *Staphylococcus* or *Pasteurella* spp. *Malassezia* overgrowth is rare in cats. Additional diagnostic tests should be performed to rule out demodicosis and eosinophilic granulomas (e.g. biopsy).

With this disease, over-treatment can cause the condition to worsen. A less aggressive approach is advised. The affected area should be clipped and cleaned. A topical antibiotic/anti-inflammatory gel should be applied or a cleansing shampoo, although shampoo choices are limited in cats. Be sure to read the label to find out if the shampoo is safe for this species. Secondary infections can be eased by hot compresses, but only in the most accommodating of cats. Systemic antibiotic therapy may be necessary. Essential fatty acid supplementation is often helpful. Severe, refractory cases may benefit from isotretinoin, but only after considering the possible side-effects and risk to handlers with this medication.

Primary seborrhoea in Persians

This is an autosomal recessive disease which can manifest as early as 2–3 days of age. The kittens are covered in a generalised greasy scale, with a wax-like build up in the skin folds and ears. Milder forms of the disease appear in more mature kittens at 6 weeks of age.

After ruling out the differentials, especially dermatophytosis, a biopsy can be performed. Findings of orthokeratotic hyperkeratosis and papillomatosis are consistent with the disease. Treatment requires a full body clip and shampooing with a mild anti-seborrhoeic shampoo licensed for use in cats.

Solar dermatitis

Ultraviolet rays alter deoxyribonucleic acid (DNA) synthesis and thus affect epidermal repair. White cats, and cats with white body parts are more susceptible to sunburn, although other genetic factors can also play a part. Exposed areas such as the ears, eyelids, nasal planum, lips and face suffer most, although it is the ears which first show clinical signs. Erythema is the primary pattern and over months to years the skin will begin to thicken, scale, erode and crust. The ear tips may curl over. Plaque-like and papillated lesions appear in chronic cases. Squamous cell carcinoma (SCC) is one sequela. Discomfort is evident.

A biopsy sample should be taken to rule out SCC, lupus, pemphigus foliaceus, mycosis fungoides, drug reactions and vasculitis. Corticosteroids can be of benefit if given early in the disease. Chronic disease is best treated by removal of the ear tips via cryosurgery or surgical excision. Antibiotics are required if a secondary infection is present. Needless to say, the cat will need to give up sunbathing. Sunscreens have been suggested but are rarely left in situ by the cat.

Tail gland hyperplasia/stud tail

In the male cat, there can be an increased number of sebaceous and apocrine glands on the dorsal tail. This increased area of glandular activity is known as the supracaudal organ and is active in intact males. A waxy secretion leads to matted hair, scale, crust, alopecia and hyperpigmentation. Secondary bacterial folliculitis also occurs.

The area should be clipped and cleaned with a gentle anti-seborrhoeic shampoo. Stud tail is rarely confused with any other problem. Treatment may need to be repeated continuously as the condition is persistent. Neutering can alleviate the signs.

Topical therapy for keratinisation disorders

Topical therapy is the main form of treatment for keratinisation disorders. The purpose of medicinal bathing is to remove dirt, which includes allergens, pathogens and toxins. By removing things such as bacteria and fungi, inflammation and pruritus can be reduced. In addition, bathing and moisturising agents give the skin direct contact with healing ingredients. Speaking particularly of keratinisation disorders, shampoo therapy should be striving to remove excess scale and debris, treat any secondary infection and normalise basal cell proliferation. Moisturising treatments should soothe and hydrate the skin.

In order for topical therapy to be effective, it must be done properly. Clients should be given a hand-out on how to bathe their dogs/cats as well as verbal instructions. It is prudent to remind the owner to wear gloves to avoid contact with the active ingredients in the shampoo. A sample hand-out is given below:

1. Prepare everything you need for the bath before you begin – shampoo, conditioners, towel, gloves, treats, etc.
2. Have some means of controlling the animal. Some cats are easier to bathe if contained in a wire basket. Dogs can be on lead with the lead tied to a handy bathroom fixture.
3. Thoroughly douse the pet in lukewarm water. Check the water on the inside of your wrist. If it is too hot for you, it is way too hot for your pet. Make sure the animal is wet all the way down to the skin.
4. Pour some of the shampoo into your gloved hands and rub your hands together. Then massage the shampoo into the pet's coat. Begin at the head and lather backwards. Avoid contact with the eyes. If you do accidentally get soap in the pet's eyes, rinse with water for several minutes. Be sure to shampoo all the nooks and crannies – armpits, under the chin, between the toes. Pets with skin folds need special attention given to cleaning between the folds. Make sure that the shampoo is actually reaching the skin and not just resting on top of the hair.
5. Once the pet is completely coated in shampoo leave the shampoo on the pet for the time recommended by the veterinarian or according to the manufacturer's instructions. Usually this is a minimum of 10 minutes. It may be helpful at this time to reassure your pet and offer it treats. In warm weather, you can walk your dog with the shampoo on to allow for full contact time. Do not let your pet lick its coat while the shampoo is on.
6. Rinse, rinse and then rinse again. When you are absolutely sure that all the shampoo has been removed from the coat, rinse one more time.
7. Conditioner can be added at this time, left on to soak and then also rinsed out.
8. Towel dry.

9. Apply lotions or moisturising sprays as directed and comb through the coat.
10. Give your pet a treat.

It is absolutely pointless to prescribe a shampoo unless the owner is going to use it properly. Decreased contact time is not only ineffective, it can cause a resistance to the ingredients over time. If the skin conditions are localised, advising the client to bathe only the affected areas may increase compliance and encourage correct technique. If the client is physically or mentally incapable of following the shampoo instructions, the pet should be booked in for regular baths at the practice or at a grooming parlour. If choosing the latter option, make sure the groomer has your shampoo instructions and is following them to the letter.

There are a confusing array of shampoo and moisturisers on the market and it can be overwhelming trying to figure out which shampoo for a particular condition. Learning what the main ingredients do can prove helpful. Each ingredient should have a specific purpose. Matching the ingredient to what you want to achieve with the skin problem and then altering choices as the condition improves is the correct way to prescribe shampoo therapy.

Keratolytics

Keratolytic ingredients are meant to increase desquamation – the process of removing scale and clearing away debris. As keratolytic ingredients can be very drying, they should be used with moisturising lotions or conditioning sprays. Conditions with increased scale, such as primary idiopathic seborrhoea, epidermal dysplasia and sebaceous adenitis, need keratolytic agents. Some of the keratolytic ingredients are: benzoyl peroxide, salicylic acid, selenium sulphide, sulphur, tar and 20% urea.

Keratoplastics

Keratoplastic ingredients have the purpose of decreasing cell proliferation at the basal layer. They achieve this by decreasing DNA synthesis and cell mitosis. The decrease in cell multiplication has the knock-on effect of decreasing scale at the surface layer. There is a big overlap in keratoplastic and keratolytic agents, with the keratoplastic ingredients including: salicylic acid, selenium sulphide, sulphur and tar. Similarly, diseases which require keratolytic treatment usually require keratoplastic treatment as well.

Barrier restoration agents

Barrier restoration is another important element in topical therapy. Emollients and moisturisers are used to help restore the skin to its normal level of hydration and suppleness. The skin acts as a protective barrier for the body and any break in that barrier makes the body vulnerable. Removing debris is all very well, but the skin layer left behind must be brought up to a level of health so that it can perform its function as a barrier efficiently. Linoleic acid, lanolin, lactic acid mineral oil, vitamin E, vegetable oil , propylene glycol, glycerine, urea and essential fatty acids are some of the many ingredients used to soothe, moisturise and hydrate skin.

Antimicrobial agents

As many keratinisation disorders have microbial agents as a secondary or underlying complaint, utilising shampoos with infection-fighting agents cuts down on the number of bottles needed in the bath. Ethyl lactate, benzoyl peroxide and chlorhexidine are some of the many antibacterial agents, while miconazole is an effective antifungal component.

Below are listed some of the commonly used ingredients with their actions:

- Ammonium lactate – keratolytic, especially at thickened stratum corneum; helps to restore normal cell turn over rate
- Benzoyl peroxide – keratolytic, de-greases, follicular flushing, antimicrobial; can be very drying; not for use on cats
- Chlorhexidine – antibacterial ingredient, non-irritating and safe for cats
- Coal tar – keratolytic and keratoplastic, de-greases; can be harsh; not for cats
- Ethyl lactate – bactericidal by lowering pH
- Glycerine – moisturising

- Hamamelis – astringent, good for pyotraumatic dermatitis (hot spots)
- Lactic acid – keratolytic, bacteriostatic, moisturises
- Linoleic acid – helps to restore epidermal barrier and thus decrease allergen and pathogen absorption
- Miconazole – antifungal agent
- Monosaccharides – immunomodulators; act by decreasing cytokine production and limiting inflammatory reaction
- Olefin sulphate – cleanser
- Piroctine olamine – antimicrobial and antifungal
- Propylene glycol – antibacterial and moisturiser
- Salicylic acid – keratoplastic and keratolytic, bacteriostatic, antipruritic
- Selenium sulphide – keratoplastic and keratolytic, antiparasitic
- Spherulites – encapsulates active ingredients allowing for progressive release
- Sulphur – keratoplastic and keratolytic, follicular flushing, can be harsh; not for use on cats
- Urea – antiseptic and moisturising, hydrates skin

Matching ingredients to skin conditions:

- Scaly, greasy skin – use a shampoo which contains sulphur, tar or salicylic acid
- Very greasy infected skin – benzoyl peroxide, followed by a moisturiser
- Dry or greasy skin with scale – sulphur or salicylic acid
- Maintenance – olefin sulphonate
- Dry skin – glycerine, propylene glycol, lactic acid, urea

Some shampoos and lotions are listed below, linked with skin conditions.

Allermyl Shampoo and lotion (Virbac). The shampoo has piroctone olamine as an antimicrobial and antifungal agent, monosaccharides as immunomodulators and linoleic acid for barrier restoration. The lotion contains linoleic acid and vitamin E, among other ingredients, to help decrease pruritus and inflammation. These products are designed for use on allergic dogs or cats with or without keratinisition disorders.

Coatex (Vetplus) has olefin sulphonate, propylene glycol, and salicylic acid among its ingredients. This shampoo is designed to remove scale and crust and has antibacterial and antifungal characteristics.

Dermacool (Virbac) contains hamemelis and benzalkonium chloride in its ingredient list. This spray is designed for drying moist lesions such as pyotraumatic dermatitis. Dermacool is also indicated for cats.

Episoothe (Virbac) has colloidal oatmeal and glycerine as ingredients. This is a soothing shampoo for mild pruritus. Safe enough for cats.

Etiderm (Virbac) includes ethyl lactate and benzalkonium chloride, which help to balance the microbial population, proving useful in cases where secondary infection has developed. Suitable for both cat and dog usage.

Humilac (Virbac) contains lactic acid, glycerine, propylene glycol and urea. It is effective treatment for dry skin conditions. It can be used after drying shampoos or as a treatment on its own. It is especially useful in decreasing pruritus. Cats and dogs can both benefit from Humilac.

Malaseb (Leo Laboratories). Miconazole and chlorhexidine act to make this an effective treatment for fungal and bacterial surface infections. Malaseb is licensed for use on both dogs and cats.

Paxcutol (Virbac). Benzoyl peroxide is a de-greasing and antibacterial agent. This ingredient is also useful for follicular flushing. Greasy, infected skin benefits from treatment with Paxcutol. A moisturising spray afterwards is advised. Paxcutol is contraindicated in cats.

Sebocalm (Virbac) contains urea and glycerine and is useful for dry, scaly conditions. It is safe for use on cats.

Sebomild P shampoo and lotion (Virbac). The shampoo is designed for use on dry or greasy skin with scale. There is also an ingredient active against secondary infections with microbes from the *Staphylococcus* and *Malassezia* genera. The ingredient list includes: ammonium lactate, piroctone olamine and essential oils. The lotion can be used between shampoos as it has keratolytic, bacteriostatic and antipruritic properties. The ingredients include salicylic acid, piroctone olamine, vitamin E and monoammonium glycyrrheginate. Both the shampoo and lotion are safe for use on cats.

Seleen (Sanofi) has selenium sulphide as its primary ingredient. This agent can be used to help control scale and inflammation. Seleen is not licensed for use on cats.

Once you have set up a topical therapy regime it is time to consider systemic treatment. If there is secondary infection, antibacterials must be prescribed. Vitamin A or zinc may be necessary if there is a deficiency syndrome. Synthetic retinoids such as isotretinoin may have to be prescribed in severe cases. However, almost all keratinisation disorders will benefit from essential fatty acid supplementation. There are a myriad of supplements available or the owner can collect their own supplementation from health food stores. A list of EFA supplements can be found in the chapter on allergic skin disease. Generally, essential fatty acid plus zinc is therapeutic for dry and greasy skin conditions. Vitamin A and zinc are helpful for dry skin conditions and essential fatty acids alone ease pruritus.

PIGMENTARY DISORDERS

Pigmentary disorders can take the form of either hyperpigmentation, hypopigmentation or altered pigmentation. Hyperpigmentation is caused by increased melanin in the epidermis. Increases in melanin can be caused by genetic factors, pigmented tumours or acquired trauma or disease. The most common cause of hyperpigmentation is chronic inflammation. Some hormonal and metabolic disorders, such as hyperadrenocorticism, can also lead to hyperpigmentation.

Hypopigmentation is caused by a complete absence of melanocytes or decreased numbers of melanocytes in the epidermis. Hypopigmentary disorders can be genetic, acquired or due to inflammation.

A few pigmentary disorders are discussed below.

Albinism

Albinism is a hereditary lack of pigment. Due to a biochemical defect, these animals cannot produce melanin. Skin, hair and mucous membranes will lack pigment. Affected animals usually have blue eyes. These animals should not be used for breeding.

Lentigo

Lentigo is a macular lesion pattern that appears in adult dogs. The lesions are caused by a localised increase in melanasomes, leading to their black colour. Lentigines (as the lesions are called) can increase in size and number over time. The macules are not pruritic and, generally, this disease is merely a cosmetic problem. If plaques form on the lesions, further investigation is warranted for underlying diseases such as nevi or papillomas (see tumour chapter). Pugs have a genetic form of lentigo known as lentiginosis profusa.

Lentigo simplex occurs in orange (ginger) cats. The lips, nose, gingiva and eyelids develop small black macules. The areas of hyperpigmentation occur at approximately 1 year of age and can increase in size as the cat ages, merging to form macular melanosis. There are no other clinical signs and the lesions do not develop into melanomas. It is prudent to biopsy to rule out malignant melanoma during the process of diagnosis.

Nasal hypopigmentation

This is also known as Dudley nose. The cause of the nasal depigmentation is unknown and it is postulated that this disease is a form of vitiligo. The dog is born with a normally pigmented nose but the colour gradually fades from the nasal planum. Affected breeds include: Afghan Hounds, Doberman Pinschers, white German Shepherds, Golden Retrievers, yellow Labrador Retrievers, Irish Setters, Poodles and Pointers. There is no treatment for the disease and affected dogs should not be bred from if the breeder is hoping for show-quality puppies.

A related disorder is 'snow nose' which manifests as a decrease in nasal pigment during the winter months. Bernese Mountain dogs, Golden and Labrador Retrievers and Siberian Huskies may exhibit snow nose, but their noses will darken again in the spring.

Periocular leukotrichia

This is a transient disease of Siamese cats. There is a patchy to complete lightening of the hair colour around the eyes, forming a spectacled pattern. Stresses such as pregnancy, poor diet or illness can set off the colour change. Hair will return to its normal colour after two growth cycles. There is no need for treatment as the cat is otherwise unaffected, although its show career may go into a tailspin.

Vitiligo

This is a hereditary disorder that affects Belgian Tervurens, Bull Mastiffs, Collie breeds, Doberman Pinschers, German Shepherds, Giant Schnauzers, Old English Sheepdogs, Newfoundlands, Rottweilers – and Siamese cats. Although the cause is unknown, it is believed that there is an autoimmune element to the disease. Lesions are macular in shape with leukoderma and leukotrichia colour changes on the nose, lips, buccal mucosa and face area. Lesions are roughly symmetrical. Footpads, claws and haircoat can also become affected. The age of onset is during young adulthood. Diagnosis is based on histopathic examination. Improvement can occur spontaneously but there is no treatment for this disease.

Wardenburg-Klein syndrome

This is a defect in the migration of melanoblasts. Affected cats, Bull Terriers, Sealyham Terriers, Collies and Dalmations will also be deaf and have blue eyes. The skin and hair is amelanotic (lacking in melanin).

References and Further Reading

Ackerman Lowell, Nesbitt Gene 1998 Canine keratinization disorders. Canine and feline dermatology. Veterinary Learning Systems, Trenton, NJ p 265–275

Ackerman Lowell, Nesbitt Gene 1988 Feline endocrine, metabolic and diseases of keratinization. Canine and feline dermatology. Veterinary Learning Systems, Trenton, NJ, p 442–450

Alhaidari Z, Olivry T, Ortonne J P 1999 Melanocytogenesis and melanogenesis: genetic regulation and comparative clinical disease. Veterinary Dermatology 10(1)

Kwochka Kenneth W, Shanley Kevin 2003 An approach to keratinization disorders. In: Foil C, Foster A (eds) BSAVA Manual of dermatology. BSAVA, Gloucester, p 43–49

Peters J, Scott D W, Erb N, Miller W H 2003 Hereditary nasal parakeratosis in Labrador Retrievers. Veterinary Dermatology 14(4):197–203

Scott D W, Miller W H, Griffin C E 2001 Pigmentary disorders and keratinisation defects. Muller and Kirk's Small animal dermatology, 6th edn. W.B. Saunders, London, p 1005–1054

Tennant B 2002 BSAVA Small animal formulary, 4th edn. BSAVA Publications, Gloucestershire

Chapter 9

Ear disease is a skin disease

CHAPTER CONTENTS

The clinical signs of otitis are familiar to anyone working in veterinary medicine. The dog or cat scratches at the affected ear, shakes its head and generally appears uncomfortable. The pinna will often show signs of excoriation and alopecia. There may be an exudate oozing out of the ear and this discharge will often smell spectacularly unpleasant. The pinna and auditory meatus will often be erythematous. In severe cases, the animal may exhibit a head tilt. Pain is often apparent and the animal is not too keen on having its ear examined. Muzzling and wrestling are often required, and a general anaesthetic or sedation may be called for to get close to the affected ear.

Getting to the bottom of an ear problem requires a thorough dermatological examination. As most vets have a consultation period of only 10–15 minutes, this is where the veterinary nurse comes in. A nurse can do a head-to-toe examination looking for skin lesions and ectoparasites. An initial ear work-up can be begun by the nurse taking a history of the problem and then passing over her findings to the vet. In this way, the animal will get the in-depth analysis it needs in order to prevent the problem from becoming a chronic pathology. An ear problem is only an isolated event when the causative factor is a foreign body. All other ear problems have to be investigated in more detail in order to treat the animal properly.

Primary causes of otitis externa are:

- foreign bodies
- fungal disease
- parasites.

Underlying disorders that can contribute to ear disease:

- allergic disorders (e.g. atopy, food sensitivity)
- autoimmune diseases
- endocrine disorders
- keratinisation disorders
- neoplasia (especially squamous cell carcinoma)
- frost bite
- miscellaneous.

To diagnose the cause of the problem you need to take a thorough history from the owner (see Chapter 2 for more details on history taking). Important questions to ask are:

- What type of parasite control is being practiced?
- Are there other in-contact pets and do they have similar ear problems?
- Have the owners experienced any lesions?
- Is the pet showing signs of pruritus? If so, for how long?
- If there is an exudate, how long has it been present? Did the pruritus occur before the exudate or vice versa?
- Has your pet gained weight in the past few months? Seemed lethargic or shown signs of heat-seeking?
- Is the pet drinking and urinating more?
- Is the pet itchy anywhere else on the body?
- Has the pet been on any medication recently?
- Does the pet swim regularly?

Be sure to note whether or not the animal has been neutered. Age is a relevant factor and breed predilections are worth keeping in mind.

After the verbal history, a full physical examination should be carried out. Weight should be recorded, along with temperature, pulse and respiration. The abdomen should be palpated, and intact testes should be examined for growths and size irregularities. Examine the eyes for any evidence of conjunctivitis.

After general physical information is gathered, the skin and hair coat should be examined for lesions and abnormalities. Are there papules, pustules or crusts on the face or pinnae? Erythema, alopecia and lesions should be recorded on a diagram. Note whether there is an active pyoderma. Keeping underlying as well as primary causes in mind, look for evidence of parasites, hypersensitivity, keratinisation or endocine disorders, as well as autoimmune diseases. Notice any hair loss, particularly if there is a pattern typical of flea allergy or an endocrine disorder. Test whether the hair is easily epilated or not. Check whether the feet are saliva-stained or if the face looks as if it has been rubbed and scratched repeatedly.

Finally, you begin examining the ear. The first thing to note is: does the animal let you touch the ear? If it is too painful to be examined you are dealing with a serious problem that needs aggressive medical management and may need surgical treatment further along the line. Note any crusting on the edges of the pinnae. These could be indicative of sarcoptic mange or an autoimmune disorder. Is the inside of the pinna inflamed? A very red pinna, without aural exudate, may indicate that the animal is suffering from an allergic condition. If there is exudate, what is it like? A dark, granular exudate is often found with *Otodectes* infestation. A ceruminous exudate can be found with endocrine disorders. Smelly, light brown exudate can be associated with *Malassezia* infection, while yellow, purulent, malodorous exudate may indicate a *Pseudomonas* infection. Although you cannot diagnose an ear problem simply by examining the exudates, you can use the discharge as a clue. The odour of the ear can also be relevant. It is not normal for a dog to have significantly malodorous ears. It can be useful, at this juncture, to ask the owner about when the discharge first appeared and whether it occurred before or after the onset of pruritus. If the pruritus occurred before the discharge the problem could be: a foreign body, hypersensitivity, atopy or food intolerance. If the discharge appeared before the pruritus, the problem could be caused by: *Otodectes cynotis*, a keratinisation defect, or an endocrine disorder.

If the dog or cat (or rabbit, for that matter) has let you get this far, you may be able to gather a few samples. If crusting is noted on the pinna, do a skin scraping for *Sarcoptes scabiei*. If you find an intact pustule, puncture it immediately and do get an impression smear. That pustule may not be there in 5 minutes time and valuable evidence will have been lost. Use a cotton bud to swab up a bit of exudate. Roll the bud onto the slide and examine it, unstained, on low power for *Otodectes*, *Demodex*, or, in the case of the rabbit, *Psoroptes cuniculi*.

Then stain it and look for yeast or inflammatory cells on a higher power. Tape strippings can also be gathered from the ear and stained for microscopic examination. If the animal is still willing, examine the vertical and horizontal ear canal otoscopically for erythema and hyperplasia. Note any accumulation of debris or hair. Most importantly, try to visualise the tympanic membrane. Normally the ear drum is translucent but a diseased ear drum will be thickened. A ruptured ear drum is extremely significant as the choice of topical treatment is severely limited in the absence of a tympanic membrane to protect the middle ear. Also otitis media may be present, which will affect the prognosis.

All of the above can be achieved in the nurse's clinic, prior to examination by the veterinarian. Even with these simple examinations, crucial information can be obtained, thus aiding the vet in an accurate diagnosis and appropriate treatment programme. A nurse's ear clinic is not only useful in the preliminary stages. Ear disease requires follow-up appointments on a regular basis. Again, in the interests of saving the vet valuable examination time, the preliminary assessment and evaluation can be done by a nurse with each follow-up appointment. Twenty minutes could be spent with the nurse, the information can be passed onto the vet, and then 10 minutes can be spent with the vet. In this way, the animal is getting a complete and accurate assessment of its condition with each visit. The nurse's time can be paid for by charging for any diagnostic tests (ear smears, et cetera) which she performs.

Ear swab sampling

1. Use a cotton bud on an uncleaned ear.
2. Roll the sample gathered onto a clean slide. Do not rub as this will damage the cells.
3. Scan under low power for mites.
4. Stain the sample using 'Diff-Quik' stains. Allow to dry.
5. Scan under low power for areas of interest and then switch to the oil-immersion lens for examination of microorganisms such as yeasts and bacteria.

If bacilli (rods) are identified, take a swab for culture and sensitivity testing.

Figure 9.1 shows rod and coccus-shaped bacteria, along with inflammatory cells, on a slide prepared from an ear swab.

Malassezia pachydermatis is a yeast that can be identified from its distinctive 'dumbbell' shape. One or two of these dark-blue-staining yeasts may be normal on a slide from an ear swab. More than two can be diagnostic of a yeast infection and the ear should be treated with the appropriate antifungals.

OTITIS

Predisposing factors

- Conformation
- Moisture
- Over-grooming
- Systemic disease
- Obstructions.

When examining ears for lesions, the knowledge of predisposing factors which contribute to ear disease is helpful. Conformation is probably the most commonly mentioned reason for predisposing a dog to ear problems. Dogs with very hairy or stenotic ears, and dogs with pendulous or concave pinnae, tend to have more problems with ear disease. To give examples of each of these ears, the Poodle tends to have an excess of hair growth inside the vertical ear canal. The hair can trap debris inside the ear, setting up an appropriate environment for

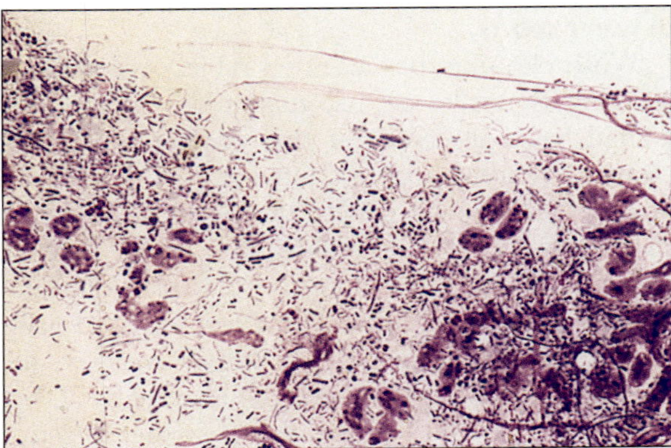

Figure 9.1 This slide, prepared from an ear swab, shows both rod- and coccus-shaped bacteria along with inflammatory cells. Photograph from L Medleau, with permission.

microbial overgrowth. As part of an investigative procedure, it is necessary to debulk the hair by scissoring it away. Unfortunately, over-zealous owners or groomers often pluck the hair from the ear canal which can lead to irritation. An irritated canal is also a favourable environment for microbial overgrowth. The Shar pei is the breed known for its narrow ear canals. Stenosis prevents adequate ventilation, creating a hot and humid environment in the ear, which is conducive to microbial overgrowth. Pendulous and concave pinnae also trap warm air and moisture in the ear, making the ear a much more hospitable place for yeast and bacteria to populate. Dogs such as Basset Hounds are known for their pendulous pinnae, but Spaniels also tend to suffer from pendulous pinnae syndrome. German Shepherd dogs have concave pinnae, and as they tend to suffer from dermatological conditions in general, they are one of the top breeds to develop ear disease.

As we have established, moisture does not belong in the ear. Dogs that are bathed often, without the precaution of preventing water entering the ear, are going to have excess moisture in the ear, as are dogs that swim a lot. In humans the condition is called 'swimmer's ear'. In dogs, it is often Gram-negative bacteria that prefer moist ears. As these are particularly difficult bacteria to eliminate, care should be taken to prevent a dog's ears becoming waterlogged. A cotton wool ball can be placed in each ear when bathing a dog. Dogs that swim regularly should have their ears cleaned, with a cleaner containing a drying agent, after partaking in water sports.

While cleaning the ears is desirable, over-zealous cleaning is not to be recommended. Unless the animal has a diseased ear that requires an acidic cleaner, the most neutral cleaner should be chosen. Strong cleaners will irritate the sensitive lining of the ear and lead to a vicious circle of self-trauma and inflammation. Even cotton buds can be traumatic to the ear and should only be used cautiously to wipe out crevices. Cotton buds should on no account be shoved down into the ear canal. All this achieves is pressing wax and debris farther into the ear. By doing this, you can create a foreign body. A cerumenolith is a mass of wax that has been pushed together inside the ear, rather than being washed to the surface and wiped away. Ear powder, or 'canker powder', as it is often called in pet stores, is another potential problem. The powder accumulates in the ear, becoming yet another foreign body. The aim of ear cleaning is to wash everything out of the ear, not put things into it.

Systemic disease is another factor in predisposing an animal to ear disease. As cats are less prone to ear problems, you should become immediately suspicious when you see an adult cat with ear disease. Testing for FIV/FeLV is practically mandatory. Hopefully, during your physical examination you would pick up any signs of pyrexia or general malaise that would remind you that the whole animal needs to be treated in order to maintain healthy ears.

Finally, obstructive ear disease is a predisposing factor for ear pathology. Polyps or tumours will affect ventilation and drainage of the ear canal, creating an unhealthy environment which is ripe for disease. Sometimes polpys can be visualised with an otoscope. Tumours are usually identified via radiography.

Primary causes

Foreign bodies can be hair, cerumenoliths or ear powder. Some foreign bodies may be difficult to locate, particularly grass seeds which can migrate up the canal, but once removed, you have eliminated the causative factor in the ear disease and the ear should heal with time and treatment.

Fungal disease is turning out to be much more prevalent in ears than once assumed. The ringworm species one associates with ear disease are *M. canis* and *T. mentagrophytes.* Any suspicious lesions on the face or pinnae should prompt fungal culture testing. *Sporothrix schenckii* causes a rare fungal disease that hunting dogs can get from interacting with moss. Again, fungal cultures can help to identify this microorganism. However, the most common fungus is *Malassezia pachydermatis.* It is believed that up to 36% of healthy dogs host this microorganism in their ears. Thus, given the right environment, this yeast can easily overpopulate and create a pathological state in the ear. *Malassezia* is identified by tape strips and swabs taken from the ear canal. Usually, infested ears are mildly malodorous and there will be a light brown, ceruminous discharge. Samples are stained and examined under the oil-immersion lens. More than one yeast per high power field is considered significant and the animal should be treated with topical antifungal drugs. Most of the polypharmaceutical ear drops contain an effective antifungal agent that can eliminate the problem.

Parasites are another fairly straightforward underlying cause. In cats under the age of 1 year, *Otodectes cynotis* is extremely common. Usually, by the time the cat is a year old it devolops an immunity to *O. cynotis* and does not show clinical signs, although a commensal population is probably residing in the ear. Some cats, however, develop a hypersensitivity reaction and will tear at their face and ears in response to these mites. The diagnosis is made by microscopic examination of ear exudate, and treatment is a spot-on version of selamectin (Stronghold, Pfizer). Some clinicians will treat with injections of ivermectin but this is off-license and not really called for when a perfectly effective veterinary product is available. Acaricidal ear drops can also be used if the cat will tolerate twice-daily treatment for the 21-day course. (One week of treatment, followed by a week of no treatment and then a third week of treatment.) Dogs can also suffer from *O. cynotis*, but not to the degree that cats do. Obviously, a dog living in a household with cats is more likely to suffer from an ear mite infestation. The presence of cat cohabitants should have been established in your general history. Diagnosis is via the same method; however, selemectin is not yet licensed for the treatment of ear mites in dogs. There are several acaricidal topical ear drops which can be given instead. The drops must be given with the life cycle of the ear mite in mind. Twice-daily treatment for a week, followed by 1 week off, then 1 week more of treatment is what is recommended to eradicate all stages of the mite's life cycle if you are using an ear drop which does not have a specific miticidal element. There are ear drops available which contain thiabendazole (Auroto, Arnolds) which will kill the eggs as well as the adult mite. According to the manufacturer, 7 days worth of treatment is all that is required; however, in practice 3 weeks of treatment is often given (with 1 week off mid-treatment). Do make sure that the pet is able to tolerate the other ingredients in the ear drops. All in-contact pets should be treated for ear mites and the environment should be treated as well because *Otodectes* can live off the host for a period of time.

Trombicula autumnalis (Harvest mite) is another mite which, in the larval stage, can cause ear discomfort. This mite will often settle in Henry's pocket, at the edge of the lateral pinnae. Harvest mites are quite irritating and an infestation will lead to significant self-trauma. Fipronil spray is considered the best treatment for an infestation. As the mites are collected from walks in chalky hills, such walks either need to be curtailed or frequent treatment with fipronil will be required through the late summer and early autumn. The spray should be applied to a swab or cotton ball and wiped onto the ear.

The mange mites, *Notedres cati* and *Sarcoptes scabiei*, can also lead to trauma and inflammation of the ear. Usually, there are tell-tale crusty lesions on the pinnal edges. Part of an ear work-up should include skin scraping from the pinna if any pinnal lesions are present. Identifying mange mites as a cause of otitis is extremely important as the use of topical treatments with corticosteroids can be contraindicated. As most ear drops do contain some sort of steroid, it is an easy error to apply steroids to a mite-infested ear, thus complicating the problem. Similarly, *Demodex* can sometimes be found on an ear swab. Steroid treatment in cases of *Demodex* infestation can lead to chronic and severe problems. Pustular lesions can develop and the infestation can become life threatening. Never skip over sampling. If you miss a *Demodex* infestation and apply the wrong treatment you could be causing the animal to suffer needlessly.

Although dog and cat fleas don't usually cause ear disease, a badly infested animal will end up scratching all over and can traumatise the ear to the point of creating a diseased state. Rabbit fleas, however, are a type of stick-tight flea that can be terribly irritating. They do prefer the ears as a home and thus will set up a self-trauma/inflammation cycle. Dogs and cats can get rabbit fleas too! Treatment with any veterinary flea product should eliminate these parasites as an underlying cause.

Underlying causes

The ear does not exist in isolation. If it is diseased, there is a reason. Without diagnosing the underlying cause of ear disease, the ear can never be completely cured. One can repeatedly treat the clinical signs, but the ear will undergo irreversible change and the client will become dissatisfied. Always ask yourself: 'Why is this dog/cat having ear problems?' and make sure you include diagnostic tests in the work-up which will help you to find an answer to that question.

Allergy is a very common cause for ear problems, with 78% of ear problems being related to an allergy problem. Over 50% of atopic animals suffer from concurrent ear disease. While food sensitivities are not nearly as common as atopy, over 50% of food-sensitive animals also suffer from ear disease. The disease can present as unilateral or bilateral. Generally, there is pruritus before any exudate is identified and in some cases exudate does not develop. The pinnae will be very erythemic and there should be other tell-tale signs of allergic disease, such as saliva-stained paws, traumatised muzzle and conjunctivitis.

Contact allergies can develop when a dog's pinna is stretched along an irritant substance, such as a carpet saturated with carpet powder or linoleum recently cleaned with an irritant substance. It is also possible for an animal to develop an allergic reaction to ear medications or cleansers. If allergy is suspected, a full work-up, including a food trial and sensitivity testing, may be performed to get to the root of the ear problem.

Endocrine disease plays a significant part in the health of the ear. Endocrine disorders are the underlying cause in 7% of ear problems. As endocrine levels affect glandular function, and the ear is lined with numerous adnexal glands, the connection is obvious. Ceruminous otic discharge is present with many cases of endocrine disorders. Hypothyroidism in particular tends to promote ear disease. Any middle-aged dog that presents with ear disease and has put on weight and seems to be slowing down should have blood tests taken for endocrine function. To a lesser extent, hyperadrenocorticoidism and sex hormone imbalances also manifest with ear disease. Noting the age and the sexual status of the dog while taking the history is very important in establishing endocrine disorders as part of the development of ear disease.

Keratinisation disorders such as primary idiopathic seborrhoea, vitamin A-responsive dermatitis and sebaceous adentis can also manifest with ear disorders. The ear is lined with epithelium and increased scale or glandular dystrophy will affect the health of the ear just as it affects the skin elsewhere in the body. As most of these diseases are managed as opposed to cured, the ear too will need to be managed with regular cleaning with cerumolytic, sebolytic cleaners.

Autoimmune disorders such as pemphigus foliaceus, bullous pemphigoid, discoid lupus erythematosus, erythema multiformae, vasculitis, alopecia areata, drug eruptions and cold agglutinin disease, may all affect the ears at some stage in the disease. Most of these diseases will manifest in blistering and scaling lesions. *Sarcoptes scabiei* should be eliminated as a differential first. Diagnosing autoimmune disease usually requires a biopsy. Treatment involves immunosuppressant drugs. Often animals with autoimmune disease are referred to specialist centres.

Neoplasia within the ear canal is obstructive and thus prevents normal ventilation. Often, the neoplasm is only a benign polyp and removal of the growth cures the condition. Malignant neoplasms are far more complicated to deal with as removal with large margins is required, which may severely alter the anatomy of the ear. Squamous cell carcinomas are one type of malignant neoplasm that frequently occurs on the ears. Cats with white ears are most susceptible to this disease. Removal of the affected pinnae can be curative.

Frostbite affects ear pinnae as they are exposed, thinly furred body parts. Frostbite causes tissue necrosis so affected tissue must be surgically excised. If not treated promptly necrotic tissue will become a breeding ground for bacteria and the microbial infection will spread into the ear canals.

The *miscellaneous* section captures any underlying cause which can affect ears. Glandular disorders and juvenile cellulitis slot into this section. Other, more common causes would be eliminated via diagnostic testing before resorting to a diagnosis of glandular disorders. Juvenile cellulitis, as its name implies, affects only puppies. Its onset is sudden and dramatic, with disfiguring swelling occurring all over the head and face. Very high doses of steroids must be given promptly in order to control this disease and prevent permanent scarring.

Perpetuating factors

- Bacterial infection
- Fungal infection
- Chronic inflammation
- Middle ear infection.

Perhaps you have successfully negotiated an animal's predisposing factors and underlying disease problem. Yet still, the ear problem persists. This is because perpetuating factors are at work. These factors are pathological changes to the environment of the ear which promote continuing discomfort for the animal. Various forms and locations of infection, along with changes in actual anatomy, can play a part in a continuing diseased state.

Figure 9.2 shows a case of chronic otitis externa.

Bacterial infections are one large group of perpetuating factors. There are commensal bacteria which live as part of the ear's normal flora and fauna. However, warm, moist conditions, hyperplastic changes and inflammation can promote the overgrowth of commensal bacteria. In this instance, you would find a larger than normal population of staphylococcal or streptococcal bacteria. Indeed, these are bacteria most commonly found when swabs are taken to investigate an ear infection. More serious is an infection with Gram-negative bacteria, often visualised on a slide as bacilli (rods). *Pseudomonas* spp are found in the soil. When an animal scratches at an inflamed ear, it passes these bacteria into the ear canal. If the temperature and humidity are right, *Pseudomonas* spp will populate that ear canal, creating an infection that will be difficult to eradicate. Other Gram-negative bacteria that are sometimes found when investigating diseased ears include *Proteus* spp and *Escherichia coli* (*E. coli*). In order to eliminate these bacteria from the ear canal, the environment must change. A clean, dry ear will not support a large population of bacteria. Therefore, the goal of treatment is to create an inhospitable environment for microbial overgrowth.

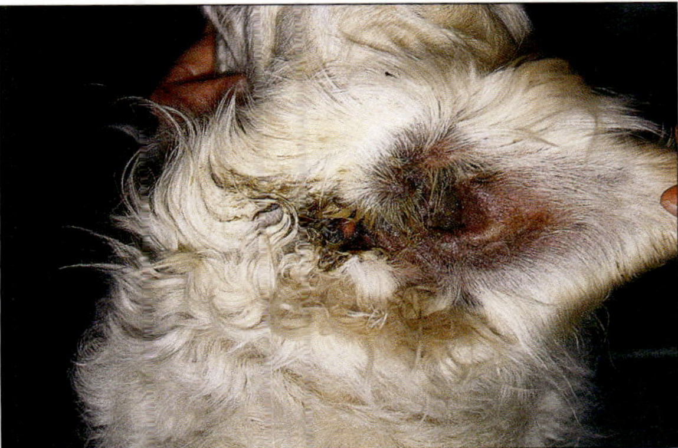

Figure 9.2 This is a case of chronic otitis externa. Notice the inflammation and hyperplasia that make it impossible to examine the ear fully. Photograph by Annette Loeffler, with permission.

Numerous topical treatments are available with antibacterial agents. If a culture and sensitivity test has been done, it is possible to pick the exact antibiotic needed. Otherwise, the choice must be based on the type of discharge and whether or not rods or cocci were identified on in-house slides. Some antibacterial agents are effective only on Gram-positive bacteria while other agents are powerful enough to take on Gram-negative bacteria. Be sure to read the packet insert and make sure you are choosing the correct antibacterial for the job. Drops containing polymyxin B or neomycin can help to eliminate Gram-negative bacteria. However, neomycin can cause a hypersensitivity reaction in some animals. In cats the reaction can be quite severe. Of course, you would never apply an ear drop without making sure the ear drum is intact. Many topical treatments, especially those containing neomycin, are ototoxic. You do not want to make the animal deaf!

Fungal infections, usually in the form of *Malassezia pachydermatis*, can also lead to chronic ear disease. *Malassezia* can be identified by samples taken from ear swabs or tape strips. The footprint or dumbbell-shaped yeasts are commensal in many canine ears but spotting more than one yeast per high-power field is a sign of overgrowth. Noting any yeast from a cat's ear is highly unusual and may indicate an immunocompromised state. There are several topical treatments containing antifungal agents such as clotrimazole or miconazole. Improving the climate of the ear is also important in eliminating *Malassezia*. A clean, dry ear is again the goal in order to reduce fungal overgrowth.

One of the more frustrating aspects of ear disease is that *chronic inflammation* leads to a change in the actual topography of the ear. The epithelium inside the ear becomes swollen and folds are created. Hyperplastic tissue can develop. All of this extra tissue blocks ventilation and creates more handholds for bacterial and fungi to attach. By reducing inflammation (e.g. with topical corticosteroids) there are fewer nooks and crannies for bacteria and debris to take a foothold. Unfortunately, if the ear has been diseased for an extended period of time, the anatomical changes become irreversible. Only surgery can remove the hyperplastic tissue and reduce the stenosis.

A final perpetuating factor is the fact that the ear infection may have spread to the *middle ear*. If this is the case, you can get the external ear as clean as a surgical site but the continuing source of bacteria or fungi from the middle ear will cause the outer ear to become re-infected. Additionally, the pain in the middle ear will cause the animal to continue to self-traumatise the area, generating the vicious circle of scratching and inflammation. The only way to know for sure that otitis media is present is to give the animal a general anaesthetic and investigate. If the external ear is gently flushed clear with saline, the tympanic membrane can be examined. The absence of a tympanic membrance or a damaged membrane is a big hint that there might be a problem in the middle ear. A swab would then need to be taken from the middle ear. It is essential to be sure that the swab samples exudate only in the middle ear and is not contaminated by debris in the external ear. This swab should then be sent for culture and sensitivity. Systemic treatment is required to treat a middle ear infection. The middle ear can also be gently flushed with saline as long as the fluid is removed later.

HOW TO DO AN EAR FLUSH

Figure 9.3 shows the ear canal in the dog and cat.

1. The owner should have been instructed to refrain from ear cleaning and using ear drops 24–48 hours prior to the procedure. If the ear was extremely swollen, a short course of corticosteroids (7 days) can be used prior to investigation in order to allow greater visualisation into the ear.
2. Place the animal under general anaesthetic. Keep in mind that the ear is probably in a

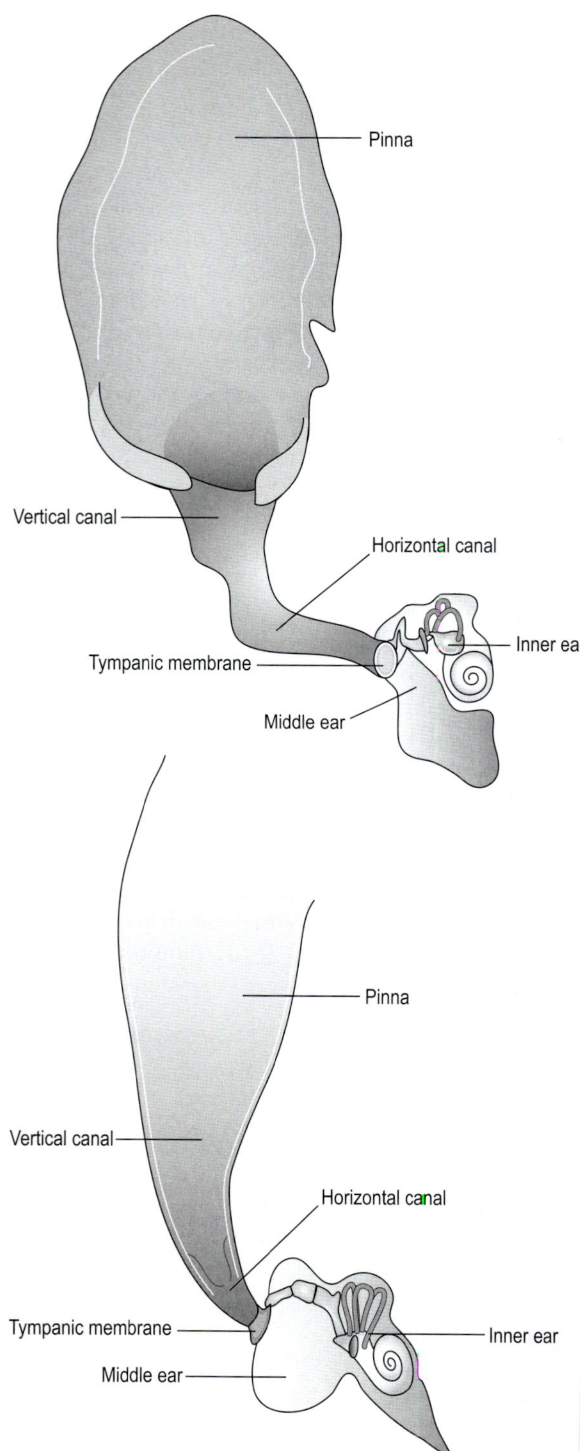

Figure 9.3 A: The canine ear. B: The feline ear.

painful state and that you will be manipulating the ear continuously. A moderately deep level of anaesthetic is, therefore, required or the animal will shake its ears, dislodging your otoscope and saturating you. Be sure that the premedication contains some form of analgesia as a pre-emptive measure.

3. With the animal in lateral recumbancy, examine the pinnae thoroughly for evidence of parasites or self-trauma. Take tape strips and skin scrapes as necessary. Biopsies of the pinnae can also be harvested if fungal or autoimmune disease is suggested.
4. Palpate the horizontal canals of both ears and compare them. Feel for possible calcification.
5. Examine the exudate for colour, consistency and odour. Take sterile swabs for mycology and bacteriology. If taking samples for culture and sensitivity, be sure to request sensitivity for marbofloxacin, as this drug is not routinely included on many sensitivity panels. Do not store the swabs in the refrigerator as low temperatures will alter results.
6. Take swab samples for in-house testing for parasites and cytology.
7. Flush the ear with 5–10 ml of saline using an atraumatic instrument such as a kwill or catheter tip. Wipe away exudate with cotton wool after each flushing. Change kwill or catheter after two or three flushes so that you are not re-introducing microorganisms into the ear. Continue to flush until the debris is cleared away.
8. Using an otoscope, examine the tympanic membrane for patency. It should be semi-transparent, with visible blood vessels. A thick, opaque ear drum is diseased. The absence of an ear drum is even worse. In some cases, a myringotomy (puncturing the ear drum) will be necessary in order to collect samples from the middle ear. If so, then a sterile nasal swab can be slid through the otoscope and through the tympanic membrane. A second swab should then be placed in the same manner, in order to gather a sample from the middle ear. Care should be taken to avoid touching the swab to the external ear canal as this will give a mixed sample. A third swab can also gather samples for in-house testing.
9. If investigating the middle ear, it should also be flushed with sterile saline. A 6 French gauge canine catheter, attached to a 2–5 ml syringe, can be used to flush saline into the middle ear. All fluid should then be syringed out of the ear. It is essential that both the middle and external ear be left dry.
10. Pain relief should be given for 3–5 days post-procedure. Cleaning with saline should be done twice daily until culture and sensitivity results are returned. At that point correct topical and/or systemic treatment can be chosen. There are no ear drops that are licensed for use with a ruptured tympanic membrane. In such cases, systemic treatment is usually relied on, along with saline flushes. Some clinicians will go ahead and use mild topical treatment even if the ear drum is ruptured but this decision is at the discretion of the veterinary surgeon. Home-made ear drops are also an option.

Radiographs are part of the evaluation of middle ear status. Dorsoventral and ventrodorsal views of the caudal skull can be taken to get an image of the external and middle ear. Rare earth screens are required because a detailed image is necessary for diagnostic purposes. Both ears should be radiographed so that a comparison can be made between the two ears. To take these views, the head needs to be extended with the hard palate parallel to the film. Sandbags or foam wedges can be used on either side of the head to prevent rotation. The beam should be centred at the axis of the two horizontal canals. The caudal edge of the frame should reach to the atlanto-occipital joint and the rostral edge should be located at the mandibular joint.

The rostrocaudal open mouth view is used for assessing the status of the middle ear (see Fig. 9.4). Again, rare earth screens should be used. The animal is placed in dorsal recumbancy and the head is flexed so that the hard palate is at a 10–15° angle from the vertical axis. The mouth should be open 10–15°, with the tongue drawn forward. Ties will be needed to maintain this position. The beam needs to be positioned perpendicular to the film and through the axis of the top and bottom lip junctions. The range of the frame is defined by the atlanto-axial joint and the mandibular rami. Extu-

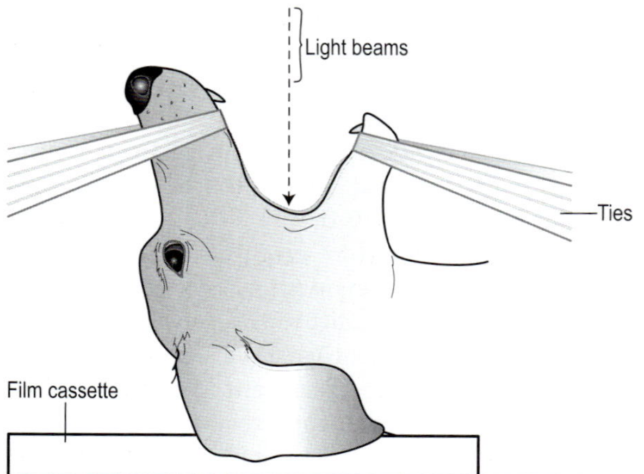

Figure 9.4 Open mouth rostrocaudal view for visualisation of tympanic bullae.

bation is necessary before taking the radiograph, followed by immediate re-intubation.

The lateral view should centre on the tympanic bullae and include the pharynx and the caudoventral skull.

When examining the radiographs you should be able to visualise some soft tissue density within the air shadow of the external ear canal. Growths should be obvious as intrusions into the shadow space. A very narrow air shadow would indicate hyperplastic change. Calcification and even ossification of the annular cartilages may be visualised in severe chronic disease.

The canine middle ear should have a half circular shadow outlined by the thin, dense bone of the bulla. The labyrinth of the inner ear is within the petrous temporal bone. Between these two regions is a bony shelf which acts as the junction between the hypo- and the meso-tympanum. The landmarks outside the middle ear are, laterally, the osseous areas of the external ear canal. Other landmarks are all skull processes, such as the jugular and mastoid processes.

The feline middle ear consists of two compartments, the dorsolateral and the ventromedial. The outline is bony and sharply defined, creating two air-shadow cavities. The tympanic ring can be seen straddling both compartments. The dense bony area is the labyrinth of the middle ear.

Tumours within the middle ear can be observed as densities within the air shadow spaces of the middle ear. Sclerosis of the middle ear can be observed as bony deposits ventral, rostral or lateral to the bullae. Any radiographic change from the normal indicates severe ear disease. However, not being able to see radiographic change does not eliminate the possibility of middle ear disease.

A thorough investigation under general anaesthetic should give you an accurate view of the ear's state of health. Using this information, you decide whether to proceed medically or surgically. There are four ear disasters which necessitate surgery:

1. Chronic proliferative otitis externa, also known as the 'fibroplastic response'. This is a constant secondary infection leading to granulation, scarring, stenosis, the formation of niches and calcification. Papillary projections can develop. The whole structure of the ear canal becomes folded, creating warm, moist niches for microbial overgrowth. The tympanic membrane thickens and may become so diseased that it ruptures. In very long-standing cases, ossification of the annular and auricular cartilages can occur.
2. Persistent ulcerative otitis externa. This condition is often indicative of a Gram-negative infection, usually *Pseudomonas* spp. There is severe pain. German Shepherd dogs are prone to this condition.
3. Middle ear disease. Disease of the middle ear create a nidus for infection elsewhere. There may be keratin plugs present which perpetuate the condition. In severe cases, the middle and external ear are occluded by debris, and draining sinus tracts form elsewhere on the head and neck. This is known as 'para-aural' disease and carries a very poor prognosis.
4. Aural neoplasia.

The vicious cycle which leads to irreversible damage begins with inflammation and the accumulation of inflammatory cells – neutrophils, lymphoid cells, macrophages and giant cells. The uncomfortable ear is scratched at and this increases the temperature in the ear canals. As the canals are inflamed and swollen, exudate is retained. The environment of the ear is altered and the commensal bacteria and yeast overpopulate, setting up a secondary infection. The microorganisms release enzymes, proteases, lipases and toxins, which further damage the ear epithelium. The cerumen itself is changed as the specialised glands of the ear are affected. The skin thickens, decreasing ventilation and drainage further and the ear becomes completely blocked. The goal of surgery is to remove irreversibly damaged tissue, promote healing of remaining tissue and avoid recurrence of otic disease.

There are two methods of surgery used to improve ear health. Traditionally, the lateral wall resection was performed when the vertical ear canal was permanently damaged. Removal of the lateral wall is supposed to change the enviroment of the ear enough to facilitate recovery and prevent further episodes of disease. Practically, this surgery is useful only if the disease is confined to the lateral wall of the external canal, which is usually not the case. Removal of the entire vertical canal can be of some worth (medial as well as lateral wall) in the treatment of otitis externa, but cannot do anything to improve a middle ear condition.

As for any surgery, the area needs to be clipped and scrupulously cleaned. In the case of ear disease, this will mean repeated ear flushing until the canal is clear and pristine. A moderate to deep plane of anaesthesia will be required while the surgeon dissects open the vertical canal and reflects back the tissue. Post-operative care includes potent analgesia and an Elizabethan collar to prevent self-trauma. Antibiotic cover is recommended. Stitches can be removed in 10–14 days but a post-operative check is recommended before removal of stitches. The owner must be fully educated on ear care and committed to keeping the remaining structure of the ear clean. Without the owner's compliance there is little hope in preventing recurrence of ear disease.

The total ear canal ablation (TECA) is a drastic surgical option, chosen only when there are no alternatives to alleviate the animal's suffering. There are risks, including: haemorrage, facial nerve damage, damage to the hyoid apparatus and damage to the labyrinth of the inner ear, which can cause severe neurological signs (head tilt and nystagamus). Any bone fragments or debris left behind will become foreign bodies and thus a nidus for infection. Wound breakdown can occur. Although the inner ear will still be functional, hearing ability will be altered. As dogs rely heavily on their hearing, an alteration of this ability may affect their behaviour.

In most cases where the TECA is opted for, there is middle ear involvement so a lateral bulla osteotomy is performed. The osseus portion of the bulla must be removed as curretting away diseased tissue is rarely a complete job. Any remaining necrotic tissue would lead to further infection. A small bone chisel or rongeurs can be used to create an opening to the lateral bulla. After curretage, flushing of the debris is required. An antibiotic solution can be instilled into the area at this time. A penrose drain is handy for retracting the facial nerve out of the field. Another penrose drain may be placed for drainage of the middle ear, ventral to the bulla. There tends to be a lot of bleeding during this procedure, which reduces visibility. Haemostatic measures need to be provided assidiously.

Chiselling out pieces of bone from the skull is inherently painful. Intense analgesia for the first 48 hours post-operation is essential. If your practice does not use morphine, don't do this operation. Send the dog to a referral centre that uses the most potent drugs available. Antibiotics also have to be on board for 5–10 days.

If surgery can be avoided, by all means avoid it. There are medical management protocols available for all but the worst ears. It is almost always worth trying the medical approach before resorting to surgery. Here is a medical protocol one can follow to treat the acute ear:

1. Clean the ear one to three times daily. Insert 5 ml of saline (or a commercial cleaner if you feel certain that the ear drum is intact) into the ear and occlude with cotton wool. Massage the ear canal so that the fluid travels down into the horizontal canal. Leave for 5 minutes. Then wipe away all the debris with cotton wool. Don't wipe too vigorously or you can cause irritation. Don't use cotton buds. If you have used an acidic ear cleaner, wait 1–4 hours before applying ear drops.
2. Apply ear drops. You can make a choice based on your cytological findings or mix up your own drops. One popular recipe is 50–100 mg enrofloxacin + 0.5–1 ml dimethyl sulphoxide (DMSO) or silver sulfadiazine. If you are concerned about the patency of the tympanic membrane, consider this carefully when choosing ear drops. Some drops are more likely to cause ototoxicity. Avoid anything containing neomycin. While this antibiotic is brilliant for getting rid

of Gram-negative bacteria, it doesn't do the middle ear any good. Home-made drops are often the best option if the ear drum is not intact. Besides the baytril recipe, one can try ticarcillin. Ear drops should be applied twice daily. Try to limit drops containing steroid to a 3-week period.

3. Severely swollen ears and ears where otitis media is present may benefit from systemic corticosteroid treatment to reduce the inflammation and pain. Prednisolone at 0.5–1 mg/kg for 2 weeks can be given if necessary.
4. At some point in treatment you may need to give the animal a general anaesthetic and thoroughly flush the ear. The earlier you do this in your protocol the better.
5. If the dog or cat has not responded within 14 days of treatment, or if you noticed bacilli on your in-house cytology, do a culture and sensitivity test.
6. Serious infections which necessitate systemic treatment do need to be treated for 6–8 weeks. Prepare the client for the cost of high doses of antibiotics (sometimes twice the normal dose for good penetration to the ear) and for the length of treatment. Cutting back on dose rates or length of the dose will not do the animal or owner any favours. The condition will either never resolve or it will recur. The ear may become permanently damaged and the client will think you are incompetent.

Most ear drops are polypharmaceuticals. The long list of ingredients can be confusing. A brief overview of what drug is supposed to serve which purpose can be helpful:

- corticosteroids: betamethasone, dexamethasone, prednisolone, triamcinolone
- local anaesthetic: amethocaine hydrochloride
- acaricide: thiabendazole
- antifungals: clotrimazole, miconazole, nystatin, thiabendazole
- antibiotics: framycetin, fucidin, genticin, marbofloxacin, neomycin, polymyxin B, thiostrepton.

Staphylococci are identified most often. They are sensitive to fucidin especially, but also to marbofloxacin, gentacin and neomycin. Miconazole and thiostrepton can also be effective against staphylococci.

Streptococci are the second most common bacteria identified in the ear. Fucidin, thiostrepton and marbofloxacin have good action against streptococci. Miconazole has a moderate effect, while framycetin, genticin and polymyxin show poor action against streptococci.

Pseudomonas spp, *Escherichia coli* (*E. coli*) and *Proteus* spp are less common. These organisms are associated with ulceration and a purulent discharge. Culture and sensitivity is always recommended if bacilli are observed in in-house cytological tests. Polymyxin B shows good activity against *Pseudomonas* spp if all organic debris is removed first. Reported resistance is developing to aminoglycosides (genticin) and fluoroquinolones (enrofloxacin). Ticarcillin has been used with some success.

There are two things to remember when dispensing ear drugs. First, even if it's going into the ear it is eventually absorbed systemically, so go easy on the corticosteroids. You don't need to use the strongest steroid if the ear isn't that swollen. Milder steroids such as prednisolone and hydrocortisone are safer. Second, BEWARE OTOTOXICITY! Signs of ototoxicity include head tilt, nystagamus, circling, falling over, eyes deviated towards the affected side and deafness. When in doubt, stick with saline. Just cleaning the ear thoroughly and drying it makes it an inhospitable place for microbes to live. Regular cleaning can make a huge difference. Make sure your clients know how to clean their dogs' ears. Make them show you what they are doing. Without the client doing the home care, the ear won't ever get better.

Use the flow chart on diagnosis of ear disease (Fig. 9.5) as a guide to making sure that you eliminate all differentials for underlying disease. In this way, you will be treating ear disease like any other skin disease and will give your patients the best chance of full recovery.

FORMULARY

Products not licensed for use in small animals in the United Kingdom are marked with an asterisk. Products not licensed for use as an otic preparation are marked with a double asterisk.

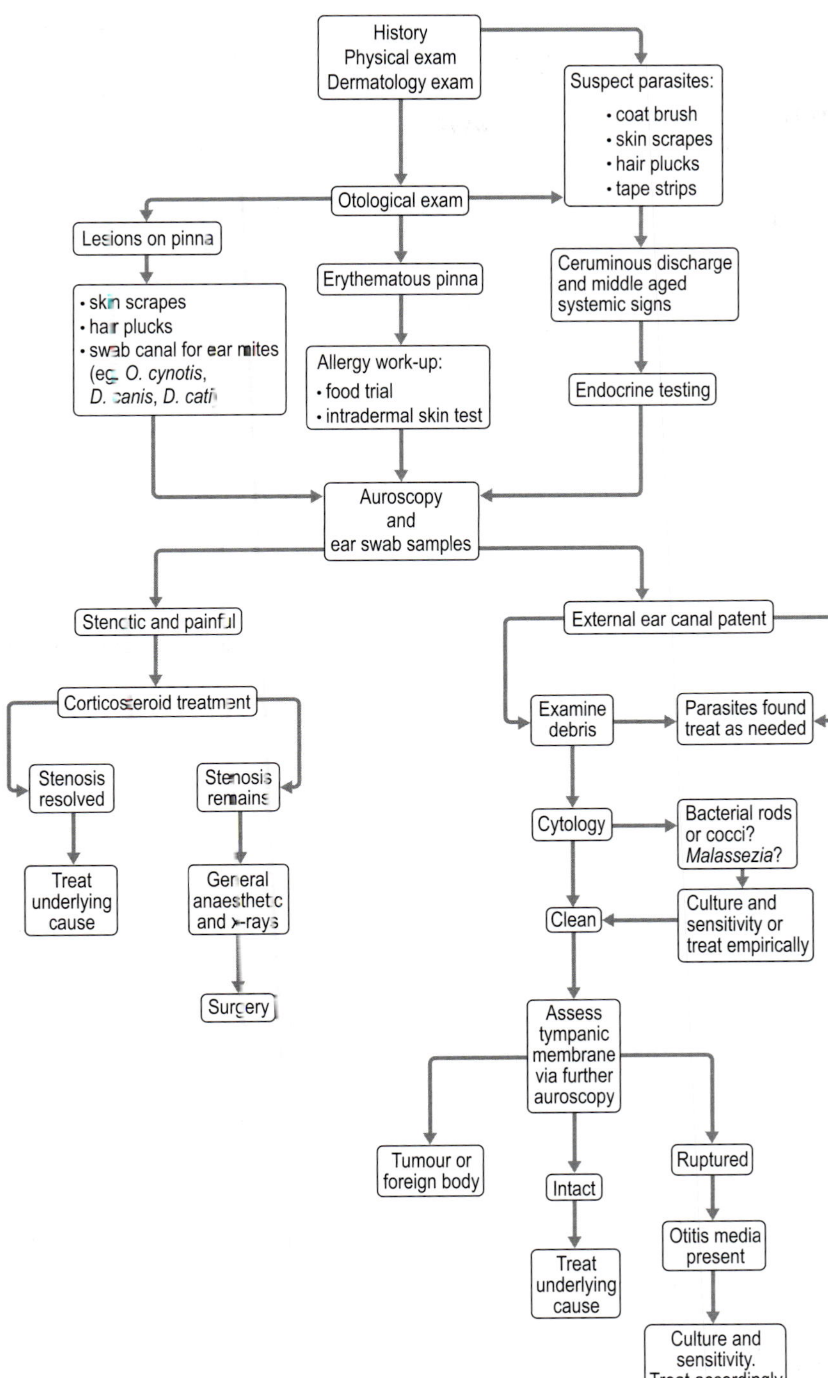

Figure 9.5 Ear disease.

Ear cleaners

Auroclens (Arnolds): coconut oil
Dermisol Cleanser (Pfizer): salicyclic acid, benzoic acid, malic acid, propylene glycol, pH 2.3 (acidic)
Epiotic (Virbac): salicylic acid, lactic acid, propylene glycol, PCMX, pH 2 (acidic)
Leo Cat ear cleaner (Leo Laboratories): glycerine, propylene glycol, polysorbate 80
Leo dog ear cleaner (Leo Laboratories): propylene glycol, emollients, boric acid, pH 6.5 (nearly neutral)
Otoclean (Janssen-Cilag): salicylic acid, propylene glycol, glycerine, lactic acid, oleic acid, ethoxydiglycol, water, plant extracts. In individual dose sizes of 5 ml each
TrisEDTA (Dermapet): EDTA, pH 8

Topicals

Aurizon (Vetoquinol): marbofloxacin, clotrimazole, dexamethasone. Once-daily application for 7–14 days
Auroto (Arnolds): thiabendazole, neomycin, amethocaine hydrochloride. For twice-daily use, 7 days consecutively. Effective against *Otodectes*
**Baytril (Bayer): enrofloxacin. Mix 1:4 with a carrier agent such as dexamethasone, dimethylsulphoxide (DMSO), or saline
*Baytril Otic (Bayer): enrofloxacin, *silver sulfadiazine. Not available in the UK but can be mixed up using injectable enrofloxacin and silver sulfadiazine ointment
Canaural (Leo Laboratories): nystatin, fusidic acid, framycetin, prednisolone. Advised usage twice daily for a minimum of 7 days. Effective against *Otodectes* if used over a 3-week period
*Flamazine: silver sulfadiazine (S&N Healthcare). Mix with Baytril or just mix with water to get a 1% solution (1.5 ml Flamazine to 13.5 ml distilled water, warm in microwave to reduce viscosity)
GAC (Arnolds): neomycin, amethocaine, permethrin. Twice-daily usage for 10–14 days. Effective against *Otodectes*
Genticin Eye/Ear drops (Roche): gentamycin
Malacetic Otic (Dermapet): 2% acetic acid, 2% boric acid
Otosporin (Dowelhurst): polymyxin B, neomycin, hydrocortisone
Panalog (Novartis): nystatin, neomycin, triamcinolone
Surolan (Janssen): miconazole, polymyxin B, prednisole acetate. Advised to use twice daily for a minimum of 7 days
**Timentin Solution (GlaxoSmithKline): *ticarcillin in 2 mg/ml strength. Reconstitute with 10 ml sterile water. Instill 1 ml into ear twice daily. Keep refrigerated. Discard after 3 days and continue treatment with new solution

Systemic treatment

Enrofloxacin (Baytril, Bayer)
Marbofloxacin (Marbocyl, Vetoquinol)
*Ketoconazole (Nizoral, Janssen-Cilag). Can also be used as a topical. Put 300 mg in one bottle of Epiotic
*Itraconazole (Sporanox, Janssen-Cilag)

Please note:

- Gentimycin, neomycin, enrofloxacin, marbofloxacin and polymyxin B are noted for their efficacy against *Pseudomonas* spp.
- Clotrimazole, nystatin, thiabendazole and miconazole are recommended for use against *Malassezia*.
- Many antibiotics are inactivated in the presence of organic debris. Make sure that the ear is clean before applying topical medication.
- Extremely acidic cleaners (7 is neutral pH; lower than 7 is acidic, higher than 7 is alkaline) can inactivate some antibiotics. Cleaning should be done at least 1 hour before medication is applied.

References and Further Reading

Bensignor E 2003 An approach to otitis externa and otitis media. In: Foster A, Foil C (eds) BSAVA Manual of small animal dermatology. BSAVA Publications, Gloucester, p 104–111

Griffin Craig 1993 Otitis externa and otitis media. In: Griffin C E, Kwochak K W, MacDonald J M (eds) Current veterinary dermatology. Mosby, St Louis, p 245–262

Harvey R G, Harari J, Delauche A J 2001 Ear diseases of the dog and cat. Manson Publishers, London

Kristensen F, Jacobsen J, Eriksen T 1996 Otology in dogs and cats. Leo Animal Health, Denmark, p 34–36

Little Chris 1996 A clinician's approach to the investigation of otitis externa. In Practice January:9–16

Little Chris 1996 Medical treatment of otitis externa in the dog and cat. In Practice February:66–71

CASE STUDY 1

Otodectes cynotis infestation

Signalment

A former rescue cat, judged to be approximately 6 years old. Female, spayed, domestic short-haired and slightly overweight at 4.2 kg.

Owner's complaint

The owner observed a dark, granular discharge from both ears. The owner explained that the cat had had ear mites previously and that she thought it was the same problem.

History

The owner formerly had dogs that had contracted ear mites while in kennels. Apparently, it took a great deal of effort to eradicate the infestation in the dogs and both dogs developed otitis media. The cat had since suffered repeated infestations, although never to the point of developing otitis media.

The cat was fully vaccinated and had tested negative for FeLV/FIV virus. However, she had had recurrent bouts of cat flu, as well as ear mites. The cat had free access to the outdoors via a cat flap. There were many cats in the neighbourhood, although there were no other pets in the household. The cat slept on the owner's bed.

Physical examination

Temperature, pulse and respiration were normal. No abnormalities were detected on abdominal palpation. No external skin parasites were obvious, although there were some dry scales present in the coat. It was noted that worming was due. Both ears did show a dark, 'coffee-ground'-like discharge. There was no particular sign of discomfort in the aural region and erythema was minimal. The owner had not seen the cat scratching at her ears or any other body parts. Licking and rubbing were not noted either.

Differential diagnosis

- *Otodectes cynotis* infestation
- Bacterial infection: *Staphylococcus* spp, *Streptococcus*, *Proteus*, *Pseudomonas*
- *Malassezia* dermatitis
- Atopic dermatitis
- Food sensitivity

Diagnostic tests

A swab was taken from both ears and a smear slide was prepared. Under low magnification, a mite was identified as *Otodectes cynotis.* Another method of isolating mites would have been to place the aural exudate on a dark background and shine a light on it. The heat of the lamp would cause the mites to become active and their white forms would be easily visible against the dark background. Still another method would be to take a serum tube with a drop of water and place some exudate in the tube and then apply heat. The heat would cause the mites to rush to the walls of the tube.

Treatment

After otoscopic examination, to make sure that the tympanic membrane was intact, the ears were thoroughly cleansed with a glycerol- and propylene glycol-based agent (Leo Cat Ear Cleaner, Leo Laboratories). Ear drops containing the antibiotics fusidic acid and framycetin sulphate, along with the anti-yeast drug nystatin and the anti-inflammatory agent prednisolone (Canaural, Leo Laboratories), were used. Although the drops do not contain any specific acaricidal, clinical trials have shown that Canaural is effective against ear mites. The owner was advised to apply the ear-drops twice daily for 7 days, stop for 7 days and then resume treatment for another 7 days. This 21-day plan would eliminate the full life cycle of the mite. The owner was also advised to clean the ears once a day, if necessary with ear cleaner, wiping away the debris with cotton wool and avoiding the use of cotton buds. The owner was also advised to treat the home with a good-quality premise spray. The cat was to be seen at the end of treatment.

Re-inspection

After 3 weeks the cat's ears were free of mites and their debris and the canals were healthy. Treatment was discontinued.

Two months later the cat was re-presented with what appeared to be a re-infestation of ear mites. Debris from a swab examined under a microscope confirmed the diagnosis. The owner was asked whether she had treated her home with premise spray but she admitted she hadn't. The owner did not want to repeat treatment with Canaural as she said it made the cat's head greasy and the cat rubbed her head all over the furniture.

A number of options were possible at this stage. The cat could have been treated with Ivermectin, (Panomec, Merial) at a dose rate of 0.2–0.4 mg/kg, repeating the injection in 2 weeks. However, this is extra-license use of the drug and the owner was not willing to sign a release agreement. Another treatment would be to apply two drops of Fipronil (Frontline, Merial) directly into the ear canal. This is also extra-license use of a product. Finally, selamectin (Stronghold, Pfizer) could be used and is licensed for the treatment of *O. cynotis* in cats. In fact, studies show a 100% efficacy rate for treatment of naturally occurring *O. cynotis* infestations treated with selamectin.

It was decided to go with the selamectin option. The owner was advised to use the product on a monthly basis as the cat has a history of ear mite infestations and the environment could or would not be treated. It was also recommended that the owner continue to clean the cat's ears on a once-weekly basis.

Final outcome

After 3 weeks the cat was seen again and was deemed free of an ear mite infestation. The owner has decided to use the product regularly and it is anticipated that the cat should remain free of *O. cynotis.*

Discussion

The adult *Otodectes* mite is extremely mobile, which is why infestation of the ears is nearly always bilateral and communication of the disease occurs readily. In the household in this case, infestation of the dogs almost certainly led to infestation of the cat, although the reverse is more often the case. The female mites have suckers on leg pairs I and II and the males have suckers on all four pairs of legs, because hind leg suckers are essential in the mating process. These suckers are excellent identification markers under microscopic examination and were certainly helpful in identifying mites in this examination.

O. cynotis causes up to 50% of otitis externa cases in cats and 5–10% of cases in the dog. In the dog, the mites are not as easily recognised as usually a secondary bacterial or yeast infection masks the tell-tale 'coffee-ground' discharge (August 1986). Most cats are exposed to *O. cynotis* at some point in their lives and this exposure can lead to later immunity, which is why most cases are seen in younger cats. In this case, the cat was fully mature, which leads one to believe that there is some sort of immunosuppression or allergic reaction. Some cats can develop hypersensitivity reactions to the mite antigen and will develop papular lesions in the neck, head and gluteal regions (August 1986). The motility of the mite often necessitates whole body treatment, especially including the tail, as that rests next to the ears when the cat sleeps (Grant 1991). Thus, systemic treatment, as used in this case with selamectin, is particularly helpful.

The mites feed on lymph and blood in the epithelial cells of the ear canal. The mite's activity tends to stimulate the ceruminous glands, leading to a build up of ceruminous debris, stained dark by the mixture of blood, epidermal scale and inflammatory exudate (August 1986).

Pruritus is variable in individuals. Some cats need a severe infestation to show clinical signs of head shaking, pawing at the ears, restlessness and distress (Georgi & Georgi 1992). The debris is an ideal breeding ground for bacterial and yeast infections, so potentially *O. cynotis* can lead to serious disease involving seizures, deafness and impaired cognition (Georgi & Georgi 1992). Severely affected cats may need treatment with glucocorticoids along with topical and even systemic antibiotic and acaricidal treatment (Grant 1991). Although this cat seemed only mildly annoyed by her infestation, obviously her previous housemates had been more deeply affected as their infestation led to otitis media.

O. cynotis is not a known vector of any other diseases. However, it can lead to transient papular dermatitis of the arm and trunk in humans who are in close contact with infected animals. Although this owner shared a bed with her cat, she remained unaffected.

REFERENCES

(for Case Study 1)

August John R 1986 Disease of the ear canal. The complete manual of ear care. Solvay Vet Inc, Veterinary Learning Systems, Trenton, NJ, p 39–40

Georgi Jay R, Georgi Marion E 1992 Ticks and mites. Canine clinical parasitology. Lea & Febiger, London, p 47–48

Grant D I 1991 Skin disease in the cat and dog. Blackwell Scientific Publishers, London, p 43

CASE STUDY 2

Chronic otitis externa

Signalment

The patient was an eight-and-a-half-year-old female, neutered Golden Retriever dog.

Owner's complaint

Discharge from both ears, accompanied by rubbing and scratching on the left side.

History

This bitch had a 5-year history of ear disease (age of onset: 3 years).

A lateral wall resection had been performed on the right ear 8 months earlier. Various ear cleaners, topical and systemic treatments had been tried on both ears over the years. The bitch had also experienced an episode of sarcoptic mange 18 months ago. This had successfully been treated with selamectin (Stronghold, Pfizer).

The owner exercised the bitch twice daily in a forest with a significant fox population. Exercise was tolerated unenthusiastically. Swimming was not allowed. No other animals lived in the household and the bitch slept in the kitchen.

Physical examination

At 36.5 kilograms, the bitch was obviously overweight. Temperature and pulse were normal on examination but panting was evident throughout the consultation. The hair coat was healthy with no areas of alopecia, scaling or ectoparasites. There was marked hyperpigmentation on the bitch's ventral abdomen and medial thighs. Mobility problems were not evident. The bitch repeatedly rubbed her left ear against her leg, intermittently shaking her head.

The left ear displayed a heavy, creamy-yellowish discharge. The right ear showed a light brown, ceruminous discharge, with a lesser degree of exudate than the left ear. Both ears had an unpleasant odour. Otoscopic examination was not possible while the animal was conscious because palpation of the left ear canal was painful.

Chronic otitis externa is shown in Figure 9.6.

Differential diagnosis

- Otitis externa of a bacterial and/or fungal nature
- Otitis media – providing a bacterial source for recurrent otitis externa
- Sarcoptes scabiei infestation
- Demodex canis infestation
- Otodectes cynotis infestation.

Underlying disorders

- Keratinisation disorder
- Flea-allergic dermatitis
- Atopy
- Food intolerance
- Drug eruption
- Hypothyroidism
- Polyps
- Foreign bodies
- Neoplasia.

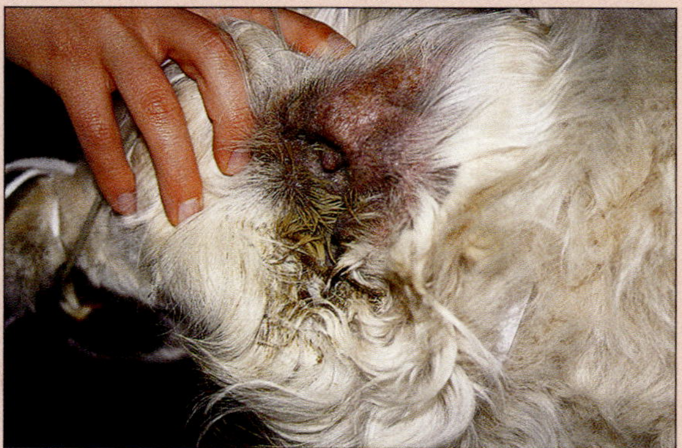

Figure 9.6 Chronic otitis externa in a retriever. Photograph by Annette Loeffler, with permission.

Diagnostic procedures

Coat brushings, tape strips, hair plucks and skin scrapes were performed, all proving negative for parasites. The bitch was admitted for a general anaesthetic. Pre-anaesthetic blood profiles were taken, which showed a slight rise in cholesterol. Blood was also taken for a T4/TSH assay.

Under general anaesthetic, several swabs were taken from each ear and tape strippings and swabs were taken from the ventral abdomen and medial thigh. Swabs collected from the middle ear were carefully removed to avoid contamination by microbes in the external ear. Samples were examined in house after Gram staining, as well as by an outside laboratory. The ears were thoroughly flushed with saline until no further debris could be brought to the outside of the auditory meatus. Otoscopy showed no evidence of a tympanic membrane on the left or the right ears. The right ear had already had surgery performed on it but hyperplastic change had occurred over the years making even a remodelled ear full of extra folds and areas for bacteria or fungal overgrowth.

The head was radiographed, with the thought that severe damage to the left ear would warrant an additional total ear canal ablation surgery. Ventral/dorsal and intra-oral rostrocaudal views were taken.

The swabs and tape strippings taken were prepared with a 'Diff-Quik' stain and examined under high power. A sterile swab from each ear was sent off for culture and sensitivity evaluation.

Diagnosis and prognosis

The thyroid function assay showed that the bitch had normal thyroid function – T4 16.0 nmol/l (normal being 13–52 nmol/l) and TSH 0.12 ng/ml (normal being <0.41 ng/ml). Radiographs showed mineralisation of both the right and left outer ears but the bullae were normal. It was not felt that the left ear was damaged enough to warrant a total ear canal ablation (TECA).

The tape strippings did not display any significant pathogens. The swabs from the right ear demonstrated a sizeable population of *Malassezia pachydermatis*. Swabs from the left ear showed heavy bacterial growth of both cocci and bacilli. These were later identified as *Pseudomonas aeruginosa*, *Proteus* spp and *Staphylococcus* spp when the culture results were returned. Sensitivity results showed no single antibiotic which all three bacteria were sensitive to.

A diagnosis of chronic, bilateral otitis externa and media was made based on swabs taken from both the external and middle ears, and on inflammatory changes visible on the radiographs. Gram-negative and Gram-positive bacteria, as well as a yeast infection, were the perpetuating factors that led to the chronic pathological state. Aggressive medical treatment was necessary to alleviate these infections. Due to the long-standing nature of the problem and the pathological changes that had taken place in the aural integument, the prognosis was guarded. Identifying an underlying cause was essential in order to make any permanent improvement.

Treatment

Cleansing the ears daily would be necessary because most topical treatments are ineffective in the face of organic debris. As the ears were already so sore, and ototoxicity was a concern, saline was chosen as a safe and soothing cleanser. The owner was instructed to flush both ears twice daily. One hour after cleaning the ears a polypharmaceutical ear drop (Aurizon, Vetoquinol) was applied to both ears. Topical eardrops are contraindicated in the absence of a tympanic membrane. However, none of the drugs in the product used are directly ototoxic and this treatment was a last resort for this patient. Oral oxytetracycline (Oxycare, Animalcare) was prescribed at the dose of 1 g per day, twice daily for 28 days (25 mg/kg). The owner was instructed to phone weekly with a progress report and to contact the dermatology nurse at any time he experienced difficulties. The bitch was also placed on a home-made diet trial consisting of rabbit and potato for 6 weeks.

Re-inspection and final outcome

There was a great deal of improvement as soon as the owner began a regular regime of cleaning and medicating. The rubbing and head shaking declined and the exudate from both ears diminished. At the end of the treatment, the ears could be said to be 'cured' but for the time being only. The search for an underlying cause was to continue. Intradermal skin testing proved negative. Later challenges with food did produce mild flare-ups. It was decided that a food sensitivity was at least one component of the underlying disease. The owner was unable to strictly adhere to a food plan for the dog so prophylactic ear cleaning was advised on a twice-weekly basis.

Discussion

Otitis externa becomes chronic when the primary cause can't be identified or is untreated (Kristensen et al 1996). As this bitch had a 5-year history of otitis externa, it was obvious that the underlying cause had not yet been eliminated. Being an 8-year-old Golden Retriever, overweight, with hyperpigmented skin areas and slight hypercholesterolaemia, she seemed a prime candidate for hypothyroidism. However, the tests proved otherwise and the early age of onset would not be consistent with hypothyroidism.

Food sensitivity with a dermatological facet begins with otitis externa in 20% of cases. When food sensitivities remain untreated, 80% of affected dogs will show signs of otitis externa (Griffin 1993). Thus, a food trail was warranted in this case and did contribute to the bitch's improvement. In cases where the dog is atopic, rather than food sensitive, a restricted diet may lower the allergy threshold and reduce clinical signs (Shaw 2001).

A drug reaction would certainly have been possible in this case as the bitch had been exposed to a variety of treatment protocols over the course of her long history of otitis. Utilising the mild cleanser saline reduced the possibility of adding irritation to already damaged and painful ears. Regardless, treatment was essential in this case due to the severity of the disease. Stopping all treatment and waiting for a possible good response would have been negligent.

Further along in this animal's treatment, an underlying cause of atopy was explored but positive diagnosis was not achieved.

Initially, it was necessary to treat the immediate case of serious infection rigorously before continuing with further diagnostic measures. While 36% of healthy ears do have a *Malassezia* population, overpopulation is evident when 5–10 yeasts per high-power field are observed (Griffin 1993). In this case, we were able to identify very large numbers of *Malassezia* per high-power field. The activity of the yeast releases lipase and protease enzymes, which cause further damage to the tissue of the ear canal (Little 1996). The heat and moisture of a narrowed canal (made stenotic by years of inflammation) created an ideal environment for infection and the infection itself perpetuated a vicious cycle of further inflammation and damage.

Likewise, *Staphylococcus* spp bacteria occur in the healthy ear but do not create an infection unless the ear becomes unhealthy. *Pseudomonas* and *Proteus* species do not occur in the healthy ear and can only proliferate once the vicious cycle of inflammation–self-trauma–exudate has begun. All of these bacteria release further damaging enzymes, leading to permanent alterations in the ear's anatomy (Little 1996). Immediate, aggressive treatment is called for when Gram-negative bacteria are present.

Unfortunately, *Pseudomonas* in particular, is difficult to treat because it is resistant to so many familiar antibiotics. If our treatment protocol had failed, we would have had to look to more exotic means of controlling the infection, in some cases risking ototoxicity. Some of the methods proposed in the literature include a 1-minute soak twice daily in 2% acetic acid (Griffin 1993). This method would definitely have been too painful for our patient. Gentimicin, amikacin (giving the injectable form as an ear drop), Tris EDTA, or silver sulfadiazene (made into a 1% solution) have all been suggested (Griffin 1993). We chose to stick with the simplest regime possible in order to guarantee the owner's compliance. When all is said and done, owner compliance is the most important part of the treatment protocol. Additionally, *Pseudomonas* cannot survive in a clean, dry ear. Changing the climate of the ear can be a cure in itself.

REFERENCES

(for Case Study 2)

Griffin Craig 1993 Otitis externa and otitis media. In: Griffin C E, Swochak K W, MacDonald J M (eds) Current veterinary dermatology. Mosby, St Louis, p 245–262

Kristensen F, Jacobsen J, Eriksen T 1996 Otology in dogs and cats. Leo Animal Health, Denmark, p 34–36

Little Chris 1996 Medical treatment of otitis externa in the dog and cat. In Practice February:66–71

Shaw Susan 2001 A practical approach to canine otitis externa. University of Bristol, Department of Continuing Veterinary Studies, p 1–10

Chapter 10

Autoimmune disease

CHAPTER CONTENTS

Autoimmune diseases with a dermatological component can be separated into two broad groups: the pemphigus diseases and other cutaneous autoimmune disorders. The locations of the lesions are one of the main factors used to help determine the specific disease.

PEMPHIGUS

Within the pemphigus group there are six diseases described: pemphigus foliaceus, pemphigus erythmatosus, pemphigus vulgaris, pemphigus vegetans (also known as panepidermal pustular pemphigus), canine benign familial chronic pemphigus (also known as 'Hailey-Hailey' disease) and paraneoplastic pemphigus. Of these six, pemphigus foliaceus is the most common in both the cat and dog, although it certainly can't be considered a common disease in general. The cat has a lower incidence of pemphigus than the dog. Pemphigus can be described as a disease in which autoantibodies act against keratinocytes. Adhesion between the keratinocytes breaks down, allowing intraepidermal pustules or vesicles to form. Desmosomes are the adhesion between keratinocytes and it is their destruction that causes the cutaneous symptoms.

Pemphigus foliaceus

In pemphigus foliaceus it is the superficial keratinocytes that are affected. Most lesions in dogs occur on the muzzle and ears. Lesions on the nasal planum are particularly indicative of pemphigus foliaceus. Nasal depigmentation will occur secondarily to the lesions and can lead to photodermatitis. Dog breeds most affected are: Akitas, Chow Chows, Dachshunds, Bearded Collies, Labradors, Newfoundlands, Doberman Pinschers and Schipperkes. In cats, the lesions start on the face or digits. Lesions can spread slowly or rapidly. One third of cases will lead to generalised lesions at the onset of the disease. Nearly two thirds of cases take over 6 months to generalise. In the dog, other areas can become involved, for example: the periocular region, the nipples, footpads and nailbed. In the cat, paronychia (nail bed inflammation) and nipple lesions occur often. Hyperkeratosis of the foot pads may occur, leading to fissured pads. Bacterial cellulitis can ensue if the case is severe. The primary lesion is an erythematous macule that develops into a pustule. The pustule ruptures, forming crust and epidermal collarettes. Pustules can occur in a group, making them appear to be a plaque. Other lesion patterns are polycyclic or arciform. The disease may wax and wane so there will be a period of pustule proliferation and then pustules will cease to form, leaving crusty skin from the earlier, now ruptured pustules. Eventually, alopecia develops and secondary pyoderma is not uncommon.

Systemic signs include lymphadenopathy, lameness, pyrexia and depression. There may be limb oedema in severe cases. Pruritus and pain are variable. The average age of onset is 4–5 years of age but cases can occur in dogs any age from 6 months to 12 years.

Within the parameters of pemphigus foliaceus (PF), there are three varieties:

1. Spontaneous PF affects Akitas and Chow Chows especially.
2. Drug-induced PF affects Labradors and Dobermans primarily.
3. Chronic dermatological disease-related PF is associated with a long history of chronic skin disease.

Diagnosis of pemphigus foliaceus is acheived by examining the clinical signs, combined with the history, especially in the third form of the disease. Impression smears should be gathered from an intact pustule, if you can find one. The pustule should be punctured and the contents expressed onto a slide and stained. A stained impression smear should reveal normal neutrophils and few to many acanthocytes. Acanthocytes are round, individual keratinoctyes from the stratum spinosum and granulosum, detached by the process of acantholysis. Acantholysis is the loss of cohesion between epidermal cells. Large numbers of nucleated acanthocytes will separate to form ‘rafts’, which divide the epidermis and create spaces where pustules can form. No bacteria should be present in a smear from an animal with an autoimmune disorder unless there is a secondary bacterial infection.

Other diseases on the differential list should be eliminated before investigating for pemphigus as it is a fairly rare disease. Folliculitis, pyoderma, dermatophytosis, sarcoptic mange and demodicosis should all be considered. Additionally, other autoimmune disorders such as discoid and systemic lupus, other forms of pemphigus, bullous pemphigoid and necrolytic migratory erythema must be included in a differential diagnosis. In fact, almost any cutaneous autoimmune disease or paraneoplastic syndrome could be included in the differential list for pemphigus disorders.

Biopsies are harvested for a definitive diagnosis. Three or four intact pustules should be collected with a 6 mm punch. Routine histology and, if necessary, direct and indirect immunofluorescence or immunoperoxidase staining should be performed on the sample. In a positive diagnosis, there will be acantholytic epidermal cells, non-degenerating neutrophils and eosinophils. Pustules will be visible in the subcorneal region, and as deep as the stratum granulosum. Hair follicles will be affected by pustules and acantholytic cells.

Once pemphigus foliaceus is diagnosed, treatment should commence with corticosteroid therapy, usually prednisolone. This alone may be sufficient to treat pemphigus in 20% of cases. Dogs should be given prednisolone at 2.2–4.4 mg/kg/day. Cats may receive 4.4–6.6 mg/kg/day as induction doses. These high doses should continue until remission takes place, usually 2–4 weeks later. Tapering then takes place over the next 8–12 weeks. Maintenance for the dog is 1.1 mg/kg/day and 2.2 mg/kg/day for the cat. If prednisolone is not enough to achieve remission, dexamethasone can be added at a dose rate of 0.1 to 0.2 mg/kg/day, tapering down to 0.05–0.1 mg/kg/day. In very mild cases, topical steroids may resolve the condition. Topical betamethasone should be used first, tapering down to treatment with hydrocortisone for maintenance.

In many cases, prednisolone on its own will not be potent enough to overcome the autoimmune process. Other drugs must be incorporated into the treatment programme. Combinations of different immunosuppressant drugs can be used to decrease the dose of steroids, thus avoiding some of the unpleasant side-effects connected with corticosteroid therapy. Azathioprine is often used in dogs but cannot be used in cats. Azathioprine (Imuran, WellcomeGlaxo) is given at a dose rate of 2–4 mg/kg once every 24 to 48 hours. As this drug can cause bone marrow suppression, pancreatitis and nephrotoxicity, haematological and biochemical blood tests should be taken every 2 weeks during induction. During maintenance, blood samples should be collected every 1–2 months initially, then each 2–3 months thereafter. If bone marrow suppression occurs, treatment should be stopped and then re-introduced later, at half the former dose.

Chlorambucil (Leukeran, GlaxoWellcome) can be used in both dogs and cats, although it is only used for dogs if they cannot tolerate azathioprine. Chlorambucil can be given at 0.1–0.2 mg/kg every 48 hours. Hepatotoxicity and bone marrow suppression are possible so the animal should be monitored as closely as it is for azathioprine. Cyclophosphamide (Endoxana, AstaMedica) is another alternative, but in dogs it frequently causes haemorrhagic cystitis that takes a long time to resolve. The dose rate is 1.5–2.5 mg/kg every 48 hours. Bone marrow suppression is, again, a side-effect of this drug.

Less frequently, gold salts (chrysotherapy) can be used with or without steroids. Intramuscular (i.m.) injections of aurothiomalate or aurothioglucose are most effective but a tablet form, auranofin (Ridaura, Yamanouchi), is also available. Dogs should receive 1 mg/kg intramuscular injection once weekly until remission every 2 weeks for a few months. Eventually doses can be tapered down to once every 1–2 months. Cats need 1–2 mg/kg i.m. every week until remission and then taper the dose in the same way as the dog dose is decreased. Side-effects include hepatotoxicity, bone marrow suppression, thrombocytopaenia, drug eruptions, proteinuria, stomatitis, sterile abscesses, eosinophilia. A complete blood count, biochemistry and urinalysis should be carried out every 2 weeks until induction treatment is completed. During remission, blood and urine tests should be run every 2–3 months. Liver enzymes in particular should be analysed.

Tetracycline (Oxycare, Animalcare) and nicotinamide (vitamin B3) are yet another treatment option. Both should be given at doses of 500 mg t.i.d. for the dog. If the dog is less than 10 kg in weight, the dose can be cut to 250 mg t.i.d. of each medication. Once remission occurs, the dose rate can be tapered down to once daily. These are relatively inexpensive drugs compared to other treatments and niacinamide can be purchased by the owner directly from a health food store. However, side-effects can still occur in the form of vomiting, diarrhoea, lethary, anorexia and increased liver enzymes. In the cat, this regime can be altered to doxycycline (Ronaxon, Merial) at 100 mg/5 kg, with, or without, the niacinamide. It is believed that this medication regime helps to interrupt the affect of the pemphigus autoantibodies on acetylcholine receptors.

Cyclosporin (Atopica, Novartis) has occassionally been used in the treatment of pemphigus but with not terribly positive effects and lots of side-effects. Dapsone (Dapsone, Alphapharma) and sulfasalazine (Salozopyrin, Pharmacia) have also been used on occasion, but again with only mild benefit despite significant side-effects.

Any drug that has been suspected of causing a previous eruption must, of course, be avoided. Unfortunately, all of the drugs used for treatment have adverse side-effects. As the treatment may need to be given for the rest of the animal's life, quality of life must be continually assessed. Perhaps 10% of owners will opt for euthanasia.

Pemphigus erythematosus

This disease is basically the same as pemphigus foliaceus but in erythematosus the lesions are predominantly on the face and ears. Occasionally the paws and genitals can also become involved. German Shepherd dogs and Rough Collies are the breeds predisposed to pemphigus erythematosus. Diagnosis and treatment is the same as for pemphigus foliaceus. Histologically, this disease is very similar to pemphigus foliaceus but there can be an interface cellular infiltrate of mononuclear cells and plasma cells, along with the neutrophils and eosinophils. Hydropic (swollen) basal cells and apoptotic epidermal cells will also be present.

Pemphigus vegetans

This occurs only in the dog. The primary lesion is a vesicle or pustule, developing into secondary lesions that are verrucous and papillomatous (types of warts). The face is most often affected. Pain and pruritus are part of the clinical signs. Diagnosis and treatment are the same as for the other forms of pemphigus. Biopsy reveals epidermal hyperplasia and intra-epidermal micro-abscesses.

Paraneoplastic pemphigus

This disease occurs in the dog only. It can occur secondarily to an internal neoplasm (e.g. mediastinal lymphoma). Paraneoplastic pemphigus is also one of the rarer forms of pemphigus. Clinical signs include vesicles on the oral mucosa and at other body orifices, or crust and vesicles on the ears and nose. These two different patterns are likened to foliaceus and vulgaris forms of pemphigus. Histologically, there will be suprabasalar as well as intra-epithelial acantholysis, kertainocyte necrosis and hydropic degeneration of basal and suprabasal cells.

Pemphigus vulgaris

This is one of the more serious forms of pemphigus because the lesions are deeper. With vulgaris, the vesicles develop into secondary lesions which are erosions and ulcers. Sites of lesions include the mucocutaneous junctions, particularly the oral mucosa. Lesions can spread to sites on the skin, specifically the axillae and groin. Half of all cases will manifest with oral lesions as the first site of the disease. Oral lesions will develop at some point during the development of the disease in 75–90% of cases. In unusual cases paronychia and onychomadesis (nail bed inflammation and loss of nails respectively) can be the only cutaneous signs. Anorexia, pyrexia and depression are systemic signs which complete the clinical picture. Diagnosis is achieved by biopsying intact lesions. As the lesions rupture so easily it is best to hospitalise the animal and examine the oral mucosa regularly. When a vesicle appears, the biopsy should be collected promptly. Histology will show deeper levels of pathology than with pemphigus foliaceus, with acantholysis appearing in the suprabasilar region of the epidermal layers. The basal cells will remain attached to the basement membrane, while clefts and vesicles form directly above the stratum basale. The attached basal cells have a 'tombstone'-like appearance. Mild to severe dermal inflammation can be observed. Treatment is the same as for foliaceus, and again, there are cases where euthanasia is the kindest option.

BULLOUS PEMPHIGOID

This is a rare blistering disorder of the dog and cat. The body creates autoantibodies to collagen in the basement membrane. This leads to the formation of vesicles, crust and erosions at the lips, pinnae, hard and soft palate, abdomen, axillae and digits. A biopsy will demonstrate subepidermal vesicles, clefts, mild to moderate lichenoid (infiltrative) inflammation, and increased eosinophils and neutrophils. Treatment is along the same lines as for other autoimmune diseases, i.e. the use of immunomodulating drugs. However, the prognosis is poor.

Mucous membrane pemphigoid is a variant on the above disease. It, too, is a subepidermal blistering disease in the dog and cat. The oral cavity, nasal planum, ear canal, eyes, anus and genitalia can be affected. Diagnosis is achieved by biopsy and treatment and should include corticosteroid therapy and steroid-sparing medications that act on the immune system. Figure 10.1 shows a lesion resulting from an autoimmune sub-epidermal blistering disease.

LUPOID DERMATOSIS

The autoimmune disease lupus comes in two forms – cutaneous lupus and systemic lupus. Lupus is caused by the formation of autoantibodies to the skin's basement membrane and/or deposits of immune complexes in affected tissue. Inflammatory infiltrate in the affected tissues consists of plasma cells, which suggests a B-lymphocyte involvement. Mononuclear cells are also present in the infiltrate and help to surround blood vessels and follicles.

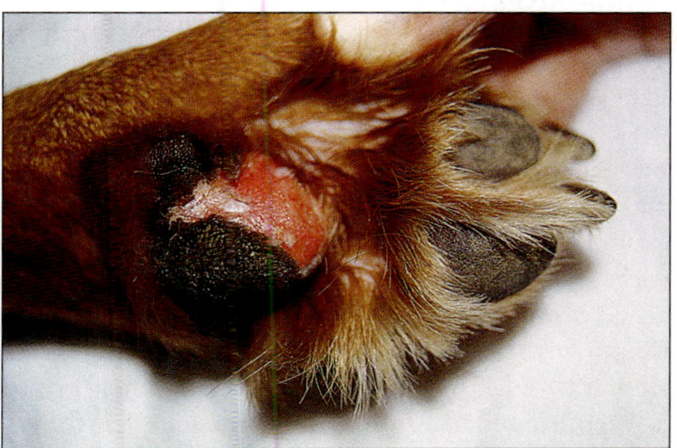

Figure 10.1 This lesion is the result of an autoimmune sub-epidermal blistering disease. Photograph by Annette Loeffler, with permission.

Keratinocyte damage is a sequel to the lymphohistiocyte infiltrate. Genetics, a virus, or an adverse drug reaction can instigate lupus. Sunlight tends to exacerbate the disease. It is believed that sunlight may stimulate autoreactive T-cells which, in turn, stimulate B cells, leading them to produce antibodies to an array of nuclear proteins found normally in the skin.

Within the definition of cutaneous lupus, there are four strains:

1. discoid lupus erythematosus (DLE)
2. lupoid dermatosis of German Shorthaired Pointers
3. lupoid symmetrical onychodystrophy
4. ulcerative Shetland Sheepdog disease.

Discoid lupus erythematosus

This disease, now also known as *photo-aggravated cutaneous lupus*, is, among autoimmune disorders, relatively common in dogs. No age or sex predilection exists but there are breeds predisposed to the disease. Smooth and Rough Collies, Shetland Sheepdogs, German Shepherd dogs, Brittany Spaniels, Siberian Huskies, German Shorthaired Pointers and Borzoi make up the list of predisposed breeds. Figure 10.2 shows a dog suffering from cutaneous discoid lupus.

The clinical signs of DLE are lesions at the borders of the nasal planum and along the dorsal nose. Depigmentation, erythema and scale occur initially, followed by a loss of cobblestone appearance as the nose becomes smooth and shiny and of a grey to white colour. Pruritus and pain are possible. Severe cases will haemorrhage at the nasal planum. There is a definite waxing and waning of the disease, often in relation to the seasons. The sunnier it is, the more acute the clinical signs will become. In later stages, the skin will show erosions, ulcers, crusts and scarring. Less frequently, lesions can affect the areas of the periocular region, the pinnae, distal limbs and the oral mucosa.

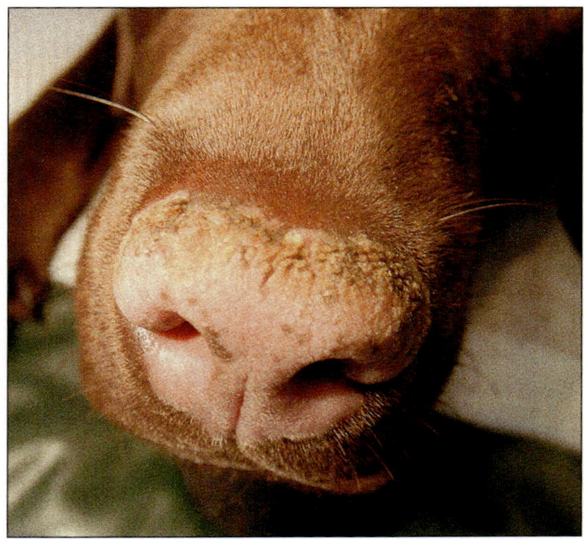

Figure 10.2 This dog is suffering from cutaneous discoid lupus. Note the depigmentation of the nasal planum. Photograph by Annette Loeffler, with permission.

The differential list associated with DLE is extensive and must be eliminated in order to achieve a diagnosis. Nasal solar dermatitis and nasal squamous cell carcinoma should be considered, along with pemphigus foliaceus and pemphigus erythematosus. Uveodermatological syndrome and epitheliotropic lymphoma are also on the differential list. Possible drug eruptions should be explored via the history. Dermatophytosis caused by fungal species less common in the dog can also cause nasal lesions, e.g. *M. gypseum*, *M. persicolor* and *Trichophyton* spp. can manifest in similar patterns to DLE.

Definitive diagnosis is attained by skin biopsy. A biopsy punch of at least 4 mm should be taken from the edge of an advancing lesion. Unfortunately, the nasal planum tends to bleed profusely so general anaesthetic is advised for this biopsy. Samples taken from other areas can be performed with a 6 mm punch. The histology of DLE exhibits a lichenoid infiltrate – this is a band of inflammatory cells running parallel to the epidermis. Deposits at the basement membrane level damage the epidermis and basement membranes, allowing the formation of subepidermal vesicles. There will be a thick basement membrane and individual cell apoptosis (controlled cell death). Remember that cell death results in the release of even more inflammatory mediators, specifically chemoattractors for lymphocytes.

The prognosis with this disease is guarded to good, but treatment must be practiced for the rest of the animal's life. Settling on the correct treatment for an individual animal may take some time. There will need to be some chopping and changing until the effective treatment for a specific dog is discovered. All affected animals should avoid the sun and sunscreen should be applied to the nose when the animal is outside for exercise. Topical steroid ointments can be used, but with care. The skin is damaged and thus absorption of the steroid will be increased. Over-zealous use of even topical steroids can cause iatrogenic hyperadrenocorticism. Topical cyclosporin can be applied by puncturing a capsule and applying it to the affected area. Handlers should wear gloves. This is an expensive treatment that may not work if it is licked off by the dog. Vitamin E, at a dose rate of 400–800 iu should be given daily; however, it takes 6 weeks before the benefits of vitamin E can be observed. The tetracycline and nicotinamide combination works as an immunomodulator. While not terribly expensive and not accompanied by severe side-effects, this combination does take several weeks to become effective. Tetracycline should be given at a dose rate of 250–500 mg three times daily. Nicotinamide should be given at a rate of 500 mg three times daily.

Further treatment options include prednisolone at 1–2 mg/kg once daily alone, or in combination with a steroid-sparing drug such as azathioprine or chlorambucil. Both of the latter drugs should be started at low doses and increased depending on the waxing and waning of the disease. Finally, severe cases may need surgical repair of the dorsal nasal planum via skin flaps.

Feline discoid lupus erythematosus

This disease is very rare. Clinical signs are periocular crusts. There may be erythema, vesicles and papules on the pinnae. Later plaques and exoriation will occur on the pinnae. Scale and crust appear on the footpads. Focal depigmentation will ensue, particularly at the nasal planum. Lesions can spread to the neck, abdomen and groin. Generalised scale and crust can develop. Biopsy should be performed for diagnosis. The histology will be similar to DLE in the dog; however, further testing is recommended. Immunofluorescence histology should be enacted. Treatment is usually oral prednisolone or dexamethasone. In recalcitrant cases injections of methylprednisolone may be used.

Lupoid dermatosis of the German Shorthaired Pointer

This is also known as 'exfoliative cutaneous lupus erythmatosus'. The age of onset is 3–36 months. Scale appears on the face, ears and dorsum, in some cases generalising over the whole body. Again, the symptoms can wax and wane. The differential diagnosis list is much different, as the clinical presentation differs greatly from DLE. With lupoid dermatosis, one should consider a keratinisation disorder, a drug eruption, sebaceous adenitis or a nutritional dermatosis. A biopsy will help to narrow the choices down. Histologically, lupoid dermatosis is quite similar to DLE. This disease is 'managed' rather than cured. Treatment should include essential fatty acids at two to three times the normal dose. Additionally, tetracycline and nicotinamide should be administered.

Symmetrical lupoid onychodystrophy

This disease occurs most frequently in the German Shepherd dog. Usually two or more claws are affected. Claws separate at the nail bed and are eventually lost. It is possible for all of a dog's claws to be lost in this manner. If the claws manage to regrow they are soft, brittle, deformed and short. Cutting claws as short as possible does not alleviate the problem. Other clinical signs include pain and lameness. Secondary infection can occur so cytology should be performed to demonstrate any bacteria present. One hopes that the affected dog has dew claws because biopsy requires removal of an entire digit. Histopathology will reveal hydropic interface dermatitis. This term refers to swollen cells causing distortion of the basement membrane.

If only one or two nails are affected, systemic antibiotics may be enough to control the disease. In more serious cases, essential fatty acids, along with tetracycline and niacinamide should be prescribed. Systemic steroids may also be necessary. Supplementation to the diet should include a mineral and vitamin supplement that contains biotin, methionine and zinc. Biometh-Z, Vetoquinol can be used at 5–10 grams per day.

Ulcerative Shetland Sheepdog disease

This disease was formerly considered a variant of dermatomyositis. Young to middle-aged dogs are affected with an ulcerative dermatitis of the ventral abdomen. Lesions can be serpigenous, annular or polycyclic. As with other forms of lupus, waxing and waning is observed and ultraviolet light can exacerbate the disease. Histopathology reveals a lymphocytic interface dermatitis with vesicles at the dermo-epidermal junction. Folliculitis occurs due to the infiltrate surrounding hair follicles. Treatment options include corticosteroids, azathioprine, tetracycline/nicotinamide combination, vitamin E and pentoxifylline. These are all various forms of immunomodulation. This form of the disease does tend to be difficult to manage.

Systemic lupus erythematosus (SLE)

This is a very rare disease that affects the musculoskeletal, haematopoietic, urinary and cutaneous systems. Affected animals should fulfil four out of the following criteria in order to 'qualify' for SLE:

- non-erosive polyarthritis
- proteinuria caused by nephropathy
- dermatopathy, including erythema, a discoid rash, photosensitivity, oral or nasopharnygeal ulcerations
- abnormal haematology, including thrombocytopaenia and leucopaenia
- serositis, pericarditis or pleuritis
- immunological disorders such as a change in the number of circulating T-cells
- a positive result on an antinuclear antibody (ANA) serology test
- systemic signs such as pyrexia, polymyositis, pneumonitis, lymphadenopathy and lymphoedema.

Cutaneous signs can be generalised or local. These signs include seborrhoea, alopecia, erythema, vesicles, bullae, hyperkeratosis of the footpads and footpad ulcers, secondary bacterial pyoderma, panniculitis and nasal dermatitis. Due to the huge number of different types of lesion possible, there is an extensive differential list. Diagnostic tests in abundance need to be put in action in order to diagnose the disease definitively. Skin tests, skin scrapes and a biopsy should be performed as well as fungal and bacterial cultures. Blood tests should start with haematology, biochemistry and urinalysis. Radiographs can follow, along with lymph node biopsy and a joint aspirate. Coombs antibody tests, serum ANA and a bone marrow aspirate are all part of the diagnostic work-up.

Concentrating on the skin, the biopsy report for an animal affected by SLE will show a lymphocyte-rich lichenoid and/or hydropic interface dermatitis. Essentially, this means swollen cells or clumps of inflammatory cells are interrupting the layers of the epidermis. The hair follicles are often involved. Vasculitis and panniculitis can occur. The histology plate will show a picture of subepidermal clefting, intrabasal and subepidermal vesicles. The basement membrane will be thickened.

If no underlying cause of the disease can be discovered (and all those diagnostic tests should be able to discover something if it's there!) immunosuppressive treatment can commence. Corticosteroid therapy, azathioprine, gold salts, chlorambucil, cyclophosphamide and tetracycline/nicotinamide medications have all been used in the treatment of lupus. As with other immunological disorders, it may take some time to find the correct treatment for a particular patient.

Feline SLE

This is similar to the canine version, and is also very rare. Clinical signs manifest with generalised seborrhoea, exfoliative erythema, alopecia, and crusts on the face, pinnae, neck, ventrum, limbs and digital pads. A biopsy of an affected cat will show a histological picture of interface dermatitis and folliculitis, epidermal and follicular basal cell vacuolation with necrosis. Treatment is achieved with corticosteroids at 4 mg/kg/day for 30 days. Remission should occur within this 30-day period.

VASCULITIS

Vasculitis is simply an inflammation of blood vessel walls. Inflammatory cells, such as macrophages, neutrophils, lymphocytes and eosinophils, accumulate in the vessels, damaging the vessel walls. Following the inflammatory influx, necrosis occurs and fibrin deposits build up along vessel walls, compromising vascular integrity. Perivascular cuffing by mononuclear cells contributes to the anoxic atmosphere. In the dermis, follicles will atrophy and collagen will be damaged. Oedema will be prevalent.

There are rare cases of primary vasculitis but most cases are secondary. A variety of conditions can cause secondary vasculitis:

- infections – bacterial, mycobacterial, fungal, viral, protozoal, rickettsial, and sarcocytosis infections
- vaccinations – rabies particularly, sera and allergen immunotherapy
- drugs – fenbendazole, itraconazole, ivermectin, metronadazole, enalapril, furosemide, imodium, metoclopramide, phenobarbitone, phenylbutazone
- allergy – to food, insects, arthropods, severe scabies, flea allergic dermatitis, eosinophilic granuloma complex
- immune-mediated – SLE, DLE, rheumatoid arthritis
- other – plasma cell pododermatitis, malignancy, ulcerative colitis, juvenile polyarthritis syndrome of beagles
- 50% idiopathic.

Some clinicians prefer to group these into infectious, non-infectious and unknown causes.

The cutaneous form of vasculitis is usually caused by a disorder of the post-capillary venules. There are several specific forms of cutaneous vasculitis: proliferative thrombovascular necrosis of the pinnae, cutaneous vasculopathy of German Shepherd dogs, cutaneous and renal vasculopathy of Greyhounds and neutrophilic leucocytoclastic vasculitis of Jack Russel Terriers. The various possible cutaneous signs are numerous. Some animals experience crusting and ulcers at extremities and bony prominences. Usually the paws, pinnae, face, lips, tail, scrotum and oral mucosa suffer lesions. Any combination of purpura, macules, plaques, haemorrhagic bullae, papules, pustules, necrosis, ulcers and acrocyanosis (lack of oxygen at skin level) can occur. Dermal oedema is inherent in the disease process, so it is not suprising that odematous plaques can form. Pitting oedema occurs on the limbs, ventral trunk, head and scrotum. Urticaria and pruritus are further cutaneous signs.

Systemic signs associated with cutaneous vasculitis are anorexia, depression, pyrexia and pain. The animal may suffer from polyarthropathy, myopathy, neuropathy, hepatopathy, thrombocytopathy, anaemia and lymphadenopathy. In other words, the systems of the body become deranged.

Cats are rarely affected, but when they are, focal ulceration occurs at the footpads, pinnae and lips. There is some anecdotal evidence linking feline vasculitis with feline leukemia and vaccination site reactions.

The differential list mostly includes diseases which are related to lack of or poor cutaneous circulation. Frostbite and cold agglutination disease figure large on the list. SLE, coagulopathies and lymphoreticular neoplasia are diseases to consider when trying to diagnose vasculitis. To further complicate the picture, vasculitis can be transitory, often followed by vasculopathy. There are many disease processes which include attack of vessel walls. Blood test results consistent with vasculitis would show lymphopaenia, leucocytosis with a left shift, leucopaenia, neutropaenia, monocytosis, normochromic anaemia, thrombocytopaenia. A biochemical analysis from serum would reveal raised liver enzymes, raised triglycerides, sub-normal albumin, raised globulins and increased fibrinogen levels.

Outside of cutaneous vasculitis, there are other forms of vasculitis with cutaneous signs. *Dermatomyositis* is a hereditary inflammatory disease that affects the skin and muscles of Rough Collies and Shetland Sheepdogs. The age of onset is usually 6 months and the disease can reach its peak as the animal approaches 12 months of age. The face, ear and tail tips, carpal and tarsal digits suffer with erythema, scale, alopecia and crust. In rare cases, the nails can also be included in the pathology.

Ulcers may evolve from earlier lesions. Myositis occurs after the dermal signs are established. The dog can suffer from dysphagia and exhibit a high-stepping gait. Atopy and necrosis of the muscles occurs – this can be ascertained via electromyogram (EMG) testing.

A skin biopsy will reveal hydropic degeneration of basal cells and hair follicles. Vasculitis will be observable on biopsy. The treatment advised is avoidance of the sun and treatment with vitamin E at 200–800 iu/day, along with a fish oil supplement. Prednisolone is also given at a dose rate of 1 mg/kg/day. Pentoxifylline may be given to decrease the required dose of prednisolone. The extent of muscle involvement determines the prognosis of the case.

Post-vaccination vasculitis occurs primarily in the United States, secondarily to rabies vaccinations. Lymphocytic inflammation and vasculitis develop in the deep dermis. Panniculitis occurs at the injection site. Surgical excision of the site is the treatment of choice.

Post-vaccination ischaemic dermatopathy can manifest with generalised lesions or focal lesions at pinnal margins, bony prominences, footpads, tail tip and periocular region. This type of vasculitis responds to vitamin E and pentoxifylline. Pentoxifylline stimulates wound healing and decreases blood viscosity. It is a very useful drug in this case as it also decreases infiltration of inflammatory cells to the skin, especially neutrophils, and inhibits pro-inflammatory cytokines. Pentoxifylline is given at 10–15 mg/kg twice or three times daily with food.

Treatment of vasculitis always has to include a search for underlying causes and treatment of these causes. Corticosteriod therapy is usually used, often with pentoxifylline to decrease the need for steroid use. Sulfasalazine and dapsone can be used as well as they decrease the damage that neutrophils cause. However, this last combination has the disadvantage of potentially causing dry eye and hepatotoxicity.

JUVENILE CELLULITIS

Juvenile cellulitis, also known as puppy strangles, is an autoimmune disorder that usually affects dogs under 6 months of age. A genetic predisposition for the disease seems to exist as multiple puppies in a litter can be affected and specific breeds, such as Dachshunds, Golden Retrievers, yellow Labradors, Gordon Setters, Lhasa apsos and Pointers, are predisposed. Clinical signs include swelling of the face and head, often with submandibular lymphadenomegaly. The lesions are nodular, and draining tracts can occur, leading to scarring if the disease is not treated promptly.

Diagnosis is attained via biopsy sampling for histopathology. Cellulitis with diffuse dermatitis and panniculitis will be reported in a positive diagnosis for juvenile cellulitis. Treatment regimes include broad-spectrum antibiotics and immunosuppressive doses (1.1 mg/kg twice daily) of corticosteroids for approximately 2 weeks. Figure 10.3 shows a puppy suffering from juvenile cellulitis.

ERYTHEMA MULTIFORMAE

This is another uncommon disease. It has a myriad of forms, appearing as flat or raised, focal or multifocal, target or polycyclic lesions. A single mucosal surface is affected in the minor form of erythema multiformae. In the major form of the disease more than one mucosal surface is lesional. The lesions are vesiculobullous in character, generally devolving into ulcers. Some cases will show maculopapular lesions instead. Lesions can also develop in the axillae, groin and footpads.

There is no age or sex predilection associated

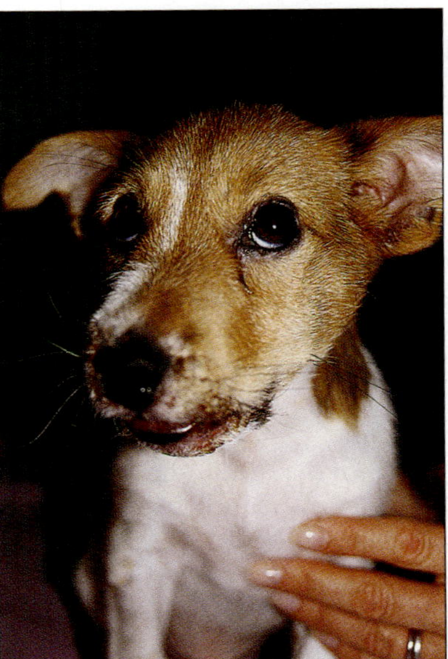

Figure 10.3 This puppy is suffering from juvenile cellulitis, which is assumed to be an autoimmune disorder. Note the oedema, erythema and alopecia. Photograph by Annette Loeffler, with permission.

with erythema multiformae. It is believed that antibiotics and potentiated sulphonamides can initiate the clinical signs. Infectious agents and neoplasia have also been considered as potential triggers. As challenge tests can aggravate the condition they have not been carried out. However, clinical signs usually manifest wthin 3 weeks of treatment with offending drugs and resolution of the pathology occurs over a 3-week period. Treatment is often deemed unnecessary.

Erythema multiformae is very rare in cats. It has been associated with the following drugs: cefalexin, amoxicillin, penicillin, griseofulvin, aurothioglucose and sulfadiazine. Lesions are similar to those seen in the dog and occur on the mucocutaneous junctions and on the trunk.

Diagnosis of erythema multiformae is obtained by biopsy. Findings would describe a full-thickness necrosis of the epidermis with subepidermal clefting in the vesicular forms of the disease. If the form is maculopapular an interface dermatitis will be found with single keratinocyte necrosis and lymphocyte and macrophage satellitosis. If the veterinary surgeon chooses to prescribe medication for erythema multiformae the standard treatment for it is prednisolone and azathioprine for the dog. Pentoxifyllin, cyclosporin and isotretinoids have also been used. Some clinicians profess the benefits of a hypoallergenic diet in case a food intolerance is the causative agent.

TOXIC EPIDERMAL NECROLYSIS (TEN)

This is a rare disease affecting the skin and oral mucosa. The type of lesion is vesicobullous, with stomatitis. Footpad lesions also occur. Pyrexia, pain and lethargy are systemic components of the disease. Biopsy is essential for a diagnosis. Full epidermal necrosis will be present. Basal cell hydropic degeneration is also possible. A history of treatment with potentiated sulphonamides or beta-lactamase antibacterials is a pertinent point in the history in some cases, although not in all. An underlying cause should be investigated. In the meantime, the animal should be given supportive treatment in the form of fluid therapy and control of secondary infection. Corticosteroid therapy may or may not help. This condition is usually fatal.

EPIDERMOLYSIS BULLOSA ACQUISITA

This is a disease which has been reported in young Great Danes. Erythema, urticaria, vesicles and ulcers can be either localised or generalised. Lesional areas include the face, groin, axillae, abdomen, foot pads, oral cavity, pinnae and mucocutaneous junctions. In the localised form, the pinnae and trunk may show scattered lesions. The autoantibody in this disease targets anchoring fibrils with the result being subepidermal blisters. Biopsies are needed to complete the diagnostic profile. Treatment is as for other autoimmune disorders discussed.

FORMULARY

Dose rates vary depending on the condition being treated and the individual animal. The BSAVA formulary can be consulted for dose rates, as can the references below. Many of these drugs are cytotoxic and should be handled with care.

Drugs marked with an asterisk are not licensed for use in small animals in the United Kingdom.

*Azathioprine (Imuran, GlaxoWellcome)
*Chlorambucil (Leukeran, GlaxoWellcome)
*Cyclophosphamide (Endoxana, AstaMedica)
Cyclosporin (Atopica, Novartis)
*Dapsone (Dapsone, Alphapharma)
Doxycycline (Ronaxon, Merial)
*Isotretinoin (Roaccutane, Roche)
*Gold salts – Auranofin (Ridaura, Yamanouchi) and Aurothiomalate (Myocrisin, JHC)
*Niacinamide/nicotinamide/vitamin B3
*Pentoxifylline (Trental, AventisPharma)
Prednisolone (various pharmaceutical companies)
*Sulphasalazione (Salazopyrin, Pharmacia)
Tetracycline (Oxytetracycline, Millpledge or Oxycare, Animalcare)
Vitamin E
Vitamin/mineral supplement with biotin, methionine, zinc (Biometh-Z, Vetoquinol)

References and Further Reading

Ackermann L, Nesbitt G 1998 Canine immune-mediated skin disease and feline immune-mediated skin disease. Canine and feline dermatology. Veterinary Learning Systems, Trenton, NJ, p 140–161, 375–387

Foster A 2002 Blistering and erosive immune-mediated disease. In: Foster A, Foil C (eds) BSAVA Manual of small animal dermatology. BSAVA Publications, Gloucester, p 197–205

Merchant S 2002 Pemphigus. In: Foster A, Foil C (eds) BSAVA Manual of small animal dermatology. BSAVA Publications, Gloucester, p 189–196

Scott D, Miller W, Griffin C 2001 Immune-mediated disorders. In: Scott D W et al (eds) Muller & Kirk's Small animal dermatology, 6th edn. W B Saunders, London, p 667–779

CASE STUDY

Pemphigus vulgaris

Signalment

Female, neutered Pointer bitch, 11 years of age, weighing 25.5 kilograms.

Complaint

Extreme redness and blistering of the gums along with salivation and severe halitosis.

History

The bitch had been treated on and off for 18 months for halitosis and gingivitis/stomatitis. Treatment had included a dental scale and polish, supplemented with home dental care with tooth brushing and a pet toothpaste. Additionally, the bitch had been treated with three different systemic antibiotics over the 18-month period. Antibiotic treatment did improve the condition for short periods of time, only for the problem to recur. Routine blood tests and thyroid function tests had been carried out showing no obvious abnormalities.

Physical examination

The bitch had a normal temperature but slightly elevated pulse and respiratory rates, possibly due to the stress of examination. Overall, her demeanour was one of depression and lethargy. Her coat was dull and greasy. Erythema and scale were visible on the cranial ventral abdomen and there was erythema interdigitally on the right forepaw. All four feet demonstrated thin footpads. The vulva was erythematous. The most obvious clinical signs were focal areas of intense, well circumscribed erythema and vesicles affecting the oral cavity. The tongue and hard palate were not affected.

Differential diagnosis

- Bacterial stomatitis (bacterial, fungal)
- Nutritional deficiency (due to overall lack of caloric intake)
- Pemphigus vulgaris
- Bullous pemphigoid

Diagnostic tests

Blood samples were taken for routine biochemistry and haematology tests. These revealed a raised cholesterol level. Swabs were taken for bacteriology. A free thyroxine (FT4) was measured by equilibrium dialysis. The result was low, at 5.8 nmol/l (normal range 7–40 nmol/l). However, the thyroid-stimulating hormone assay was within the normal range, thus likely to be consistent with euthyroid sick syndrome. Under general anaesthetic, several biopsies were taken from the oral mucosa and one from the ventral chest. The chest biopsy confirmed the scaling observed on clinical examination as hyperkeratosis. Intact vesicles were sampled from the oral cavity (see Fig. 10.4) and histopathology revealed suprabasilar clefting and epidermal separation, consistent with pemphigus vulgaris.

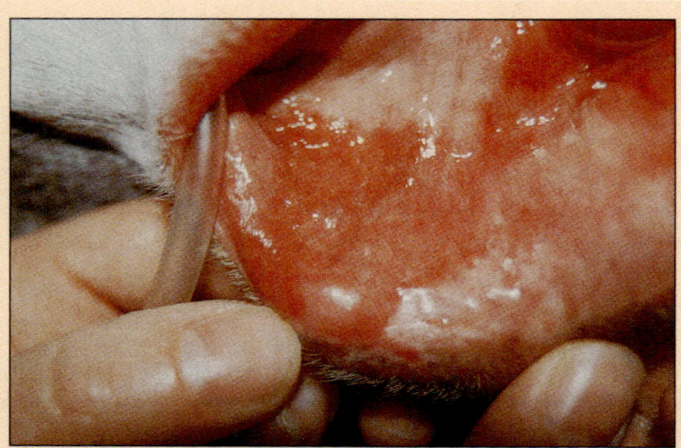

Figure 10.4 Pemphigus vulgaris. An intact vesicle is prepared for sampling. Photograph by Annette Loeffler, with permission.

Diagnosis and prognosis

The diagnosis was pemphigus vulgaris. Pemphigus vulgaris warrants a guarded prognosis because it is the most serious of the pemphigus diseases. Without treatment, pemphigus vulgaris can prove fatal, and even with aggressive treatment remission can be difficult to achieve.

Treatment

The owners' main concern was the powerful halitosis, generated by the oral ulceration and necrosis. The strength of the halitosis was prompting the owners to consider euthanasia for their pet. It was thus necessary to decrease the severity of the ulceration and secondary infection as soon as possible. Therefore, even prior to biopsy, the bitch was placed on two antibiotic therapies: clavulanate-potentiated amoxicillin (Synulox, Pfizer) at a dose rate of 15 mg/kg, twice daily for 21 days, and metronidazole (Metronidazole, Millpledge) 8 mg/kg twice daily for 10 days. The antibiotics were extended through the first month of steroid treatment because the corticosteroid doses were at their highest during this period. Further treatment was given for the scaling skin in the form of essential fatty acid supplements (Efavet, Schering-Plough). Three 550 mg capsules were to be given once daily with food.

Most importantly, the pemphigus vulgaris had to be attended to. It was decided to use prednisolone (Prednisolone, Millpledge) at an anti-inflammatory dose rate of just under 2 mg/kg twice daily (20 mg total) for 4 weeks, then 15 mg twice daily for 2 weeks, followed by 30 mg once daily for 2 weeks. The lowest therapeutic dose achieved was 10 mg every other day as a long-term maintenance treatment.

Re-inspection and final outcome

The patient was re-examined 2 weeks after diagnosis had been made. The erythema was greatly reduced, although still redder than the adjacent mucosa. The owners were pleased with the alleviation of the halitosis. Often, pemphigus vulgaris needs a more aggressive approach, such as azathioprine (Imuran, Glaxo-Wellcome). In this case, the ulceration had subsided considerably on steroids alone, so no additional drugs were added to the regime.

One week later, the bitch presented with ptyalism and a green discharge staining her ventral chin. Clinical examination pointed towards oral discomfort because the bitch had a heavy tartar growth throughout her dental arcades. It was decided that a full dental scaling should be undertaken as soon as the bitch was stabilised. An antibacterial/antifungal shampoo (Malaseb, Leo Laboratories) was prescribed as a preventative measure to keep the chin free from erythema and malodour. A swab from the chin was taken to be sure that the current antibiotics covered this infection. Culture and sensitivity revealed that there was a growth of *Pseudomonas aeruginosa*, sensitive to gentamicin and marbofloxacin. Marbofloxacin (Marbocyl, Vetoquinol) was prescribed at a dose rate of 3 mg/kg once daily.

One week later, the erythema and ulcers had completely resolved and there was no ptyalism present. Four more days of antibiotics were prescribed and the steroid dose, at this point, had reached the level of 15 mg twice daily.

Discussion

Pemphigus vulgaris is the second most rare – and the most dangerous – of the pemphigus complex. If left untreated, the disease can prove fatal

(Paterson 1998). Primarily focussed on the intra-oral region, pemphigus vulgaris can also attack the lips, nostrils, eyelids and vulva. In this bitch, the disease was sited in the vulva as well as intra-orally. Fifty percent of the afflicted will show oral lesions at the first presentation for veterinary treatment (Scott et al 2001). This was certainly the case with this Pointer, as her treatment from day one had been concentrated on regaining oral health and the reduction of halitosis – another signalling clinical sign. The depression and anorexia associated with the pemphigus complex can be overlooked as a sign of mouth pain, as can secondary bacterial infections. Clinical signs of pemphigus vulgaris can be misleading because the vesicles are transient. Biopsy is essential for diagnosis.

The difficulty with diagnosing pemphigus vulgaris is the need to biopsy a fresh lesion (Ackerman & Nesbitt 1991). It is suggested that the animal be hospitalised and examined every 2–4 hours in order to locate an intact lesion (Scott et al 2001). We were fortunate to be able to do this and our biopsies were thus diagnostic. Other methods of diagnosis include the presence of Nikolsky sign where firm, sliding pressure can cause the epidermis to separate from the basal skin layer (Ackerman & Nesbitt 1991); and the appearance of acantholytic cells on an impression smear (Harvey & McKeever 1998). However, neither of these procedures is diagnostic on its own. Histology is needed for confirmation.

Strict monitoring is required when an animal is on immunosuppressive doses of corticosteroids. Side-effects can range from the inconvenience of polydipsia and polyuria to vomiting, diarrhoea, gastric ulcers, nephrotoxicity and iatrogenic hyperadrenocorticism. Haematology and biochemistry can show raised plasma glucose and decreased T3 and T4 values. Of specific interest in dermatology patients, cutaneous atrophy and slow wound healing can occur. Side-effects can affect the quality of life such that euthanasia becomes necessary. As the owners of this pet were already considering euthanasia, and the bitch had endured 18 months of unpleasantness, aggressive treatment was a valid option.

REFERENCES

(for the Case Study)

Ackerman L, Nesbitt G 1991 Immune-mediated disease. Dermatology for the small animal practitioner. Veterinary Learning Systems, Trenton, NJ, p 89–98

Harvey R, McKeever P 1998 Skin disease of the dog and cat. Manson, London, p 98, 165

Paterson S 1998 Skin disease of the dog. Blackwell Science, London, p 167

Scott D, Miller W, Griffin C 2001 Immune-mediated disorders. In: Scott D W et al (eds) Muller & Kirk's Small animal dermatology, 6th edn. W B Saunders, London, p 669–679

Chapter 11

Neoplastic and non-neoplastic tumours

CHAPTER CONTENTS

A tumour is defined as any swelling. Cutaneous tumours can present as nodules, solid masses or fluid-filled cysts. Tumours can exist solely in the epidermis or extend deeper through the subcutis into the panniculus and into muscle tissue. There are three main categories of tumour: inflammatory tumours such as abscesses or granulomas, non-inflammatory tumours such as cysts, nevi, keratoses, cutaneous horns, and neoplasms, both benign and malignant. Figure 11.1 maps out the different types of tumour.

SKIN LUMPS COMMONLY SEEN IN PRACTICE

Abscesses

The most common lesion seen in general practice is an infectious abscess. This is an inflammatory-type lesion, caused by infection. The abscess can be identified via history ('My cat gets into fights') and empirically. In some cases diagnostic methods such as aspiration or punch biopsy are called for. The usual treatment is to lance the abscess, flush out the purulent debris and prescribe systemic antibiotics. As abscesses may contain zoonotic mycobacteria, it is wise to wear gloves and a protective apron when draining the lesion. Most lesions are left open for draining purposes. A large abscess may require a Penrose drain to reduce the dead space. Straightforward cases will heal fairly rapidly. With recurrent or non-healing abscesses, an underlying cause should be investigated (e.g. FeLV/FIV). There may be a foreign body promoting

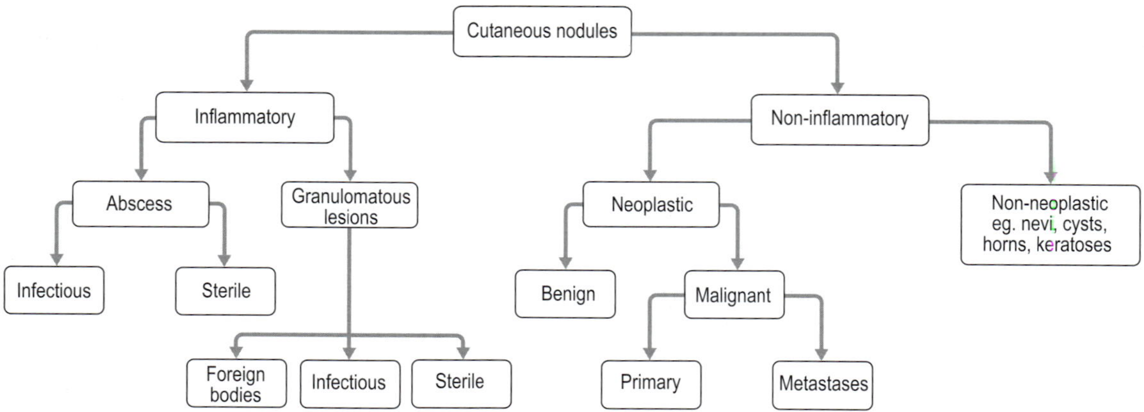

Figure 11.1 Types of tumour.

continuous infection or the type of antibiotic chosen may not be appropriate for the organism in the wound. A swab can be taken for culture and sensitivity testing. Some wounds need extensive nursing care, which cannot be carried out at home. These patients require hospitalisation or daily examinations in order to resolve their abscesses.

Lick granulomas

Lick granulomas are another common inflammatory lesion. These lesions are the result of self-induced trauma, occurring repeatedly in a specific location. Most lick granulomas occur on the anterior carpis. The underlying causes of lick granulomas include parasite infestation, allergy, joint pain and behavioural problems. The dog responds to a site of irritation by licking it obsessively to the point that granulation tissue develops as a response to the self-trauma. Unfortunately, the continuous licking creates further irritation, setting up a vicious circle of repeated injury.

The aim of treatment is to break the itch–lick cycle. Identifying an underlying cause is important, but immediate treatment is required to prevent further damage. Plastic buster collars are recommended to limit access to the site. The use of an anti-inflammatory, antibiotic cream (e.g. Fuciderm, Leo laboratories) is soothing. Additionally, creating some form of distraction can keep the animal from resorting to constant worrying at its lesion. The use of interactive toys and increased exercise can be substituted as an alternative to the self-destructive behaviour. In serious cases, the lesion will need to be removed and a long course of antibiotics prescribed. However, lick granulomas will recur if the underlying problem is not addressed.

Non-inflammatory and non-neoplastic lesions

Non-inflammatory and non-neoplastic lesions consist of hyperplastic accumulations of keratinised cells, or an excess of non-cellular material, such as collagen. There are numerous non-infllammatory cutaneous lesions which will be described briefly. Most can be treated with benign neglect, unless the location of the lesion inhibits a normal activity, such as eating. Often, owners will request removal of the growth for aesthetic reasons, or because the growth gets scratched and occasionally bleeds.

Cysts

Epidermoid (sebaceous cysts) are common in the dog, although rare in the cat. They exist in the dermis or subcutis and can be located on the head, neck, trunk or proximal limbs. Usually the cysts consist of epithelial cells and are often located at a plugged hair follicle. If opened, the cyst will discharge a thick, grey to yellow material. Avoid discharging the contents of any cyst into the dermis as this can set up a foreign body reaction. Squeezing is not recommended.

Dermoid cysts are congenital/hereditary lesions that consist of lamellated keratin, hair and sebaceous secretions. Some dermoid cysts discharge via a sinus directly to the surface of the skin. Rhodesian Ridgebacks are particularly prone to dermoid cysts.

Keratoses

The keratoses are a relatively rare group of dermatoses that often present as alopecic plaques and are non-pruritic and non-painful. These would be diagnosed on histopathological examination and are important to assess as they can be confused with squamous cell carcinomas.

Cutaneous horns

Cutaneous horns occur in the dog and the cat and can grow up to 5 cm in length. In the cat, multiple footpad horns can be a sign of FeLV. Horns can be surgically excised or removed via cryosurgery.

Hygromas

Large-breed dogs suffer from hygromas, which are acquired bursae on bony prominences. In some cases a hygroma is trauma-induced but often it is the end result of a large, overweight dog resting on hard surfaces. The hygroma is soft and fluid filled but can often become infected and ulcerate. When this occurs, it is extremely difficult to manage as you cannot tell the dog to stop resting on the limb. The lesion should be drained and bandaged and the dog provided with padded bedding. Wound breakdown is a common occurrence.

Calcinosis circumscripta

Another, albeit rare, condition that affects pressure points is calcinosis circumscripta. This is a white, gritty lesion on the elbow, tarsus joint, phalanges or tongue. German Shepherd dogs are prone to this affliction. Sometimes an underlying renal problem is the cause of these deposits. These deposits can also occur with hyperadrenocorticism.

Specific test procedures

Non-neoplastic and inflammatory lesions can easily be mistaken for skin neoplasms and vice versa on initial examination. Therefore, further investigations are necessary. History and clinical examination may give clues and point towards broad categories of tumours but owners should be made aware that tumours cannot be diagnosed on gross examination.

The first diagnostic test usually performed with growths is a *fine-needle aspirate* (FNA) for cytological examination. Not all tumours lend themselves to aspiration, but in many cases you can get useful information quickly and cheaply by employing FNA. For the anxious owner, being able to give them some information on the same day is very important. No one can diagnose the type of tumour by just feeling it. An FNA should not be used to completely rule out neoplasia because only a small part of the lump is being sampled and examined. For example, there are cases reported where a mast cell tumour existed within a lipoma. However, FNA can help to narrow the list of differential diagnoses. Early diagnosis usually leads to a better prognosis. If an animal is older or too debilitated for other reasons, choosing not to do any diagnostic tests is probably appropriate for that pet and owner. However, every owner should be given the opportunity to make a choice about whether or not they want a lump tested. The procedure for a fine-needle aspirate is listed below. This test can be conducted by a veterinary nurse but the slides should be examined by someone experienced in identifying neoplastic cells. It is always wise to send two slides to an outside laboratory for analysis, in addition to keeping another slide or two for in-house examination.

Figure 11.2 gives guidelines on interpreting cytology of lumps and swellings.

1. Gently clip or scissor away hair on lesion. Wipe the lesion once with spirit.
2. Insert a 23 gauge needle, with or without a syringe, into the lump and re-direct it several times. A very firm lesion may require a bigger gauge. Remove the needle from the lump.
3. Attach a 5 ml syringe, half filled with air, onto the needle and blow the contents of the needle onto a slide.
4. Gently squash the sample with another slide or smear the sample along the slide as if making a blood film. You are trying to create a layer that

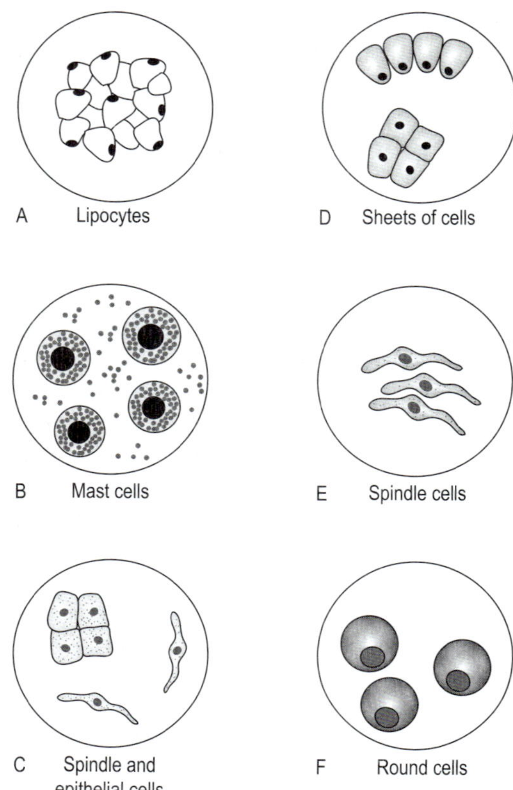

Figure 11.2 Guidelines on interpreting cytology of lumps and swellings.
A: Large, foamy cells with small, unusually placed nuclei. No cytoplasm to speak of. This is a fine-needle aspirate consistent with a lipoma.
B: Mast cells are large, with a single, large nucleus. The cytoplasm is full of purple-staining granules when Diff-Quik is used. A slide with several mast cells, some degranulating, is indicative of a mast cell tumour.
N.B. Cells can be easily damaged, causing degranulation; thus, degranulation can be genuine or forced.
C: This fine-needle aspirate has produced a slide with both epithelioid cells (rectangular cells) and spindle cells. Both types of cell are full of melanin granules. This could indicate a melanoma.
D: Sheets of cells joined together is suggestive of an epithelial cell tumour such as basal cell, squamous cell carcinoma, hair follicle or sweat gland tumour.
E: A uniform population of spindle cells with extended arms and poorly staining cytoplasm may be a spindle cell tumour. These include fibromas, haemangiomas and haemangiopericytomas, among others.
F: This fine-needle aspirate is of round cells. If the population is primarily round cells, a tumour such as a histiocytoma, lymphoma or plasmacytoma is possible.

is one cell thick. Do not press so hard that the cells are damaged.

5. Repeat the procedure until you have four slides of sample material. Allow slides to air-dry or heat fix.
6. Use 'Diff-Quik' stains to prepare the slides. If the slides have been heat-fixed, you can skip the first solution (the fixative stain). Prepare two slides for in-house viewing. Two slides should be left unstained to send to a professional laboratory if you wish to extend the test to that level.
7. Examine the slides under low power first, then with the oil-immersion lens. Some authors recommend the use of a coverslip for a better image.

Other stains can be used if looking at particular structures. Methylene blue is used for nuclear details and Leishman's, Wright's and Giesma stains are helpful for examining cellular detail.

Mast cells are large, round cells with granules. Benign cells are more uniform in their nuclear size and the manner in which they take up stain. There will be more variation in the size and shape of malignant cells. The size of the nuclei vary with malignant cells and multinucleated cells can occur. Numerous mitotic figures are commonly associated with malignant cells.

Epithelial cell tumours are well-defined cells with good cell-to-cell adhesion. They aspirate into sheets on a slide for easy viewing. Spindle cell tumours have medium to large cells which clump and do not aspirate easily. There is poor cell adhesion and cells may show indefinite margins. Identifying the exact cell type is difficult. Round cell tumours exfoliate well and create a slide of well-defined, often distinctive cells. Mast cells, plasma cells, lymphocytes, monocytes and melanocytes can be identified from round cell tumours.

By using the FNA technique, you can narrow your list of differential diagnoses. Usually, you can identify round cell tumours. Sometimes you can identify a specific type of tumour. For example, if you find multiple mast cells, you are likely to be dealing with a mast cell tumour. Mast cells are large, round cells with granules. If you suspect a mast cell tumour, you can plan the surgery needed to remove this type of tumour – wide margins of at least three centimetres in each tissue plane. Further investigations into metastasis should also be initiated.

If you find lipocytes, you are probably dealing with a lipoma. Lipomas, on aspiration, will generate a thin, oily smear of fatty cells. Cells must be examined for the slight possibility of a malignant liposarcoma. Lipomas are the most common cutaneous tumours. However, it is possible for a mast cell tumour to exist within a lipoma. Thus, it is important that you make sure your aspirate is representative, drawing material from deep within the growth. Your diagnosis can only be as good as the sample taken. If it is a particularly large growth, excision biopsy or a tru-cut biopsy is a better course of action if you hope to get a representative sample. Aspirates from lymph nodes are indicated if any nodes feel swollen or hard. Evidence of any cell other than lymphoid cells is very often an indication of metastasis.

A variation on the fine-needle aspirate is the impression smear. This is done when the tumour has an ulcerated surface, exposing deeper layers of tissue. One can gently remove any surface crust and debris and then lightly swab the area. A glass slide is then placed directly onto the tumour. The slides are prepared in the same manner as for fine-needle aspirates.

Although cytology from an FNA or impression smear can be useful to identify some tumours and tumour types, in most cases, biopsy for *histopathological examination* is required to make a diagnosis. Two types of biopsy can be collected: incisional or excisional. Incisional biopsies are done with biopsy punches, tru-cut blades, or as wedges or ellipses. The technique depends on the location of the tumour, its density and size. Small tumours are best assessed by punches and deep tumours by tru-cut. Wedges are usually taken from larger tumours, often when a margin between healthy and diseased tissue is required. Incisional biopsies can usually be harvested under sedation and local anaesthetic except for at the head and paws. Lignocaine is one local anaesthetic that can be used, reducing the cost for the owner and stress for the patient. The area should be gently clipped or scissored and then wiped lightly with a spirit swab. It is important not to do a full surgical scrub as this will eliminate surface cells that may be needed for diagnosis. One millilitre (1 ml) of lignocaine can be injected around the site of the intended incision. The sample is taken after the lignocaine has been given a few minutes to be absorbed. Once obtained, the sample should be placed in 10% formalin. The ratio of solution to mass should be at least 10:1. Great care should be taken when handling formalin solution. Soluble suture material can be used to close the wound edges.

Incisional biopsies are used for histology and grading and can, therefore, be helpful in giving a prognosis and plan for what surgery is required. Excisional biopsy allows histology and grading, while also removing the tumour and allowing assessment of margins within the healthy tissue. Margins will vary in size depending on the tumour being excised. Mast cell tumours require a 3 cm margin at every plane of the tumour. In many cases, excisional biopsy is curative, but not in all cases. Owners must be told before the surgery that removing the tumour does not always mean removing the cancer. Margins can be messy, or metastasis may have already occured. Recurrence is common with some types of tumour.

Excisional biopsies generally require a full anaesthetic, particularly if the lump removed occurs on the head or feet. Older animals and animals with systemic signs should be blood tested to assess their ability to tolerate a general anaesthetic. Some types of tumour bleed excessively (e.g. haemagiocytomas) and it is possible for a patient to bleed to death in extreme cases. Mast cell tumours, when manipulated, release vasoactive substances that can make monitoring the anaesthetic a nightmare. Do not take lump removal lightly. This is a surgical procedure. Owners should be well informed regarding the risk of anaesthetic, wound breakdown and haemorrhage.

Preparation of the area is the same as with incisional biopsy, without the administration of local anaesthetic. Preservation of the lump is, again, in formalin. Large lumps should have parallel cuts in them so that formalin can reach into the deeper tissue. All samples should be fully labelled with the date, patient's name, and location of the lesion. The jars should be tightly sealed and taped over once. Sufficient absorbent material should be wrapped around each jar so that if the formalin should leak it will be absorbed by the cotton wool provided in the packing and will not contaminate post office personnel. Pots and packing should be placed in a jiffy envelope or box marked 'pathological samples' and posted on a weekday. Avoid the weekend post. Make sure laboratory forms are filled out as completely as possible with any relevant history. The more details the laboratory has, the more accurate the diagnosis.

Some types of neoplasms can be graded by the pathologist. The higher the grade, the worse the prognosis. As an example, grades one to three for mast cell tumours are as follows:

Grade One: Large, plentiful granules with deep purple to red staining. Clearly defined cytoplastic boundaries. Regular spherical nuclei. Rare or non-existent mitotic figures.

Grade Two: Even more plentiful granules. Cells so closely packed that they are beginning to lose differentiation. The nucleus-to-cytoplasm ratio is lower. A few mitotic figures are observed.

Grade Three: Few granules appear but there are frequent mitotic figures. The cell boundaries are irregular. Nuclei are large and irregular.

Grading, combined with the location of the tumour and the presence or absence of systemic signs, helps to decide which diagnostic tests to do next. A plan of action can be created and a preliminary prognosis can be established, even at the first consultation. This saves valuable time and may be the difference between life and death. Some tumours, for example, aggressive grade 3 mast cell tumours, grow very quickly.

In order to get a fuller picture of how the tumour has behaved so far, or whether it has spread from its primary site, staging needs to take place. Staging involves histopathological analysis of the tumour and adjacent lymph nodes or nearest internal organ. Biopsies are taken from the tumour and usually aspirates from the lymph nodes are harvested. Biopsies can be taken from nodes and adjacent tissue, however, if this is deemed to be necessary. The World Health Organisation (WHO) has five levels of staging for neoplastic tumours:

0: one tumour completely excised from dermis
1: one tumour in dermis with no lymph node involvement
2: one tumour in dermis with lymph node involvement
3: multiple tumours or a large, infiltrating tumour with or without lymph node involvement
4: a tumour with distant metastasis or a recurrence of a tumour with metastasis (Hendrick et al 1998).

NEOPLASTIC CUTANEOUS LESIONS

A neoplasm is literally a 'new growth'. Neoplasms develop faster that the tissue surrounding them. Neoplasms also grow in a continuous but inconsistent pattern. History and clinical examination can help to guide one towards the category of neoplasia from which to seek a diagnosis. For example, a previous history of neoplasia with subsequent appearance of lumps in the same area raises suspicion of recurrence. A button-like tumour on the extremities of the head of young dogs is often a histiocytoma, but should still be investigated because a definitive diagnosis can be made only with histopathology of biopsy samples or, occasionally, with a fine-needle aspirate. Examining a tumour clinically may give you an indication of whether the tumour is benign or malignant. If the growth has characteristics of a malignant tumour, it is important to begin diagnostic procedures immediately. However, all tumours should be investigated as a clinical examination cannot provide a definitive diagnosis. A brief chart of tumour characteristics can be consulted (see Table 11.1).

Neoplastic cutaneous lesions are grouped in a variety of ways. The cytological grouping includes the categories of epithelial tumours, round cell tumours and spindle cell tumours. An alternative method of categorisation is histopathologically. These groupings are the epidermal tumours, mesenchymal tumours and haematopoietic tumours. In this chapter we will use the first method of organising tumours – see Table 11.2.

Epithelial tumours

Papilloma

This is a common canine tumour, often referred to as a wart. There are many different types of benign, exophytic skin tumours caused by the papilloma virus. They consist of hyperkeratotic stratified squa-

Table 11.1 Tumour characteristics

Benign neoplasia	Malignant neoplasia
Slow growing	Rapid growing
Growth limited or encapsulated	Growth unrestricted
Growth by expansion into local tissues	Infiltrates into local tissue
Mobile attachment to underlying structures	Firmly attached to underlying tissue
Does not easily ulcerate unless traumatised	Ulceration common
Does not create systemic signs	Metastasis possible
	Systemic signs co-exist

mous epithelium and may have a fibrovascular stalk. In the young dog, this tumour often appears in the oral cavity and usually will regress spontaneously although they can be contagious for up to 30 days. In older dogs and cats, the papilloma usually appears on the face, eyelids, conjunctiva and footpads, but can appear anywhere. Although the papilloma is usually benign it can ulcerate, in which case it should be removed. Papillomas are also removed if they get in the way of normal function such as eating, or blinking. Surgical excision, cryosurgery or electrocautery can be used to remove papillomas. Papillomatosis is shown in Figure 11.3.

Table 11.2 Classification of tumours

Type of tissue	Example of tumour
Epithelial	Papilloma Squamous cell carcinoma Basal cell tumours Hair follicle tumours Sweat gland adenomas and carcinoma Sebaceous adenoma and carcinoma Hepatoid adenoma and carcinoma Melanocytoma and malignant melanomas
Round cell	Canine Langerhans cell tumour (histiocytoma) Lymphoma (cutaneous and epitheliotropic) Plasmacytoma Mast cell tumour
Spindle cell	Lipoma and liposarcoma Fibrosarcoma Haemangiopericytoma Haemangioma, haemangiosarcoma Lymphangioma, lymphangiosarcoma
Tumours metastatic to the skin	Various

Squamous cell carcinomas (SCC)

These malignant tumours are common in both the dog and cat. Animals that live in sunnier areas tend to have a higher incidence of this tumour than do residents of more northern climates. There are two forms – a protruding or proliferative version that has a cauliflower-like appearance, and a destructive type than invades the dermo-epidermal junction. In the dog, the tumour usually appears on the ventral abdomen, nasal planum or nail bed. Dalmations, English Bull Terriers, Boxers and Poodles are more prone to SCCs than are other breeds. In the cat,

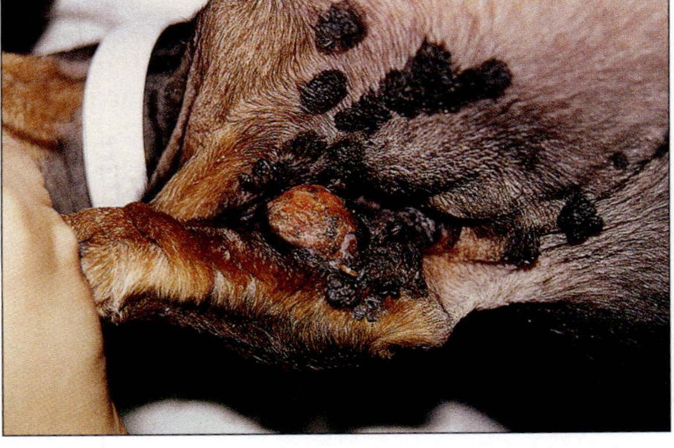

Figure 11.3 This dog is exhibiting papillomatosis, the disease state of multiple papillomas. Photograph by Annette Loeffler, with permission.

favoured locations are the ear tips, lower eyelid and nasal planum. White cats and cats with white areas of fur are several times more likely to develop SCCs. The average age of onset is 9 years. Squamous cell carcinomas rarely metastasise, unless the tumour has initially occurred at the nailbed. However, they are locally invasive.

Histopathologically, this tumour looks like cords of epidermal cells infiltrating into the dermis. The nuclei are large and there is significant mitotic activity. Some of the tumour cells are surrounded by a ring of keratin with a necrotising tumour cell at the centre. Neutrophils are attracted to these areas of necrosis.

Surgical excision and/or radiation therapy are used to treat squamous cell carcinomas.

Basal cell tumours

This term is a misnomer as it is used to describe a large group of common benign tumours of the dog, that are not strictly basal in origin. Most so-called 'BCTs' are solid lobules separated by fibrous stroma. Histopathologically, there are several different forms possible: cystic, medusa pattern, garland, adenoid, cystic, basosquamous and solid. Large basal cell tumours will ulcerate, and alopecia commonly occurs at the tumour site. However, most are encapsulated, so are easy to remove by surgical excision.

Benign feline basal cell tumours originate in basal cell tissue. These tumours can be multiple, and even invasive but are rarely diagnosed. The common sites of occurrence are the head, neck, dorsum and limbs.

Basal cell carcinomas occur at the basal cell layers of the epidermis and adnexa. Although malignant, these tumours grow slowly. Metastasis and recurrence does not often take place. Basal cell carcinomas are common in cats but rare in dogs.

Fine needle aspirates can be used to differentiate BCTs from Mast Cell tumours but histopathology for all types of basal cell tumours is recommended for definitive diagnosis. Treatment is by surgical excision.

Hair follicle tumours

Hair follicle tumours are common in the dog, with Cocker Spaniels, Poodles and Kerry Blue Terriers being predisposed to this type of tumour. These tumours are usually benign in nature. Types of hair follicle tumours are: trichoepithelioma, pilomatrixoma, tricholemmoma, trichoblastoma and intracutaneous keratinising acanthoma. Surgical excision often solves the problem but multiple tumours may require retinoid therapy.

Trichoepitheliomas are slow growing but can begin as 0.5 cm tumours and expand up to 10 cm growths. They do tend to ulcerate, so should be removed, despite their benign behaviour. Cocker Spaniels and Basset Hounds can be prone to this type of tumour.

Pilomatrixoma is a tumour of the hair matrix. In rare cases it can metastasise to the lungs. Poodles and Kerry Blue Terriers may succumb to this type of tumour.

Tricholemmomas are rare tumours which occur in middle-aged to older dogs. The tumour develops from the root sheath of the hair follicle into a firm, round mass of up to 7 cm. Sites generally occur on the head and neck.

Trichoblastomas originate from the hair germ and usually occur in dogs older than 5 years. These tumours are solitary, firm, dome-shaped lesions of 1–2 cm in diameter. The lesions can become alopecic and may ulcerate, and the skin may darken. In the dog, common sites of occurrence are the head (especially the ear base) and the neck. In the cat, these lesions tend to occur on the cranial trunk. A trichoblastoma is shown in Figure 11.4.

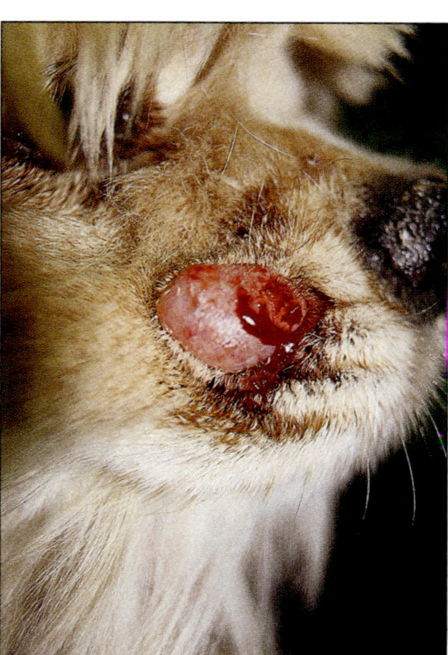

Figure 11.4 Trichoblastomas are an example of a hair follicle tumour. Photograph by Annette Loeffler, with permission.

The *intracutaneous keratinising acanthoma* (formerly known as the intracutaneous cornifying epithelioma) is a rare tumour that affects Norwegian Elkhounds. Typically, it is 1–4 cm in size with a central pore containing a keratin plug. Benign in nature, these tumours only need excision for aesthetic purposes.

Melanomas

Melanomas are common in the dog and rare in the cat. These types of tumour can be benign or malignant. Scottish Terriers, Boston Terriers, Airedales, Cocker Spaniels, Boxers, Chow Chows, Dobermans and Chihuahuas are prone to melanomas. The disease occurs more often in older animals and more often in males. Usually, there is a single lesion which occurs on the face, feet, trunk or scrotum. Malignant lesions tend to appear on the lips, eyelids, digits or scrotum. Melanomas in the cat tend to be malignant more often than benign. Benign melanomas appear as small, pigmented nodules that grow slowly. Malignant melanomas grow rapidly and ulcerate. Metastasis takes place early on and transfers the disease to the lymph nodes, liver and lungs. Surgical excision should be wide and chemotherapy can be given as adjunctive treatment; however, the prognosis for malignant tumours is poor, especially if they occur in the oral region.

Sweat gland tumours

Epitrichial adenomas are solitary, slow-growing tumours that affect older animals. The tumour tends to be well-circumscribed and will appear on the head, neck, back or flanks. The usual size is 1–4 cm. They are common tumours in dogs that can generally be cured via surgical excision. On the other hand, epitrichial adenocarcinomas are rapid-growing and invasive and tend to metastasise. They are poorly defined and infiltrate into deeper layers of the skin. There is a high incidence of ulceration and haemorrhage. In the cat, the tumour appears at the base of the ear, on the dorsal skull, neck and the tailbase. The usual size is 1–2 cm. As the disease progesses, metastases to the lungs and local lymph nodes occur. The prognosis depends on how early these tumours are caught.

Atrichial adenomas and adenocarcinomas are uncommon tumours of the eccrine sweat glands. Eccrine glands exist on the footpads so one can expect to see swelling of the foot pads and digits. In the cat, there can be multiple tumours in this region. It can be difficult to differentiate these tumours from SCCs. Sweat gland tumours often ulcerate and can also cause lysis of bone. The adenocarcinoma version is very aggressive, leading to local infiltration and metastases. Treatment requires amputation of the affected toe(s). Chemotherapy can be helpful but the prognosis given should be guarded to poor.

Sebaceous gland tumours

Cocker Spaniels, Kerry Blue Terriers, Boston Terriers, Beagles, Dachshunds and Basset Hounds are prone to the three types of sebaceous gland tumour. The first, the adenoma, is a slow-growing tumour, usually appearing at multiple sites. The average size is 0.5–2 cm. Haemorrhage can occur when removing these tumours, or when the dog traumatises the site. These are very common tumours in older dogs.

Sebaceous epitheliomas are similar in appearance and behaviour to basal cell tumours. Sebaceous adenocarcinomas are rapidly growing tumours but they rarely metastasise. Surgical excision or cryosurgery is recommended.

Hepatoid/perianal gland adenoma and hepatoid/perianal gland adenocarcinoma

The perianal gland adenoma is very common in the older dog, especially entire male dogs. Cocker Spaniels, Beagles, English Bull Terriers, Afghans, Dachshunds and Samoyeds tend to be over represented in the afflicted breeds. The tumour can appear in the perianal area, on the ventral tail, on the prepuce, or in the lumbosacral region. In appearance, the tumour is firm and nodular with a tendency to ulcerate and bleed profusely. Typically, growth is slow. Castration can resolve the problem in the majority of cases. All ulcerated tumours should be removed. Unfortunately, local recurrence is common.

Perianal adenocarcinomas are rare. These are rapidly growing, malignant tumours with a high tendency to metastasise. Excision is often not curative as recurrence is common with metastasis. Radiation therapy has proved to be of some use in treating these tumours.

Round cell tumours

Mast cell tumours (MCT)

These tumours comprise 8–15% of all malignant neoplasms in dogs. Mast cell tumours can appear anywhere on the body, although they more often occur on the perineum, prepuce and distal limbs. Tumours occurring at the scrotum, prepuce and perinanal region tend to be highly malignant. The average age of onset is 8 years and the breeds predisposed to this type of tumour are: Boxers, Boston Terriers, Bull Terriers, Fox Terriers, Dachshunds, Labradors and Weimaraners.

Grossly, MCTs create alopecia and erythema at the site of the tumours. Nodules of oedema are also possible. The tumour can be a few millimetres to 10 cm in size. In fact, mast cell tumours can resemble any other tumour. A fine-needle aspirate reveals large, round cells with granulated cytoplasm. The granules stain dark red to purple. Aspirates are used for identifying the tumour, which helps the clinician to set up a treatment plan. Biopsy and histopathology are used to grade the tumour, while fine-needle aspirates and excisional biopsies of lymph nodes and other organs are required for clinical staging. Surgical excision is performed to remove the tumour, but requires a 3 cm margin at all planes. This is not possible in some anatomical locations. Incomplete margins, lymph node involvement and metastases require further treatment past excision. Radiation therapy is the best option but in the UK this is available only at Cambridge University. The use of vinblastine as chemotherapy can be of some use, but is not tremendously successful. Prednisolone is commonly provided as adjunctive therapy.

The systemic effects of MCTs must also be considered. Mast cells release heparin, histamine and other vasoactive substances. These chemicals cause local and generalised inflammation, as well as changes in blood pressure which complicate any procedure requiring anaesthetics. Bruising and bleeding are more likely to occur intraoperatively. Even if the tumour is merely palpated, significant bruising could occur. This is referred to as Darier's sign and is a useful diagnostic measure, albeit an unsightly one. The gastrointestinal system may also be adversely affected by MCTs, leading to increased acid secretion and hypermotility. Affected patients require a drug such as cimetidine to counteract the gastrointestinal effects of MCTs.

MCTs in felines appear in older cats (average age: 10 years) as firm nodules or papules with alopecia. Pruritus is variable and ulceration is possible. The most common locations are the head and neck. The tumours are sometimes multicentric. If there is a single, well-differentiated tumour, surgical excision can lead to a more positive prognosis. However, the majority of feline MCTs metastasise early and present a poor prognosis.

A sub-type of feline MCT tumour occurs in Siamese cats aged 6 weeks to 4 years. Multiple cutaneous nodules appear on the head but often resolve without intervention.

Figure 11.5 shows an ulcerated mast cell tumour.

Cutaneous histiocytomas

These are now referred to as canine Langerhans cell tumours. They occur in dogs aged between

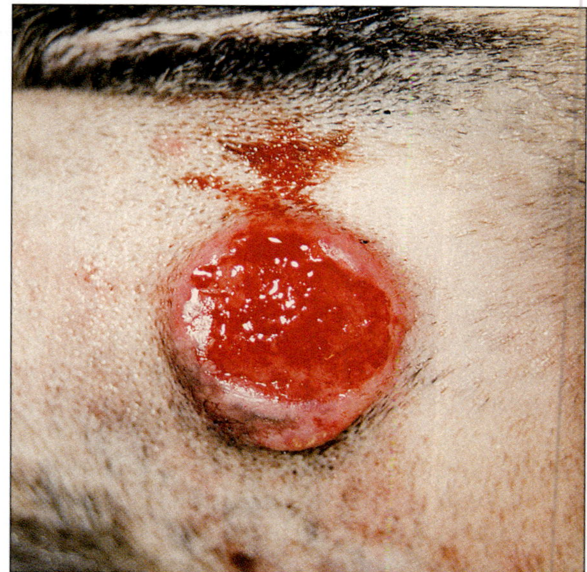

Figure 11.5 This mast cell tumour has ulcerated. Photograph by Annette Loeffler, with permission.

3 months and 13 years, but most often occur in younger dogs. Histiocytomas are very common in dogs and quite rare in cats. Boxers, Labradors, Great Danes and Cocker Spaniels have a breed predisposition to histiocytomas. Histiocytomas are usually about 2 cm in diameter, creating erythema and alopecia at the site of the growth. Commonly affected sites include the ears and feet. This is a benign neoplasm; however, cytology will, perversely, show high numbers of mitotic figures. Metastasis of this type of tumour is not recorded, and the growth usually resolves spontaneously within 3 months. However, surgical excision is often performed for diagnostic purposes or because the lump is pruritic and is ulcerated by patient interference.

Figure 11.6 shows reactive histiocytosis.

Fibrous histiocytomas occur in dogs and cats but are rare. Younger dogs, especially collies, are predisposed. The tumours are firm nodules which are well-circumscribed and usually multiple, with an average diameter of 0.5–7 cm. The common sites of occurrence are the face and feet, although they can occur on the cornea. A malignant form of this tumour also exists in cats and dogs but again is rare. The malignant fibrous histiocytoma is a solitary, firm tumour which tends to occur on the limbs and neck. The growth pattern is invasive.

Lymphoma

Cutaneous lymphosarcoma is an uncommon tumour in both dogs and cats. There are epitheliotrophic and non-epitheliotrophic forms. The epitheliotrophic form is actually a collection of diseases, of which mycosis fungoides predominates. Four types of lesions present within the mycosis fungoides disease state. A) Generalized pruritus, erythema and scale. B) Erythema, depigmentation and ulceration at mucocutaneous sites. C) Solitary or multiple plaques or nodules. D) Ulceration of the oral mucosa often with hyperkeratinization of the footpads. Due to the broad spectrum of the dermatological lesions, more common skin diseases should be eliminated first, particularly allergy and autoimmune diseases.

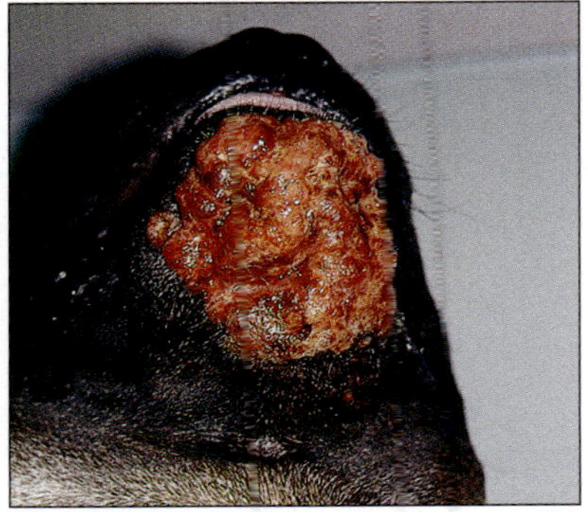

Figure 11.6 Reactive histiocytosis with severe secondary bacterial infection. Photograph by Annette Loeffler, with permission.

Definitive diagnosis is attained through biopsies. The prognosis is poor, with an average life expectancy of five to ten months. Combinations of chemotherapy can be used to extend life span but are not terribly successful. Chemotherapy protocols tend to be expensive and require repeat blood testing to ascertain the animal's white blood cell count. Therapy needs to be adjusted if neutropenia (a common side effect of chemotherapy) develops. Usually prednisolone is given as a palliative treatment.

The non-epitheliotrophic form of cutaneous lymphosarcoma is a multifocal or generalized disease showing erythema, exfoliative dermatitis and nodules at the dermo-epidermal junction. Single or multiple plaques, nodules and ulcers occur with acute or chronic pruritus. In some cases, pathological signs occur in the eye as well as the skin. Diagnostic procedures should include fine needle aspirates and skin biopsies at the lesional sites and, also, fine needle aspirates of the lymph nodes and bone marrow aspirates. A complete blood count should be taken, along with thoracic and abdominal radiographs. A thorough ophthalmology exam is also in order. Single tumours can be excised but most treatment modalities require chemotherapy protocols. The prognosis is poor.

Treatment again involves extensive chemotherapy regimes, which can be costly to the owner and stressful to the patient. The owner needs to be carefully educated regarding chemotherapy. Many owners believe that chemotherapy is curative, as it is meant to be in humans. However, in pets, chemotherapy is given at much lower doses. The side effects are much less devastating than in humans, however the dose level is not sufficient to effect a full cure. Chemotherapy in animals is designed to achieve remission, not cure.

Secondary cutaneous lymphosarcoma can also occur as a metastasis from internal lymphoma. However, this is very rare. The dermatological signs are the same as for primary cutaneous lymphosarcoma and the treatment protocol is as for other lymphosarcomas.

Plasmacytoma

These tumours are common in dogs but rare in cats. Usually older dogs, of no particular breed predilection, are affected. Common sites of occurrence include the feet, trunk, ears and oral cavity. Sometimes tumours can appear at mucocutaneous junctions. The lesions are raised and erythematous, often with ulceration. They can range in size from 2 to 5 cm.

The cutaneous and oral forms of plasmactyoma tend to be benign. However, the tumour should be thoroughly investigated as it is difficult to differentiate from other, more sinister, round cell tumours. Excisional biopsy is curative if the lesion is found to be a plasmacytoma.

Spindle cell tumours

Lipoma and liposarcoma

Lipomas are very common in the dog (especially older dogs), but rare in the cat. A lipoma can be anywhere from 0.5 to 30 cm in size. When palpated, they usually feel well-defined and moderately mobile within the subcutaneous tissue. Palpation should not be painful. They can occur anywhere where there is adipose tissue. Obesity is a risk factor with this type of tumour. Specific breeds, namely Labradors, Cocker Spaniels, Dachshunds and Weimeraners, are more at risk for developing lipomas.

Lipomas can be diagnosed by fine-needle aspirate. A thin sheen of fat will appear on the slide. The primary differential for lipomas is the MCT, as they both feel soft and fleshy on palpation. When collecting material for an aspirate, make sure that it is a sample representative of the whole tumour. It is not unheard of for MCTs to exist within lipomas.

Lipomas are slow growing but can reach a considerable size. Large intramuscular growths can lead to lameness. The tumour should be measured with calipers and the location and size recorded in the patient's chart. Lipomas are well encapsulated and have a poor blood supply – so that surgical excision tends to be uncomplicated. Large masses may leave behind dead space, which will need to be managed with a Penrose drain.

Liposarcomas are rare spindle cell tumours. Wide surgical excision is recommended but metastasis is rare. Liposarcomas are usually solitary tumours of the ventral abdomen or thorax. Dachshunds and Brittany Spaniels are predisposed.

Fibroma and fibrosarcoma

Fibromas are common in the cat, though less common in the dog. Dog breeds most affected are the Boxer, Boston Terrier and the Fox Terrier. Females tend to suffer more than males. The limbs, flank and groin are areas where growths appear. If the neoplasms are unsightly or uncomfortable they can be removed.

Fibrosarcomas are malignant tumours common to both the dog and cat. Again, female dogs are more prone than males and Cocker Spaniels are the breed most affected. Solitary lesions occur on the trunk or limbs. Fibrosarcomas show rapid growth and infiltration, with a quarter of all tumours metastasising to other regions. In cats, the tumours can occur at injection sites, particularly rabies vaccines. Wide surgical excision is recommended, which is not easy if the injection site chosen was the thorax. It has been suggested that injections may be better given in the proximal limbs, as amputation of a limb is simpler than removing a tumour from the dorsal neck region. Local recurrence is a frequent phenomenon. Radiation and chemotherapy have been used in treatment but are not effective if metastasis has already occurred.

Fibrosarcomas can occur in kittens less than 4 months old as a FeLV-related disease. These sarcomas are multicentric.

Haemangiopericytoma

These tumours are common in the dog but rare in the cat. Affected dogs are usually older and often from the following breeds: German Shepherd dogs, Boxers, Springer Spaniels, Cocker Spaniels and Fox

Terriers. The tumour is generally a solitary, firm lesion of 2–25 cm in diameter. The lesion is well defined and is most likely to occur on the limbs. As these tumours can grow so large, surgical excision with adequate margins can be difficult. Therefore, recurrence is common.

Haemangioma and haemangiosarcoma

Haemangiomas occur often in the dog but rarely in the cat. Boxers are often prone to this type of tumour. A benign tumour of the endothelial cells of the blood vessels, this tumour can appear pigmented due to its vascularisation. Haemangiomas are actinic (caused by UV rays) in origin. Usually single lesions, these often occur on the flanks, limbs and head. They are slow growing, firm and well-defined growths of 0.5–3 m in size. Surgical excision can be practised but haemorrhage is a risk.

Haemangiosarcomas are rare tumours in both the dog and cat. German Shepherd dogs, Boxers and Bernese Mountain dogs suffer from these malignant tumours. Appearing as a single lesion, haemangiosarcomas are rapidly invasive and tend to ulcerate. Metastasis occurs early in the dog, although not quite so quickly in the cat. Wide surgical excision is required as recurrence is common. Radiation therapy and chemotherapy have been offered as complements to surgery but the prognosis is poor and death ensues rapidly.

Lymphangioma and lymphosarcoma

These tumours originate from the endothelial cells of the lymph vessels. Both dogs and cats can be affected with no particular age, breed or sex predilection. The benign version appears as a poorly circumscribed, fluctuant swelling of up to 18 cm. These swellings tend to occur in the axillae, inguinal region and on the limbs. A serous to milky substance can be drained from the sites of occurrence. Treatment is by surgical excision, or even amputation in extreme cases.

The malignant lymph tumour in the dog is a solitary area of pitting oedema. Purpura and ulceration may also occur at the site. A serosanguineous fluid can be drained from the lesion. Areas most affected are the limbs and ventral abdomen. In the cat, the lesion appears as a plaque-like oedematous mass with erythema to purpura at the site. The mass will feel soft and spongy on palpation. In the cat, the lymphosarcoma grows rapidly, may recur after excision, and is known to metastasise. In both the dog and cat, surgical excision or even amputation is recommended once the tumour has been identified via cytology and histopathology.

METASTASISED LESIONS

Metastatic lesions are neoplastic and malignant. Diagnostic tests will reveal the nature of these tumours. These types of tumour underline the importance of taking a thorough history and performing a full clinical examination. Lymph node palpation and abdominal palpation are particularly important. Sexual status should be questioned. Intact males should have their testes examined and owners should relate any particulars about the oestrus cycles of intact females. Unusual growths should always prompt a top-to-toe examination with all findings recorded. The lesion in question should be described with respect to its location and the size should be measured with calipers. Any other lesions should be noted along with the primary concern. Owners should be asked relevant questions regarding the length of time the growth has been visible/palpable, how quickly it has grown and whether the animal has a history of previous growths. The nodule should be palpated, and whether it is fixed or mobile, defined or diffuse, should be observed. Note whether the tumour exists in the epidermis, dermis or subcutaneous regions.

If systemic disease is indicated by the history and/or clinical signs, further diagnostic tests should be instigated promptly. Blood samples should be obtained for haematology and biochemistry and either radiographic or ultrasonagraphic imaging should be sought out. In cases where metastasis has already occurred to the skin, treatment may be involved and expensive, possibly including chemotherapy or radiation therapy. If the disease is at an advanced stage, the prognosis may be poor and the owners must be prepared for the worst. It is important when dealing with tumours to explain carefully the difference between diagnostic testing and curative procedures. It is easy for an owner to want to believe that removing a tumour will cure the pet of cancer. Unfortunately, this is not always the case. The owner must understand that growths are removed for staging and grading, helping the clinician to choose an appropriate treatment modality. Lump removal may help with treatment, but, if the disease is widespread or aggressive, treatment may not be advisable. Removal of a lump is only the first step, and may not even give a full diagnosis. Excisional biopsy can be curative in some cases, so it is worthwhile to remove a lump. However, the sample does not need to be sent to an outside laboratory for analysis if the owner does not wish to proceed with treatment. The reason for every procedure and the costs involved at each step along the way should be explained fully and given to the owner in some sort of written format. Pet owners are being asked to make emotionally difficult and financially costly decisions. They need to be given as much information as possible with which to make informed decisions. Following this procedure prevents misunderstandings and eases the process for an owner dealing with a seriously ill pet.

References and Further Reading

Ackerman L, Nesbitt G 1998 Canine cutaneous neoplastic and non-neoplastic tumours and cysts. Canine and feline dermatology. Veterinary Learning Systems, Trenton NJ, p 279–313

Ackerman L, Nesbitt G 1998 Feline cutaneous neoplastic and non-neoplastic tumours and cysts. Canine and feline dermatology. Veterinary Learning Systems, Trenton NJ, p 451–470

Dobson J, Shearer D 2002 An approach to nodules and draining sinuses. In: Foil C, Foster A (eds) BSAVA Manual of small animal dermatology. BSAVA Publications, Gloucester, p 55–65

Dobson J, Morris J 2001 Skin. Small animal oncology. Blackwell Science, Oxford, p 50–68

Goldschmidt M.H, Shofer F S 1992 Skin tumours of the dog and cat. Pergamon Press, Oxford

Grant D 1991 Neoplastic skin disease. Skin disease in dogs and cats. Blackwell Science, London, p 126–145

Hendrick M J, Mahaffey E A, Moore F M et al 1998 Histological classification of mesenchymal tumours of skin and soft tissues of domestic animals, Second Series, Vol II. Armed Forces Institute of Pathology and The World Health Organisation Collaborating Center, Washington DC

Vail D 2002 Mast cell tumours. In: Foil C, Foster A (eds) BSAVA Manual of small animal dermatology. BSAVA Publications, Gloucester, p 220–228

CASE STUDY

Multiple trichoepithelioma

Signalment

Nine-year-old Gordon Setter bitch, neutered. Weight: 35 kg.

Complaint

Recurrent multiple skin tumours, with ulceration and malodour.

History

The bitch had a history of recurrent cutaneous masses. One lesion had been biopsied 5 years earlier, which identified the growths as trichoepitheliomata. More recently (1 year earlier) a further biopsy was done to identify a number of new nodules. These were also confirmed as trichoepitheliomata. In both biopsy reports, a good prognosis was offered providing the tumour margins had been wide because hair follicle tumours are usually benign.

Physical examination

The bitch was of a normal weight for the breed and exhibited healthy vital signs. Popliteal lymphadenomegaly was noted on palpation. Multiple cutaneous nodules of approximately 5 cm were visible over the head and trunk. There was a large, ulcerated lesion at the dorsal tail base. The hair was clipped away from the tail base and profuse exudate was cleaned from the site. There was an obvious pain response on palpation of the lesions

Differential diagnosis

- Infectious granulomata (bacterial, fungal, mycobacterial)
- Follicular tumours:
- Trichoepithelioma
- Infiltrative trichoepithelioma
- Malignant trichoepithelioma
- Tricholemmoma

Underlying problems:

- Internal disease
- Internal malignancy with metastic spread to the skin

Diagnostic tests

Swabs were taken from the ulcerated lesion at the tail base and culture and sensitivity testing were requested Biochemistry, haematology and thyroid function blood tests were carried out. None of these yielded abnormal results.

Bacteriology revealed a heavy growth of: *Pseudomonas, Staphylococcus intermedius, Enterococcus faecalis* and *Escherichia coli* sensitive to marbofloxacin (Marbocyl, Vetoquinol), which was prescribed prior to surgery to help prevent dehiscence and to resolve the secondary infection of the ulcerated masses.

Under general anaesthetic, surgical removal of the larger tumours was performed and excisional biopsy samples were taken from nodules at the tail base, lateral neck, right lateral thigh, and right caudal thigh. When the large mass at the tail base was surgically excised, a drain was placed to enhance wound healing and a skin graft was utilised at the site of the large tail-base tumour. The biopsies were submitted for histological examination. A radiograph was taken of the patient's chest in case of metastasis. No abnormalities were present on the radiographs.

Diagnosis and prognosis

All biopsies confirmed the suspected diagnosis that the nodules were a recurrence of the earlier trichoepithelioma. Trichoepithelioma is a non-malignant neoplasia (Fig. 11.7). However, the disease had progressed to penetration of the basement membrane, indicating that the growths were now in the infiltrative phase. The biopsy report advised checking for metastases because infiltrative and malignant trichoepitheliomata are difficult to distinguish between. Metastases to the chest are most commonly reported, and this had been recently radiographed.

Generally, the prognosis is good with trichoepithelioma, as long as the growths have been excised with wide margins. However, this bitch was unusual in exhibiting multi-focal lesions with recurrence. It was impossible to remove every growth, or continuously repeat surgery, so the prognosis for cure was guarded.

Treatment

The primary treatment had already taken place with the removal of masses on the dorsal head, dorsal neck, right thigh and the tail base. The bitch was placed on antibiotic therapy marbofloxacin (Marbocyl, Vetoquinol) at a dose of 80 mg once daily (2 mg/kg) for the 10 days post-surgery. The

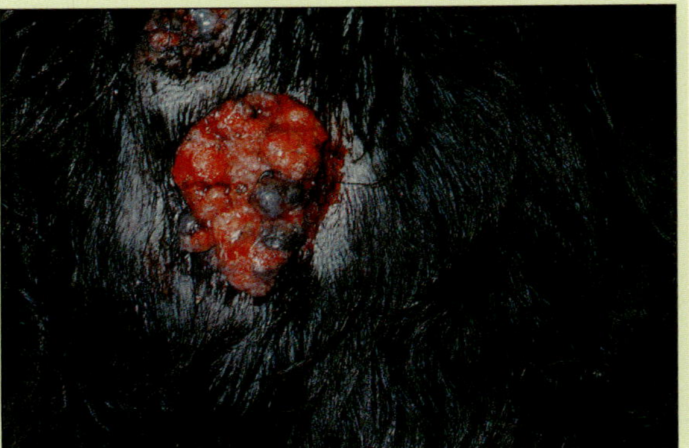

Figure 11.7 Trichoepithelioma is a non-malignant neoplasia. Photograph by Annette Loeffler, with permission.

sutures were removed following the 10 days of antibiotic therapy.

Re-examination and final outcome

As not every nodule had been removed, and recurrence had been the pattern with this patient, further treatment was called for. As this was an exceptional case in that the tumours were recurrent and multiple, retinoid therapy was discussed with the owners. This type of therapy is not entered into lightly as the side-effects are extensive: pruritus, erythema of pedal and mucocutaneous junctions, stiffness, diarrhoea/vomiting, hyperactivity and keratoconjunctivitis sicca (KCS), along with raised cholesterol, triglycerides and liver enzymes (Harvey & McKeever 1998). The main risk is the extreme teratogenicity of the drug – both to humans and animals. The owner must take great care when handling the drug, and women of childbearing years should not be in contact with retinoids at all. Retinoid therapy is a last-resort treatment for intractable cases.

As the bitch's haemogram had been normal, it was felt that she was well enough systemically to proceed with a potentially toxic therapy. A Schirmer's tear test was performed to measure tear productivity because KCS is one of the most common side-effects of retinoid therapy. The bitch had been neutered and the owners were past childbearing years so the risk of teratogenic complications was minimised. Gloves were distributed with the medication.

Retinoid therapy is not licensed for use in animals so a release form had to be signed by the owners. The drug also needs to be obtained directly from the pharmaceutical company on a named patient basis. Isotretinoin (Roaccutane, Roche) at a dose rate of 40 mg once daily, commenced 3 weeks post-surgery (1–2 mg/kg). Two months later the dose was lowered to 40 mg every other day for 2 months. No recurrence had occurred at this point but it was felt that it was necessary to maintain the bitch on isotretinoin due to the many recurrences she had already suffered.

Discussion

This case was an unusual manifestation of what is usually a benign, relatively common hair follicle tumour, easily cured by excision. However, as this case shows, some cases with multiple lesions can recur and can be difficult to manage. Lesions are more often small, but again, this bitch was unusual in that her lesions were large and appeared multifocally, rather than just on the dorsum, which is the more common presentation (Ackerman & Nesbitt 1991).

The disease was not only epidermal but also involved infiltration to the basement membranes. It is an unusual histological finding for there to be follicular encroachment of the basement membrane. Infiltrative growths have a 10% likelihood of recurrence (Goldschmidt & Shofer 1992), thus requiring a more aggressive approach to treatment. Additionally, the similarity in histology between infiltrative and malignant trichoepitheliomas causes one to treat infiltrative disease with some respect. It is only possible to differentiate between malignant and benign tumours by the clinical behaviour of the neoplasm. Metastases to distant organs indicate a malignant growth.

All of the complicating factors in this case supported the need for therapy beyond the norm. While retinoid therapy can cause significant side-effects, it was still considered worth the risks, as long as a Schirmer test is performed every two weeks. Regular monitoring of biochemistry, tear production and urinalysis are advised to prevent any serious problems developing. Monitoring should occur every 1–2 months till the treatment is concluded (Harvey & McKeever 1998). Yet, it should be noted that retinoids are reported to be less of a problem in dogs than in people (Hill 2002). Owners must be compliant with the therapy and well educated on the possible toxic effects to themselves, agreeing in full to practice all safety precautions.

REFERENCES

(for the Case Study)

Ackerman L, Nesbitt G 1991 Cutaneous neoplasia and cystic disease. Dermatology for the small animal practitioner. Veterinary Learning Systems, Trenton, NJ. p 155–163

Goldschmidt M H, Shofer F S 1992 Trichoepithelioma. Skin tumours of the dog and cat. Pergamon Press, Oxford, p 115–123

Harvey R, McKeever P 1998 Skin disease of the dog and cat. Manson Publishers, London, p 57–79

Hill P 2002 Small animal dermatology. Butterworth-Heinemann, London, p 288–289

Chapter 12

Wounds

CHAPTER CONTENTS

Wounds, while not caused by a disease process, are nevertheless a dermatological condition. Various forms of trauma can affect the skin and these traumatic events go through a healing process which can be enhanced by good nursing care. Choosing the correct bandaging material and applying good bandaging techniques are essential skills for any nurse, and especially so for the dermatology nurse.

Wounds are classified in two ways: by the type of wound and by the degree of contamination. It is important to understand wound classification in order to decide how to treat each specific wound. The reconstructive techniques utilised vary greatly from one type of wound to another. However, initial first aid treatment is similar for all wounds.

TYPES OF WOUND

Different types of wound are going to heal in significantly different ways. It is not only the level of contamination and severity of the injury that defines the course of treatment. The type of wound encountered must play an important part in the decision-making process regarding wound management.

Incision

This is the type of wound one would create with a scalpel blade. There is not a lot of tissue damage and the wound has not been inoculated with microbes. Generally, this type of wound heals by primary closure, i.e. suturing the wound closed.

Laceration

This is a tear to the epithelium and possibly deeper tissues. It is usually a traumatic wound, possibly caused by something like glass or barbed wire. There can be a lot of bleeding, which reduces the level of contamination, though it is usually not heavy enough to be life threatening. Paw lacerations, however, can be very difficult to deal with as any continued pressure on the paw causes the wound to re-open. Paw wounds also tend to be quite contaminated from their contact with the ground. These wounds need thorough exploration and lavage. The dressing needs to help prevent pressure on the wound. Cotton wool should be placed between the toes to prevent pressure sores developing there. Often boots are utilised.

Punctures

These wounds look small and may not bleed much but they can be very serious. If a puncture wound is deep enough it can perforate an internal organ, leading to life-threatening difficulties. Puncture wounds require deep investigation. One would not want to miss a punctured lung, which would develop into a pneumothorax, or a punctured peritoneum, causing a haemoabdomen. Additionally, bacteria are inoculated deep into the wound with puncture wounds. Typical causes of puncture wounds are bite wounds, where there may also be extensive bruising and even crushing to surrounding bones and tissue. Radiographs are recommended with bite wounds. Both sides of the animal should be clipped in preparation for exploration as there are often bilateral wounds.

Stick injuries and insect bites fall within this category.

A gunshot wound is also a type of puncture wound. Bullets do a great deal of damage passing through tissue as they are moving with speed and force.

As puncture wounds cannot drain easily and do not bleed freely, there is a great risk of infection – think of cat bite abscesses. Seromas occur frequently within a puncture wound and typically infections with staphylococci, streptococci and *Pasteurella* spp will occur. If the wound closes completely, anaerobic bacteria, such as *Clostridium* spp, can grow inside the wound tract.

Abrasions

An abrasion occurs when the top layers of the skin are rubbed away. In severe abrasions, the epidermis and parts of the dermis can be lost. A common abrasion is wear on the pads from long walks. A more serious abrasion would occur when an animal is dragged along the road in a traffic accident. Abrasions tend to be extremely contaminated. As they are also very painful, the animals tend to lick at the wound, causing further contamination. Extensive lavage is called for in the treatment of abrasions.

Avulsions

With an avulsion wound, skin tissue is forced away from its attachments. A de-gloving injury is a type of avulsion. In the instance of de-gloving, the entire epidermis is torn away from the animal, leaving the underlying structures exposed. The tail and extremities are prone to de-gloving injuries in road traffic accidents. It is not possible to re-attach the outer layer of skin as the vascular system has been damaged beyond repair. In smaller avulsions, if there is some vascular vitality, the tissue can be sutured back in place. However, with a de-gloving injury, there will either be a long healing process via second intention or reconstructive surgery will be required.

Contusions

These are bruises. There is no break in the skin but there is pain and the animal may need analgesia, especially if loss of function is observed.

Burns

Burns can be caused by frictional, thermal (hot or cold), electrical or chemical causes. Thermal scalds, due to an animal getting a hot drink spilled on it, are frequently seen. Burns on recumbent patients can be caused by heatpads. Any hospitalised patient on a heatpad should have a notice placed on his cage so that he is constantly checked. Thermal burns require cooling of the area with cool, not cold, water and supportive therapy, definitely including fluid therapy. An enormous amount of fluid is lost through the skin when a thermal burn occurs.

Handling the animal with gloves and sterile drapes prevents contamination of the wound, an important consideration as burn wounds are very prone to secondary infection.

The classification of thermal burns via degrees is no longer used. Now burns are referred to as full or partial thickness burns. The percentage of the body area affected is what is most prognostic, in terms of survival. Burns that cover 25% or more of the body surface area are life-threatening.

Frostbite is typically found on the tail, ears and nose but is usually confined to extremely cold climates. Gentle warming of the area with tepid fluid is recommended, along with supportive treatment.

Chemical burns can be caused by caustics, for example: acids, alkalis, or phenols. The animal may have had the substance spilled on it or it may have walked through the chemical. With chemical burns, the initial act of treatment is copious flushing. The quicker the treatment is enacted, the better.

Electrical burns can be a contact burn, for example, a puppy chewing an electric cord, or a flash burn, as when an animal comes into contact with high-voltage cables. The person finding the animal should not put himself or herself at risk. Hence the electricity source should be shut off before rescue can take place. Treatment for shock and stablising the animal are required before the wound can be treated.

CONTAMINATION

The level of contamination is a major factor in determining how the case will be handled. There are specific levels of contamination defined as follows:

1. Clean: A clean wound is a surgical incision made under aseptic conditions. A clean wound can be sutured closed and should heal without complication.
2. Clean-contaminated: A clean-contaminated wound is a surgical wound into a body cavity or organ. Contamination is controlled in these cases and the procedures are carried out under aseptic conditions
3. Contaminated: A contaminated wound is a surgical wound into a body cavity or organ where gross spillage has occurred. For example, urine from the bladder or intestinal contents have not been contained within the organ and have spilled out into other areas of the surgical field. A contaminated wound can also be a traumatic wound that has been presented for treatment within 6 hours of occurring.
4. Dirty: A dirty wound is a traumatic wound that has been presented for treatment more than 6 hours after the wound has occurred. Any wound with obvious infection is also considered a dirty wound.

Defining the level of contamination is necessary in order to decide how to proceed with treatment. Obviously contaminated and infected wounds need far more extensive lavage and debridement. These wounds are not usually closed initially and must be repeatedly debrided until they are deemed clean enough for closure. This is termed 'delayed primary closure'. In some cases, these wounds will not be closed surgically at all, but will heal via second intention, or at a later date, by reconstructive techniques.

HEALING

There are three stages to wound healing:

1. inflammation
2. repair
3. remodelling.

These stages can be further subdivided into six phases:

1. Inflammation. The wound is swollen, hot, red and painful, There may be loss of function if the wound is on a weight-bearing site or joint. It is the release of histamine that causes the erythema, vasodilation and blood vessel permeability that manifests as redness, swelling and pain. While uncomfortable, it is this process that allows the inflammatory exudate to rush to the site of the trauma and begin to clean up the mess. In the inflammatory exudate you will find neutrophils, phagocytes and macrophages which destroy or digest bacteria and debris. Plasma, proteins and antibodies accumulate at the site to help fight off infection and promote the healing process.

2. Repair/phagocytosis. This phase begins minutes after the initial shock and may continue for several weeks, depending on whether or not the wound becomes infected. It is during this phase that the process of removing debris and bacteria from the wound takes place. Macrophages will even digest necrotic tissue! Additionally, fibroblasts are attracted to the wound; this stimulates the production of collagen which is needed to re-build the injured area. Cell division is increased and angiogenesis is instigated.
3. Fibroplastic/granulation. This is the phase in which granulation commences. Collagen is deposited and a matrix is created from new capillary buds and inflammatory cells. The framework is laid for the wound edges to grow back together. This phase usually begins about 24 hours after the initial insult.
4. Epithelialisation. This phase overlaps with the granulation phase as the epithelium re-grows and re-surfaces the lost skin area.
5. Wound contraction. After about 48 hours, the skin edges surrounding the wound begin to contract due to increased skin elasticity. This helps the wound close together more easily.
6. Remodelling. After a few days, the initial epithelialisation is replaced by more permanent collagen. This is where scar formation begins. This phase can go on for months.

EMERGENCY TREATMENT

When an animal is first presented to a veterinary surgery with a wound the most important thing to do immediately is assess the vital signs. Airway, breathing and circulation (ABC) must be attended to as a priority. Often animals with wounds have suffered from road traffic accidents or have been bitten. The injuries can be alarming and the first instinct may be to start treating the wound. Avoid this tendency and make sure you have a patent airway, adequate respiration and circulation before proceeding to the lesser problem of wound treatment. Stabilising a patient may require introducing an endotracheal tube for oxygenation, or control of haemorrhage. As well as applying pressure, there are new methods of haemorrhage control utilising polysaccharide beads or calcium alginate.

Once ABC has been sorted out you can attend to the wound. The first thing you should do is cover the wound with a sterile drape to prevent a nosocomial infection. If the wound cannot be covered then cover the examination table you are placing the animal on for assessment and, by all means, make sure that you are wearing gloves! If you cannot treat the wound immediately, pack it with sterile swabs soaked in saline, wrap it and then deal with more pressing needs. Once you have finished setting up your drip or taking radiographs, then you can get back to the wound, assured that it did not become further contaminated in the intervening period.

To begin wound treatment, fill the wound with sterile lubricating jelly (KY, Johnson & Johnson), then clip wide margins around it. If you have a bite wound or a bullet wound be sure to clip both sides of the animal – there may be wounds from the opposing set of teeth or an exit wound. Cleanse the area around the wound with ordinary surgical scrub, making sure not to get any of the scrub into the actual wound as antiseptic solutions are not good for open wounds! They are not isotonic and act as an irritant. Additionally, surgical scrub solutions in an open wound can lead to cell destruction and delayed wound healing.

Once the area is prepared, begin lavage. Firstly, the jelly with its loose hairs will be washed away. Then debris from the wound and bacteria should be sluiced off. Seriously contaminated wounds (for example, road abrasions, full of bits of grit and mud) can be flushed with tap water initially. The best lavage solution is compound sodium lactate (Hartmann's) with 0.9% saline coming in as a second preference. Hartmann's is isotonic and the least likely solution to cause cellular damage. Lavage should be applied at 8 pounds per square inch of pressure. This can be achieved by using a 20 ml syringe, 18 gauge needle, three-way tap and a giving set attached to the bag of fluids. Place the three-way tap between the needle and syringe and attach the giving set. In this way, you can repeatedly refill the syringe without breaking sterility. This set-up will provide the correct pressure to irrigate the wound without damaging tissue. Lavage should continue till all debris is removed. At least 15 minutes of lavage is required for even the simplest of wounds.

Once the wound has been freed from debris and surface bacteria, debridement can begin. Any and all necrotic or devascularised tissue should be excised away. Devitalised tissue left in the wound will lead to infection and wound breakdown, so if in doubt, cut it out. When finished debriding, the wound edges should be bleeding freshly. If there has not been too much contamination and the wound edges are close enough together, primary closure can take place. If there is gross contamination and/or too much tissue loss, the wound must be dressed for delayed primary closure or healing by second intention. In cases of extensive tissue loss, planning for reconstructive surgery must commence. Infected/dirty wounds will most likely require several days of debridement before a time of closure can be considered. Rarely, en-bloc debridement is used, where the entire wound area is removed from the animal. Layered debridement is preferred in veterinary wound management. The careful removal of devitalised tissue in a sequential manner usually creates the desired result.

Pain relief cannot be overlooked at any point in the wound treatment process. There are a lot of nerve endings in the skin and the animal will be distressed regardless of the depth of the wound. Opioids are recommended for serious wounds, but even minor wounds warrant some level of analgesia. Some clinicians recommend local as well as systemic analgesia. Pain will slow wound healing. Pain relief should be provided for as long as the animal is experiencing discomfort, as observed by clinical signs such as licking at the wound, restlessness, anorexia and resistance to handling.

Emergency treatment of wounds

- ABC! Airway, Breathing, Circulation + cover wound with sterile drape.
- Pack wound with sterile saline-soaked swabs while stabilising patient and examining serious injuries.
- Under sedation or general anaesthesia, fill wound with KY jelly, clip area generously, then flush away jelly and debris.
- Lavage wound copiously with isotonic solution (preferably Hartman's).
- Debride all devascularised, necrotic tissue. Create freshly bleeding edges to wound.
- Close wound if possible or dress for second intention healing.

DRESSING OPTIONS AND SECOND INTENTION HEALING

There are three levels of dressing: the primary layer which is next to the wound, a secondary or absorbent layer and a tertiary, protective layer. The primary layer can consist of plain sterile swabs, gel-impregnated gauze, antibiotic-impregnated gauze, occlusive swabs, alginates, hydrocolloids or hydrogels. Secondary dressings are much more simple, consisting primarily of cotton wool or a related material. The protective layer can be a plaster cast or a self-adhesive wrap.

The type of dressing depends on what function you want the dressing to perform. Simply covering the wound is only one aspect of dressing. A simple incision probably doesn't need any dressing, or perhaps just a protective semi-permeable film, whereas a dirty/infected wound may need a dressing that assists healing by mechanical debridement. Formerly, dry-to-dry dressings were used to debride. Dry swabs were placed in the wound to soak up exudates. A secondary, absorbent layer and a protective layer were placed on top of the swabs. These dressings were removed, sometimes on a daily basis to clear away the necrotic tissue. Dressing changes of this sort were painful and usually required sedation or even general anaesthetic.

We have learned through research, and from human studies, that moist wounds heal signifigantly more quickly, and that dressing changes with a moist wound dressing are not nearly as painful as dry-to-dry dressings. It was feared that moist wounds would promote bacterial growth but this has not proved to be the case; in fact, moist dressings are a vast improvement on dry dressings with respect to healing. The old-fashioned wound powders are also to be avoided as the body interprets the powder as a foreign body and this potentiates inflammation, thus further delaying the healing process.

Therefore, most wounds requiring debribement are now dressed in a wet-to-dry format. This can be done simply with sterile swabs soaked in saline. Excess fluid should be squeezed from swabs to prevent maceration of healthy surrounding tissue. The swabs should be changed daily until a granulation bed is established.

In common use now are hydrogels and hydrocolloids, which can be used instead of soaked swabs. Some examples of these products are: IntraSite gel (Smith & Nephew) and Collamend (Genitrix). The gels and colloids do not create a risk of too much moisture and have other advantages – they are able to absorb water while promoting autolysis of devitalised tissue. Most of the gels and colloids can be left in place for 3 days before a dressing change is necessary. For some wounds, that may be enough time to establish a granulation bed. In severely infected/traumatised areas, repeated debridement may be necessary. It is safe to continue re-applying gels or colloids as needed.

Alginates are also hydrophilic and thus useful for moist wounds. Alginates are made from calcium and seaweed and are very well tolerated by the body but should not be placed in deep wounds as they will be treated as a foreign body. They should be changed every 2–3 days. There is no pain on removal. Algistite M (Smith & Nephew) is one example of this type of product.

Foams are also very useful at this early stage in wound repair. Foams, by their nature, are very absorbent and non-adherent. Some types of foam can be packed into deep wounds, for example Alleyvn cavity (Smith & Nephew). They should not remain in situ for any length of time due to the possibility of a foreign body reaction. Other foams in the Alleyvn range can be cut into the appropriate shape needed. Foams are recommended for wounds with heavy exudation.

Antibiotic-impregnated gauzes are used in infected wounds. Nanocrystalline silver releases silver ions on interaction with skin fluids. The silver ions bind to tissue proteins and cause changes to bacterial and yeast cell walls. The dressing Acticoat (Smith & Nephew) has proved effective in fighting a variety of both bacteria and yeast infections. There are different versions of the dressing, depending on the frequency of bandage changes. Silver sulphadiazine cream is an another source of silver as an antibacterial agent.

Once the wound is free of devitalised tissue and infection the process of debridement can stop. In some wounds, closure can take place at this point. This is termed *delayed primary closure* and usually occurs 3–5 days after the initial trauma.

More complicated wounds will require more than 5 days to complete the debridement process fully. It is absolutely essential that a wound is fully debrided in order for it to heal cleanly. Some wounds will need mechanical and surgical debridement repeated at frequent intervals. However, once a granulation bed appears, and provided there is sufficient tissue available, *secondary* closure can take place.

If there is no hope of secondary closure, the wound must heal by *second intention*, that is, granulation and re-epithelialisation. This is a lengthy process that will also be a considerable expense to the owner. If at all possible, owners should be warned of the cost and time commitment at the outset of wound treatment.

If a wound is healing by second intention it is necessary to use a dressing that will not disturb the granulation bed. Semi-occlusive, non-adherent swabs are needed and foams can also be used. If some exudate is still present, or padding is needed, a foam is the correct choice. The secondary layer of absorbent dressing may be decreased as the exudate diminishes. The protective layer is still important to prevent contamination and interference with the fragile wound bed.

As re-epithelialisation progresses the wound edges will contract. Eventually scar tissue will develop and the wound will be considered healed. In some instances scar tissue may inhibit movement. It is in these cases that reconstructive techniques should be used instead of second intention healing.

Table 12.1 shows the right dressing for a given type of wound.

SURGICAL REPAIR TECHNIQUES

Primary, or delayed primary, closure is achieved by suturing a wound closed. The suture pattern most often used is simple interrupted. The bites should be 5 mm from the wound edges and 5 mm apart from each other. It is best to slightly evert the wound edges as they will flatten with healing. Over-tight sutures devitalise tissue and encourage self-trauma. Mattress stitches tend to tighten so should be used with caution.

Wounds are rarely simply closed, however. Often it will be necessary to pre-suture the wound closed, debride and then suture closed more permanently.

Table 12.1 The right dressing for the wound

Type of wound	Gel or colloid	Foam	Calcium alginate	Non-occlusive swab	Antibacterial swab	Semi-permeable film
Surgical						x
Contaminated, low exudate	x					
Contaminated, moderate to high exudate	x	x	x		x	
Infected/necrotic, low exudate	x				x	
Infected/necrotic, high exudate	x	x	x		x	
Laceration, low exudate	x					
Laceration, high exudate	x	x	x			
Abrasion	x				x	x
Burn	x			x		
Avulsion, partial thickness	x					
Avulsion, full thickness	x	x	x		x	
Granulating, low exudate				x		
Granulating, high exudate		x		x		

Skin stretching devices can be utilised if it is necessary to cross across tissue deficits. One method of stretching is to tie in very tight sutures, leave them for a few hours and then close the adjusted skin with less stringent sutures.

Intradermal sutures can be placed and tightened daily until the wound edges are apposed and the wound can be properly closed. One stretching method used requires an adjustable horizontal mattress pattern pulled through buttons on either side of the wound. Split shot or fishing weights are used to hold the tension of the suture at the top and bottom of the wound. Button sutures are shown in Figure 12.1.

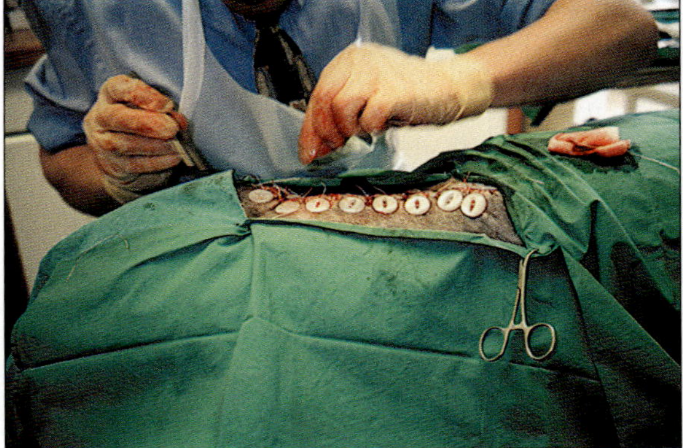

Figure 12.1 Button sutures are being used to stretch the available skin for later wound closure. Photograph by Frances Gaudiano.

Other methods of stretching the wound edges include injecting a tissue expander of saline into the region or creating punctuate relaxing incisions parallel to the wound edge. Velcro patches have also been glued to the wound edges and tightened with elastic bands. Clinicians will have their favoured method of adjusting a wound towards closure but it must be remembered that every wound is unique. Flexibility in approach is recommended.

Large wound deficits require advanced reconstructive techniques. These might include the harvesting of omentum to be placed in a wound to create a new vascular bed. This is particularly useful with axial wounds.

Skin grafts can be split or full-thickness. Grafts need to be placed onto a sterile wound bed with a good blood supply; thus, grafts occur after complete and thorough debridement. The face and muscle tissue are good locations for a graft to take. There are a variety of graft forms, including: sieve, punch, mesh and strip grafts.

Pedicled muscle flaps are used to cover vital areas and pad bony areas. This very vascular tissue helps to decrease the risk of infection and allows healing at both a cellular and humoral level.

Microvascular free tissue transfer is an extremely advanced surgical technique that requires anastamosis of microvessels. Only specialist referral centres would attempt this very difficult wound reconstruction technique.

NEW APPROACHES

There is continuing research centred on wound healing techniques and new methods are constantly being developed.

Collagen is available as a suspension or a dressing and is useful for minor to major wounds. It helps to absorb exudates and provides a good environment for cell growth and granulation. It is a bridge for the epithelial cells to migrate across the wound edges, helping to reduce healing time.

Dermal grafts made of porcine small intestine are also in use. These also act as a scaffold for the skin cells to grow across and are absorbent and help to protect against bacteria. They reportedly help to reduce scarring.

Low-level laser therapy is used to reduce inflammation, provide analgesia and promote regeneration of tissues. Lasers operate at a cellular and a secondary, systemic level by stimulating chemical processes and activating enzyme activity needed for the healing process. The immune response is altered so that there is an increase in T and B lymphocytes, increased phagocytosis and an inhibition of prostaglandin, among other functions. It is a non-invasive therapy but is very expensive as repeated sessions are required for the therapy to be effective.

One new treatment that is actually very old is the use of maggots for debridement. The skin surrounding the wound is protected by a hydrocolloid sheet and ten fly larvae per centimetre squared (cm^2) are held in place by nets. Moist swabs are placed over the larvae to keep them from desiccating. They are left in place for 48–72 hours. As well as devouring dead tissue, the maggots secrete enzymes which enhances their debridement achievements.

Honey is another old-fashioned re-discovered treatment. With a pH of 3.7, honey is capable of killing some streptococcal and coagulase-positive staphylococcal bacteria. It is less expensive than antibiotic impregnated swabs if budget is an important factor in the treatment protocol.

SYSTEMIC ANTIBIOTICS

The question of whether to medicate systemically or not must be dealt with in every wound dilemma. Many texts recommend a prophylactic dose for the first 24 hours for any wound. If the wound is contaminated, systemic antibiotics are indicated. Ideally, a culture for sensitivity should be performed to enable the correct antiobiotic to be chosen. However, if empirical judgement is required, a broad-spectrum antibiotic active against coagulase-positive *Staphylococcus* or *E. coli* is a safe bet. Usually, clavulanic acid-potentiated amoxicillin, a second-generation cephalosporin or a fluoroquinolone will serve the purpose. It should be remembered that potentiated sulphonamides have poor efficacy in the face of abscesses and gross necrosis and that anaerobes resist fluoroquinolones and aminoglycosides. *Pseudomonas* spp are resistant to β-lactamase-based antimicrobials and first- and second-generation cephalosporins. If the wound is not healing as it should, repeat the culture and sensitivity. The bacterial species colonising the wound may have changed.

References and Further Reading

Anderson D 1996 Wound management in small animal practice. In Practice March:115–128

Anderson D 1997 A practical approach to reconstruction of wounds in small animal practice, Part 2. In Practice November/December:537–545

Conner J, McKennell J 1995 A guide to small animal bandaging. Retford, Notts, p 5–7

Fowler D, Williams J M (eds) 1999 BSAVA Manual of canine and feline wound management. BSAVA Publications, Gloucester

Garden C, Hotson-Moore A 1999 Surgical conditions and surgical nursing. In: Moore M (ed) Manual of veterinary nursing. BSAVA Publications, Gloucester, p 142–147

McGehee R, Taylor R 1995 Manual of small animal post-operative care. Williams & Wilkins Media, PA, p 36–73

Tracy Diane L 1994 Small animal surgical nursing. Mosby, St Louis, MO, p 274–276

CASE STUDY

Wound management

Signalment

The patient was a 9-year-old, female neutered German Shepherd-Crossbreed dog.

Complaint

A laceration of 15–20 cm to the left flank. Wound gaping significantly and showing significant sepsis and necrosis. A purulent exudate was draining from the wound. An attempt at suturing had been made but the wound was breaking down. (See Fig. 12.2.)

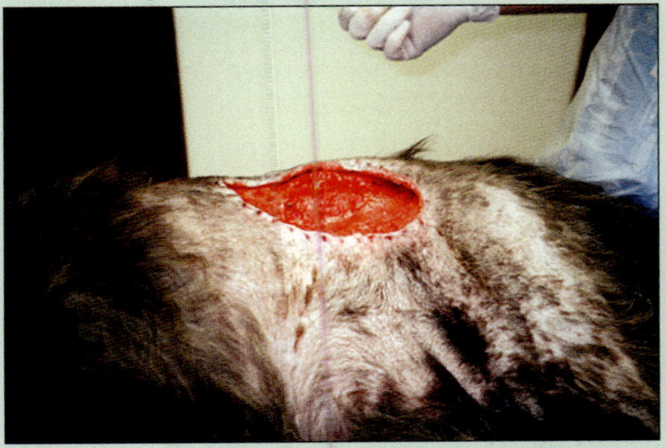

Figure 12.2 Wound management. This gaping wound required extensive treatment and time in order to heal. Photograph by Frances Gaudiano.

History

The dog had been staying with relatives, had run off, and had been missing for several days before being recovered by an animal charity. The charity had sutured the wound but the wound had broken down almost immediately. Re-suturing had taken place shortly thereafter (exact number of days not stipulated in notes). The owner had then recovered the dog and was seeking assistance from the dog's primary veterinarian. The owner reported that the dog was anorexic.

Physical examination

The dog appeared slightly underweight at 25.6 kg. Respiration and heartbeat were normal. The temperature was slightly elevated at 39.5°C. The dog's demeanour was depressed. The wound itself reached across the caudal lateral abdomen. The wound was of full thickness, exposing the underlying muscle mass. The stitches that had been placed were severely stretched across the centre of the wound. The wound edges had become necrotic and infection was obvious in the exposed cavern and by the overwhelming smell and nature of the exudate. Wound breakdown was imminent.

Differential diagnosis

The cause could have been a road traffic accident, an animal attack or an interaction with barbed wire. Significant contamination had taken place. When a rescue agent had collected the dog the wound was certainly more than 6 hours old and could be identified as a dirty/infected laceration wound of full thickness.

Diagnostic tests

A biochemistry panel was done to ascertain the dog's systemic health status and a swab was taken from the wound site. The swab was sent to an outside laboratory for analysis.

Biochemistry revealed slightly elevated ALT: 103 U/l (normal range 10–100 U/l) ALKP: 597 U/l (normal range 23–212 U/l). These levels would be consistent with septicaemia and starvation. We awaited the laboratory results regarding the infection in the wound.

Diagnosis and prognosis

The wound was diagnosed as infected and with necrotic tissue present. The current sutures were inadequate and there was no evidence of healing. The owner was advised that the area would need to be re-sutured but that the possibility of further wound breakdown was very high. She was also informed that the wound would need to heal primarily by second intention and that this would be both time consuming and costly.

Treatment

Marbofloxacin (Marbocyl, Vetoquinol) was prescribed for antibiotic cover and meloxicam (Metacam, Boehringer, Ingelheim) was administered for pain relief. The owner was instructed to find tasty treats and hand-feed the dog in order to boost her dog's nutrition. After 2 days, further breakdown was apparent. Metronidazole (Stomorgyl, Merial Animal Health) was added for additional antibiotic support and the analgesic treatment was changed to carprofen (Rimadyl, Pfizer) along with paracetamol/coedine phosphate (Pardale V, Arnolds). By the fourth day of treatment the dehiscence had increased to the point of creating a deep cavern beneath the wound edges (5–10 cm deep). It was necessary at this point to intervene surgically.

Five days after the initial consultation the dog was admitted for wound repair. The remains of the former stitches were removed and the wound was protected with sterile petroleum jelly (KY, Johnson & Johnson). A large area around the wound was clipped and cleaned with a dilute chlorhexidine solution (Hibiscrub, Medicam).

The wound was then flushed with metronidazole (Torgyl, Rhone Merieux) and co-amoxiclav (Augmentin, Smith Kline Beecham) – 10 ml of each along with copious amounts of sterile saline. Flushing was performed with a 20 ml syringe attached to an 18 gauge needle, creating the correct lavage pressure of 8 pounds per square inch (p.s.i.). Once the wound had been flushed enough to remove debris and dilute the bacteria present, the wound areas were prepared with a surgical scrub and the area was draped with four sterile drapes.

Dehiscence in itself had created a skin flap for wound edge advancement. After thorough debridement, the surgeon assisted wound advancement by placing tension sutures into the underlying muscle structures using 4 metric braided synthetic absorbable suture material (Vicryl, Janssen). A swaged on 30 mm half circle, taper cut needle was used. The wound cavern was so deep that this procedure had to be repeated on a more superficial layer.

At this point, a collagen suspension (Collamend, Genitrix) was inserted into the wound to assist with granulation and speed the reconstruction process. Further tension sutures were placed along the superficial wound edges. The surgeon then used sterile buttons to decrease dead space and add pressure to the wound, thus preventing seromas, haematomas and cavernous areas. Superficial and button sutures were placed with 4 metric Polyamide (Supramid, SMI). The wound was finally closed with a simple interrupted suture pattern. A 26 mm curved cutting edge needle was used for the closing sutures.

Before waking the animal, a pressure bandage was applied. A non-adherent, absorbent dressing (Melolin, Smith & Nephew) was used for the primary layer. The secondary layer was cotton wool to provide absorption, thus keeping the area less hospitable to bacteria. The tertiary layer was made of a cohesive, protectant dressing (Vetwrap, Smith & Nephew). The dog was injected with marbofloxacin (Marbocyl, Vetoquinol) and pethidine (Pethidine, Arnolds) and sent home on marbofloxacin, metronidazole and pethidine tablets. A buster collar was prescribed to prevent self-trauma and the owner was instructed on bandage care.

Re-inspection and final outcome

Day 3. After the procedure, the wound was re-dressed. Paraffin gauze (Jelonet, Smith & Nephew) was used along with a hydrocolloid (Intrasite gel, Smith & Nephew) covered by Melolin and then the padding and cohesive layers. Granulation tissue was appearing. The owner was still having trouble getting the dog to eat.

Day 5. The swab results came back with the wound testing positive for *Escherichia coli*; this required a change in treatment to cephalexin (Ceporex, Schering-Plough). Pain relief was changed to paracetamol and codeine (Pardale V, Arnolds). On re-dress, the mid-section of the wound looked healthy but the edges were not healing as quickly.

Day 7. The far edges of the wound seemed to be healing by second intention. Exudate was still evident in the Melolin swabs. Two stitches were removed at either end of the wound. The dog's appetite was beginning to recover.

Day 10. The wound showed a healthy serous exudate. The owner was advised that dressings would need to continue until scarring had begun.

Day 13. The dressing was removed and the dog was given a good brush. The wound was cleaned with a dilute antiseptic scrub (1:80) and re-dressed using intra-site gel, paraffin gauze, non-adherent swabs and cotton and cohesive layers. The buttons were removed at this point, as were the cutaneous sutures.

Day 16. The cranial and caudal edges were creeping together. The exudate had reduced to a minimal level. A light dressing of non-adherent swabs, thin padding and cohesive dressing was applied.

Day 22. The dog was given another 10-day course of cephalexin. A light dressing was applied.

Day 27. The final dressing was removed. The wound was remodelling well and the dog had full mobility in the area.

Discussion

The trauma of being lost and injured, along with poor nutrition, did not put this dog in a good state for healing. It is likely that the wound was already infected when the animal was brought into the shelter – suturing at that point was perhaps not the best option. Infection leads to collagen lysis and not remodelling (Anderson 1996)! Iatrogenic causes of breakdown can include poor surgical technique, poor pain control, incorrect support bandaging and even incorrect suture material (Anderson 1996). Additionally, the stress of a shelter situation and the likelihood of self-trauma occurring contributed to the failure of the initial attempts at repair.

While under the primary vet's care, the dog was in obvious pain – to the point of developing anorexia. Additionally, pain can slow wound healing. Analgesia had to be given, although non-steroidal anti-inflammatory drugs (NSAIDs) can contribute to poor wound health (Womak 2001). It was fortunate that a swab was taken because the initial choice of metronidazole was not correct. Topical antibiotics were not considered as these are more useful in preventing rather than destroying infection (Womak 2001).

Reconstruction of a large wound needs to be planned carefully. Unfortunately, this wound stretched across, rather than parallel to, the dog's natural tension lines (Anderson 1996). Careful preservation of the vascular bed is also important in surgery as oxygenation of the tissues will greatly enhance healing. However, the damage was already done with this wound and the best that could be hoped for was to reduce necrotic tissue and use dressing to continue debriding. The technique used was secondary closure alongside second intention healing.

REFERENCES

(for the Case Study)

Anderson D 1996 Wound management in small animal practice. In Practice March:115–128

Womak B H 2001 Wound management: healing and assessment. Veterinary Technician 22(11):588–592

Chapter 13

Dermatological conditions in exotic pets

CHAPTER CONTENTS

Poor husbandry is a major element that can lead to disease in exotic pets. Skin diseases are no exception to this rule; thus, a thorough history of the animal's care and the standard of husbandry is essential in order to ascertain the root of the problem. Ideally, an owner of an exotic pet should be asked to fill out a questionnaire prior to the appointment (see example below). Bringing the animal along in its usual abode is also helpful, when appropriate.

Dealing with small mammals can be frustrating due to the fact that the pets often belong to children. Care of the animal may be less than desirable, and getting full, accurate descriptions from a child can be hard work. Additionally, the finances set aside to care for a child's pet are usually minimal. Luckily, most skin conditions can be diagnosed with fairly inexpensive diagnostic tests and treatment does not tend to be prohibitively expensive.

A useful questionnaire for gathering history on small mammals might be as follows:

1. Please list the species, breed, age and gender of the pet.
2. Where was the pet purchased and how long has it been owned by yourself?
3. Are any other pets kept in the same cage with this pet? Please list the species, breed, age and gender of these pets.
4. Are there any other pets in the household?
5. Who is the primary caretaker for this pet?
6. Is this pet housed indoors or outdoors? If outdoors, do wild animals (rabbits, foxes, hedgehogs) enter your garden? If indoors, in which room of the house?
7. Describe the pet's enclosure – type of cage, flooring, bedding, toys, etc.
8. What do you feed the pet? Include brand of food, treats and supplements.
9. Is there any previous medical history?
10. Describe the current problem – when did it start? Has it got progressively worse? Is the pet itchy? Are other, in-contact pets affected? Have people who handle the pet developed any rashes or lesions? Where is the skin problem located and what does it look like?

If you are unable to get a questionnaire to the client by post, or filled out in the consulting room, do be sure to ask these questions during the consultation. Once the preliminary questions have been answered it is time to do a physical examination. As with any species, the physical should be as complete as possible, although adjustments are necessary in order to adapt to smaller species. Sensitive scales are required to get an accurate weight. This should be recorded in the patient's file in grams/kilograms. Pulse and respiration rates may be difficult to count as most small mammals have extremely rapid rates. Observing the animal in its container before handling is a good way to assess whether or not the respiratory rate is normal. Using a thermometer is quite stressful in smaller species and the technique would be considered invasive, although rabbits and ferrets may tolerate having their temperature taken. The general demeanour of the animal – bright, alert, responsive, versus lethargic and depressed – can be observed and recorded. Look for any nasal or ocular discharges, obvious lameness or paresis (weakness).

Before handling the pet, you can observe its coat condition. Is it glossy and smooth or does it appear patchy and unkempt? Are there any gross skin lesions detectable? Eventually though, you will have to pick the animal up and begin a more intimate inspection. Please be confident in your handling techniques of small mammals! Hamsters can give a very nasty bite and it is our natural instinct to shake them off as they sink their teeth into our flesh. More than one hamster has come to a sudden end after being flicked off a finger onto the floor. Scruffing all along the dorsum is one way of avoiding being bitten by a hamster. Rabbits need to have their hind legs controlled. Chinchillas need careful handling or furslip can occur (complicating your dermatological picture!). Gerbils should not be gripped by the tail, while rats and mice can be restrained by the tail and scruff of the neck. When in doubt, ask the owner to restrain the animal while you examine it. Owners can get quite upset if they feel that their small creatures are being overly restrained.

As with any dermatological examination, note the location of the lesion or lesions. Note whether the animal is showing signs of pruritus and/or self-trauma. Describe the type of lesion and its colour and diameter. From the initial assessment, decide what type of diagnostic tests need to be done.

Suspicion of ectoparasites would indicate the need for hair pluckings, skin scrapings and tape strippings. If a fungal infection is suspected, samples should be collected for a fungal culture. Ear swabs may be indicated if debris is noted in the outer ear canal or a head tilt is observed. An ulcerated lesion may warrant a swab for culture and sensitivity and certainly an impression smear for cytology. Lumps can be assessed via fine-needle aspirates. Keep in mind that pus from rabbit abscesses tends to be quite thick so use a 21-gauge needle to aspirate. Biopsy or surgical excision may be warranted in some cases. In ferrets, endocrine disease is a problem that can manifest as alopecia so blood testing may be required or ultrasonograpy of the adrenal glands. Be sure to quote the cost of each procedure before proceeding as you may be dealing with quite limited funds. People may be happier to have the vet choose an empirical course of treatment rather than reach a definitive diagnosis.

RABBITS

Rabbits are the third most popular pet in the United Kingdom and are now covered by insurance plans. Formerly considered a children's pet, many adults now own rabbits and they are quite concerned about the health and wellbeing of their pets. Problems relating to husbandry may be the easiest to identify, but not always the easiest to correct.

Abscesses

Occasionally abscesses are the result of fight wounds. The owner should be questioned about the other in-contact animals and dominance issues should be discussed. The pets may need neutering and/or separation. In many cases, abscesses are related to dental problems. The underlying dental problem needs to be corrected and the owner needs to be educated on the addition of roughage to the diet and adding tooth-wearing blocks to the pet's environment.

Initial diagnosis of an abscess can be established by fine-needle aspirate of the mass. Use a 21-gauge needle and use Gram stains for cytology. If bone involvement is suspected a radiograph should be included in the diagnostic work-up. Once diagnosed, the abscess itself should be lanced and flushed thoroughly. Rabbit pus is extremely viscous and a curette may be required to scoop out all the purulent material. Extensive flushing with saline should be carried out, taking care to keep the animal as dry as possible. Rabbits aren't the best anaesthetic candidates and getting them cold and wet will not enhance recovery. Once the area is clean, some vets advocate packing the pocket with a topical antibiotic cream or even opening a capsule of parental antibiotic into the wound. Systemic antibiotics for a minimum of 2 weeks are recommended. Enrofloxacin (Baytril, Bayer) is the current drug of choice and is licensed for rabbits. However, rabbits can also tolerate amoxicillin, clindamycin and trimethoprim/sulphonamide, to name a few other choices. If deemed necessary, a swab can be taken of the pus for culture and sensitivity. Rabbits carry *Pasteurella multocida* in their nasal cavity so this is a likely bacterium to take advantage of a wound and multiply. However, *Staphylococcus aureus*, *Pseudomonas aeruginosa*, *Proteus* spp and *Bacteroides* spp have all been identified from rabbit abscesses.

Although relatively simple to diagnose and treat initially, rabbit abscesses are a real challenge to eliminate entirely. Owners need to be informed that a rabbit abscess may never completely resolve. The rabbit may need life-long antibiotic therapy and a lot of nursing and extra care from the owner will be involved. The rabbit owner should be fully informed of the time and financial considerations involved in treating rabbit abscesses. Does the owner have the stomach to clean out the abscess site two to three times a day or does the pet need to be hospitalised during this stage of treatment? As rabbit abscess pus is too thick for drains, manual lavage is required. Additionally, the underlying cause must be addressed. The rabbit may need extensive dental work. If a joint is involved, amputation may need to be considered. Recurrence is common. If an abscess recurs more than twice, the animal is a candidate for lifelong antibiotics, albeit at lower than the normal dose rates (2.5–5 mg/kg s.i.d. of enrofloxcin has been suggested for chronic cases). Giving the client the full picture, with all the possible scenarios, will help the owner to make the appropriate decision for his/her lifestyle and financial situation.

Barbering

This husbandry issue often relates to the problem of which rabbits are housed together. A dominant rabbit will pull fur from more submissive rabbits. Alopecia will appear on the head and back. A trichogram will show fractured hair shafts, indicating traumatic hair loss. The solution to this problem is to separate the rabbits. Neutering may help if separation is not possible.

Rabbits on low-fibre diets have also been known to self-barber. Increasing the amount of hay fed can decrease the amount of fur pulled out. Oestrus can stimulate barbering in does, and pregnant does will pull fur from their forelegs, chest and hips to line their nests.

Matted fur

Long-haired rabbits should be groomed daily from kittenhood. This accustoms them to the process of grooming and gets the owner into good habits. Long fur is not natural in a rabbit and the rabbit is not equipped to sort out his grooming problems on his own. Owners who opt for the glamorous breeds must also opt for the extra work involved. Matted fur is an invitation for maggots! Faeces get caught in matted fur, urine collects and it become a site for bacterial overgrowth. Physically demonstrate how to properly brush out a long-haired rabbit. Some people do believe brushing out the top layer of fur is enough. They need to be taught otherwise.

Faced with an already-matted rabbit, all you can do is clip it. Brushing out tight mats will be too stressful for the rabbit and may tear the skin. Be sure you are working with clean, sharp clipper blades and proceed with caution. Rabbit skin is very easily damaged. Generally speaking, only anaesthetised rabbits will tolerate clipping. This is a two-person procedure, as one person must clip while the other carefully monitors the anaesthetic. Do charge accordingly for the time the procedure takes and the personnel needed. Gently remind the client how much money he/she will save if he/she grooms the pet regularly instead of waiting until it is matted again.

Pododermatitis

This problem is nearly always directly related to poor husbandry. In the early stage of this condition, the rabbit presents with ulcers of the plantar metatarsals and palmar metacarpals. The infectious agent is usually *S. aureus*. As the condition becomes chronic, the secondary lesions are elevated, hyperkeratotic and usually annular. This can be described as granulomatous dermatitis. Abscesses can develop and affect the bone.

The causes of pododermatitis can be trauma from rough flooring, such as wire, or lack of movement from confinement in a small cage. Obesity can aggravate the condition. The most important aspect in the treatment regime is to improve the husbandry. The housing needs improvement, the animal should be given free exercise on a daily basis and the weight should be monitored. The lesions should be cleaned twice daily with an antiseptic solution (2% chlorhexidine diluted 5:1 with water is adequate). Topical antibacterial ointment can also be applied twice daily. A check-up 1 week later should include a thorough review of husbandry suggestions.

Scent glands

It is normal for there to be a waxy, brownish secretion around the scent glands. Some owners find this offensive. The secretion can be cleaned away with a cotton bud for aesthetic reasons. Note that rabbits have three sets of scent glands – under the chin, at the anus, and the perineal glands, which are located in the inguinal region. Bucks mark more often in general, while does tend to use their chin and perineal (inguinal) glands to mark their kits.

Slobbers

Rabbits with dental problems will salivate profusely, creating a moist dermatitis on their chin and ventral neck. Drinking from water bowls, rather than dropper bottles, can also promote moist dermatitis. Rabbits with large dewlaps are particularly prone to this condition. There will be a green staining to the fur and *Pseudomonas aeruginosa* can be identified if a swab is taken (cytology will indicate the presence of Gram-negative bacteria). The area should be clipped and cleaned with an antiseptic solution and thoroughly dried. Drinking arrangements should be changed and any dental problems investigated. The condition should resolve if these alterations are made.

Urine scald

Dirty bedding can cause moist dermatitis in the perineal region. Bedding should be changed twice daily if moist dermatitis has occurred. Urinary tract disease is also a major cause of urine scald so the rabbit must be examined for urinary problems as an underlying disorder. Overweight rabbits may also suffer from urine scald as they are unable to groom themselves properly. Gently cleaning with an antiseptic solution twice daily and applying a barrier cream – e.g. nappy cream – will treat the condition until the underlying problem is resolved.

Dermatophytosis

Rabbits do not suffer greatly from ringworm infections. If exposed to dogs and cats, rabbits can contract *Microsporum canis*, but may or may not exhibit clinical signs. *Trichophyton mentagrophytes* occurs more commonly in the rabbit, although it can also sometimes be in an asymptomatic form. In the clinical form, the rabbit will have scaly sites of alopecia which start as a small area that gradually enlarges. Typically, early lesions begin on the head and forelimbs. A dermatophyte infection is more likely to occur in the young or debilitated rabbit. Any adult rabbit appearing with dermatophytosis is a probable victim of poor husbandry and the owner will need tutelage on proper nutrition and hutch cleaning. Dermatophytosis is best diagnosed via a fungal culture. Because *T. mentagrophytes* does not fluoresce, a Wood's lamp is relatively useless with lagomorphs. Owners should be told that ringworm can be zoonotic but *T. mentagrophytes* tends to be less communicable to humans than *M. canis*. Nevertheless, children may be handling the rabbit and as a child's immune system is not fully mature zoonotic infection may occur. Treatment for dermatophyte infections can be griseofulvin at 25–50 mg/kg once daily or divided into two doses given with a fatty acid supplement to enhance absorption. However, this drug is not licensed for rabbits and is teratogenic. Keeping in mind that the rabbit is often a young family's pet, the likelihood of a pregnant woman having to medicate the rabbit is fairly high. Therefore, the use of enilconazole (0.2% w/v, Imaverol, Janssen) is a safer option. This rinse can be applied every third day to the obvious lesions for a minimum of 3 weeks. Treatment should continue until a negative fungal culture is achieved. Some vets propose the use of topical antifungal creams as used in humans. Itraconazole (Itrafungal, Janssen) is only licensed for use in the cat but anecdotal evidence has supported its successful use in other species.

The rabbit should be given high-quality nutrition and kept in a clean hutch that has been thoroughly scrubbed with either enilconazole or a household bleach solution. Any in-contact animals should also be treated.

Ectoparasites

Fleas

Rabbits can be infested with *C. felis*, especially if living in a house with a cat population. *C. felis* can lead to pruritus in the rabbit. They can also be infested by the rabbit flea, *Spilopsyllus cuniculi*, a stick-tight flea which can be passed on from wild rabbits. Rabbit fleas can often be found attached to the margins of the pinnae, although they will infest other areas of the body. *S. cuniculi* can be a vector for myxomatosis virus so infestations should be dealt with promptly. Imadicloprid is licensed for use on rabbits for the elimination of fleas (Fipronil, however is contraindicated in this species). Pyrethrin-containing flea powders that are safe for feline kittens can be used on rabbits to treat *S. cuniculi*. Stick-tight rabbit fleas should be removed manually to ensure hasty eradication. Environmental treatment is also required, especially in the case of infestations with *C. felis*. The rabbit should be removed from the environment while spraying is taking place.

Lice

The rabbit louse, *Haemodipsus ventricosus*, is a sucking louse that can cause anaemia in severe infestation. It may also be the cause of pruritus and scaling along the dorsum. However, it is considered to be a rare cause of dermatological problems.

Coat brushings are the best way to gather samples to identify this six-legged creature or its eggs under the microscope. The eggs tend to be larger than the fur mite's eggs and are operculated. Treatment with ivermectin subcutaneously or per os, at a dose rate of 0.2–0.4 mg/kg on three occasions, at 2-week intervals, is recommended for elimination of lice. Ivermectin is, of course, not licensed for use in small animals and the owner must be aware that an extra-license drug is being used on his/her pet.

Mites

There are two main mites that infest rabbits, an ear mite and a fur mite. *Psoroptes cuniculi* is the ear mite. The rabbit will present with inflamed pinnae, encrusted with thick exudate made up of mites, mite faeces, desquaminated epithelial cells and inflammatory exudate. The condition is pruritic so self-trauma may complicate the clinical signs. In a debilitated rabbit the mite can spread out onto the legs, feet and perineum. Some severe infestations cause inner ear infections, which may manifest in a head tilt.

P. cuniculi is a member of the Psoroptid mite family. These are round-bodied, relatively long-legged mites with numerous setae extending from their legs. Three of the four pairs of legs have suckers, while the fourth pair of legs is quite short and without suckers. In general appearance, *P. cuniculi* is not unlike *Otodectes cynotis.* The rabbit ear mite can be identified via an ear swab rolled onto a glass slide. Magnification under low power will reveal the mite, eggs and often mating pairs of mites. The life cycle lasts 3 weeks so treatment must take that into account. Subcutaneous injections of ivermectin at 0.4 mg per kilogram should be given every 8 days for a total of three treatments. Ivermectin is not licensed for use in small animals. An alternative to ivermectin is to use a topical miticidal eardrop, such as is used in the treatment of *Otodectes* infestations. Instructions would be the same as for *Otodectes* treatment – 1 week twice daily, stop treatment for 1 week, repeat treatment as done in the first week. Anecdotal evidence supports the use of selamectin (Stronghold, Pfizer) on rabbits for the treatment of ear mites. The kitten or cat strengths (15 mg or 45 mg) should be used, depending on the weight of the rabbit. One or two treatments, 28 days apart at dose rate of 6–18 mg/kg, has been used successfully in a recent study (Mc Tier et al 2003).

While it is very tempting to leap in and clean out the crusty ears, cleaning should be delayed until the mites have died and the crusts fall out easily. Removing the encrusted exudate right away is painful for the rabbit and can cause bleeding. General anaesthetic would be required. If the client is willing to wait, the cleaning can be done a few days after the injections.

Figure 13.1 shows the rabbit ear mite, *Psoroptes cuniculi.*

Cheyletiella parasitovorax is a surface mite. It is sometimes referred to as a fur mite but the true fur mite of the rabbit is *Leporacarus gibbus* (see later). C. *parasitovorax* can be briefly zoonotic, a point to remember as rabbits are often children's pets. In addition, *C. parasitovorax* can be transferred to other pets, particularly cats and dogs. In humans, the infestation appears as erythematous, pruritic papules on the areas in contact with the rabbit, usually the arms.

The clinical signs in the rabbit are white scale with thinning of the fur on the dorsal cervical region. The scaling can spread along the dorsum to the rump. Pruritus may or may not be present. Rabbits are usually not much bothered by this mite but owners do become concerned by the appearance of the scale and fur loss.

Diagnosis can be achieved by taking tape strips along the dorsal spine. Coat brushings and skin scrapings are other methods of collecting samples. Identification can be made by visualising the hook-like accessory mouth parts typical of this family of mites.

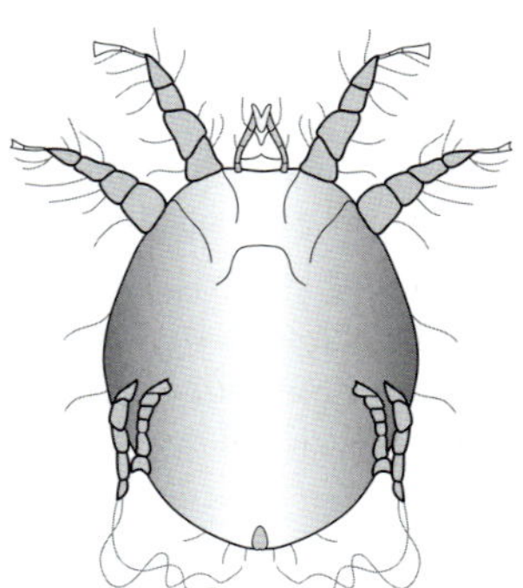

Figure 13.1 Rabbit ear mite (*Psoroptes cuniculi*). Notice the forward extension of the first pair of legs and the suckers at the ends of the legs.

The life cycle of this mite requires treatment every 2 weeks for three doses of ivermectin at 0.4 mg/kg, as a subcutaneous injection. Environmental treatment is a must with this mite as it can live off the host for up to a month.

Leporacarus gibbus is a fur mite that is known to infest rabbits. However, it can be present in large numbers without creating any clinical signs, although it occasionally causes pruritus. Treatment can be achieved with ivermectin injections or selenium sulphide baths. Both treatments would need to be repeated twice at intervals of 7–10 days.

Myiasis/Fly strike

The maggot-infested rabbit is most often seen during the summer months. It is primarily outdoor rabbits that become flyblown and there are predisposing factors, such as obesity or poor husbandry. Yet, even conscientious owners can be caught out. It takes a horrifyingly short period of time for fly eggs to hatch into larvae and begin eating away at a live rabbit. Well-meaning owners that let their rabbits out onto grass to exercise and forage can unwittingly be exposing their beloved bunnies to the ravages of myiasis.

There are different types of fly strike caused by different families of fly. The Cuterebra family of flies spawn large larvae that mutate through three larval stages. The adult fly is rarely seen as it has an extremely short life span in this form. The eggs are laid and then pupate in the subcutis of the ventral neck, axilla, inguinal area, or rump. There is one larva within each subcutaneous swelling, breathing out of an air hole in the nodule. A rabbit can have one to several nodular swellings. There may be no clinical signs at first but the rabbit will later lose weight, perhaps become lame and may die of toxic shock.

Diagnosis is made by opening a nodule and exposing the larva. Treatment is to clip and clean each nodule, enlarge the larva's air hole and carefully remove the entire larva from each nodule. Necrotic tissue should be debrided away. If the area has abscessed surgical excision will be required. In such cases, systemic antibiotics will be required and general supportive care (fluids, warmth, good nutrition) will be necessary in any case of fly strike.

The more common type of fly strike seen in the United Kingdom is usually caused by *Calliphora* spp and involves multitudes of smaller larvae writhing over the perineal region and rump. Sedentary, overweight rabbits, with clinging caecotrophs, attract flies and fall prey to this form of myiasis. Urine scald can also be a major attraction. There is no need for diagnostic testing as the problem is all too obvious. The rabbit needs to be clipped and cleaned. Flushing with copious amounts of saline can help to remove some of the maggots but there is no avoiding the tedious job of plucking away at maggots with a pair of forceps for what seems like hours on end. As the rabbit is not in top condition to begin with, be sure to place warming bags all around it while flushing away the maggots. It may be necessary to debride necrotic tissue, in which case an anaesthetic will need to be given to an animal that is, frankly, a very poor anaesthetic risk. Owners should be informed that the prognosis is poor.

Several follow-up visits, at first on a daily basis, should be made to check that all maggots have been eliminated. Often, you will find that they have not. Hospitalising the patient is often the best option. Antibiotic therapy, utilising a drug with good skin penetration (e.g. trimethoprim-sulphates), may be useful adjunctive therapy. Warmth, fluids, and good-quality nutrition all play an important part of the nursing picture.

If the rabbit recovers, the owner should be advised to help the rabbit lose weight, improve the grooming regime or do whatever needs to be done to prevent a recurrence of this unhygienic event. Sometimes, the rabbit is unable to groom itself properly due to dental problems. Any and all underlying problems should be addressed. Finally, prevention is always the best option. Cyromazine (Rearguard, Novartis) is now available to help prevent fly strike. It is applied directly to the rabbit every 8–10 weeks, especially during the summer and autumn. There are also products for reducing fly populations in the rabbit hutch. Owners should be educated on the use of these products.

Other dermatological conditions affecting rabbits

There are a collection of viral and bacterial diseases which have dermatological symptoms. Probably the most well known is myxomatosis. The infected rabbit will have swollen eyelids, erythema and swelling at the facial area. Similar swelling and erythema also occurs at the perineum. Other clinical signs include red eyes with an ocular discharge, pyrexia and lethargy. There is no cure for this disease, only supportive care can be offered. Rabbit owners should be encouraged to keep their pets' myxomatosis vaccines up to date with reminders. Venereal spirochaetosis is also known as rabbit syphilis. This is a bacterial infection that has the dermatological signs of ulcers and crusting at the nostrils, lips, eyelids, chin, genitalia and perineum. Diagnosis must eliminate any possible parasitic causes. Biopsy should be performed to obtain a definitive diagnosis. Once identified as syphilis, penicillin can be used in rabbits to treat this condition. It should be given subcutaneously at a dose rate of 42 000–84 000 iu/kg. Three injections should be given at 7-day intervals (Hillyer 1997).

Acute cellulitis is an oedematous swelling of the head, neck and sometimes thorax. Pyrexia occurs in conjunction with the oedema. A bacterial infection of *S. aureus* or *P. multocida* is the cause. An abscess may eventually form, which should be treated accordingly. In some instances a necrotic eschar will form. Treatment with systemic antibiotics is recommended. Emergency treatment may be required if the airway is inhibited by the swelling. *S. aureus* infection can cause an exudative dermatitis with pustules, plus or minus subcutaneous abscesses. Young rabbits are particularly susceptible to this type of infection. Occasionally the disease is associated with mastitis or pododermatitis. Clipping and cleaning the area and treating with systemic antibiotics are the appropriate response. Swabs can be taken for culture and sensitivity when choosing the antibiotic but most clinicians prefer empirical choices for small furries.

Skin tumours in rabbits are uncommon. A firm mass can usually be assumed to be an abscess. Fine-needle aspirates are a diagnostic method for determining what a mass actually is. If cytology does not reveal pustular exudate then it is possible that the mass could be a skin tumour. Biopsy can be both the diagnostic tool and the treatment. Complete excision, with wide margins, should be practiced just in case. Papillomas and basal cell carcinomas do occur in rabbits. Melanomas tend to appear on the ears and can metastasise quickly. Rectal bleeding can be a complication of rectal polyps, or the rabbit can be asymptomatic. Removal is advised if bleeding occurs.

There are no studies regarding the use of chemotherapy in rabbits. Treatment of tumours, whether malignant or benign, is via surgical excision.

Abrasions and lacerations are common occurrences in rabbits. Territorial fights between two intact males can lead to bite wounds around the eyes, ear and testes. The area around a wound should be clipped carefully and flushed with saline. Surgical glue can be used if the laceration is fresh and there is little traction in the area. Otherwise, general anaesthesia and suturing is required.

FERRETS

The questionnaire at the beginning of this chapter should apply to ferrets and all small mammals. Particularly with ferrets, one must pay attention to age, gender and reproductive status. There are some important systemic conditions in ferrets which are closely related to hormonal levels. In some systemic ferret diseases alopecia is one of the clinical signs. As ferrets should be routinely vaccinated for canine distemper, vaccination status should also be queried as this disease has dermatological signs. A complete physical examination is incredibly important when examining ferrets with skin disease.

Ferret skin is replete with sebaceous glands, with the male having even more glands than the female. This plethora of sebaceous glands is one of the contributing factors in that particular ferret smell. On the other hand, ferrets have minimal sweat glands and are thus vulnerable to hyperthermia. Neutering can reduce the odour of ferret but not eliminate the musk entirely. Anal glands are another contributing factor but do not warrant removing unless impacted, a rare occurrence.

The coat is thick and coarse, showing thinning in the warmer months. This change is known as 'pelt cycling'. Bilateral, symmetrical alopecia of the tail, perineum and inguinal areas often concurs with the breeding season of March to August for jills and December to July for hobs. Even neutered ferrets will show a thinning of coat during breeding season. Red to brown waxy deposits can also appear within the coat as secretions from the sebaceous glands.

Abnormal coat changes can occur due to poor nutrition. An inadequate diet leads to a dull, dry coat. Ferrets need to be fed ferret diets preferentially, or good-quality cat or kitten food if ferret diets are unavailable. The feeding of raw eggs used to be a popular practice. However, the avidin in raw egg binds to biotin, leading to bilateral, symmetrical alopecia. Some traditional ferret keepers may still be using old-fashioned diets and should be warned that salmonellosis is a risk with raw egg.

Ferrets without hidey-holes in their enclosures may become stressed and show signs of self-mutilation. Intact females may tear out their own fur for nesting material. Ferrets can also lose coat through rough play and mating.

Endocrine alopecia

The most common pathological reason for alopecia in the ferret is hyperadrenocorticism. This can be referred to as 'endocrine alopecia' or 'adrenal gland disease'. This disease is much more common in the United States than in the United Kingdom. It has been suggested that the early neutering policy in the United States may be partially responsible for this as the reproductive hormone imbalance induced may be a causative factor in the disease. Unlike the dog, in the ferret this condition is pruritic. Also unlike the dog, serum cortisol levels are not raised so a simple blood test will not diagnose the disease. Adrenal gland disease usually occurs in middle-aged to older ferrets, showing no sex preference.

Diet, housing, the photoperiod the ferret is exposed to, or the gene pool may be factors in stimulating adenomas, adenocarcinomas or adrenocortical hyperplasia that are the causes of the hormonal imbalance. Clinical signs begin in the late winter to early spring with hair loss starting at the rump and progressing forwards. Complete alopecia can occur. The coat may grow back in the autumn but will be lost again the following spring. This cycle can take place two to three times and then further hair growth stops altogether.

Hair loss is a clinical sign in 90% of ferrets affected with adrenal gland disease. The coat is easily epilated and loss is symmetrical – both strong indicators of endocrine disease in any species. One third of afflicted animals experience pruritus and erythema along the dorsum and between the shoulder blades. Females show vulva enlargement with or without a mucoid discharge. The enlarged adrenal glands, especially the left gland, can be palpated in a fat pad cranial to the kidney, but ultrasound is needed for an accurate assessment. Haematology may show anaemia or pancytopaenia, and biochemistry may show raised alanine aminotransferase (ALT), but not in all cases. As mentioned before, an adenocorticotrophic hormone (ACTH) stimulation test is not useful nor is a dexamethasone suppression test. Instead, plasma steroids should be measured. The dehydroepandrosterone steroids to measure are: oestradiol, 17-hydroxyprogesterone and androstenedione. The diseased animal will show markedly raised levels of these compounds.

An intact jill in oestrus, or even a neutered female with an ovarian remnant, can also have vulva enlargement with hair loss. To ascertain whether she is showing normal hormonal fluctuations or is suffering from adrenal gland disease, she can be injected with human chorionic gonadotrophin. This will cause the vulva to decrease in size within 10 days. If this does not occur, then adrenal gland disease should be investigated.

Medical management of endocrine alopecia is not usually as successful in ferrets as it is in dogs. Mitotane has been used but is not nearly as effective in ferrets since their hyperadrenocorticism is caused by the adrenal glands, rather than the pituitary gland. Additionally, mitotane can lead to severe hypoglycaemia if there is concurrent insulinoma. Unfortunately, insulinoma is often subclinical in the ferret so mitotane can be given inadvertently to an affected pet. Mitotane is best used as a palliative, rather than curative measure if surgery is not an option.

Surgery is the preferred method of treatment. The animal should be fasted for eight to twelve hours, intravenous access attained and fluid therapy given throughout surgery. Feeding can resume six to twelve hours post-operatively. More careful management during surgery is thus required with concurrent insulinoma. Debulking the pancreas can take place along with adrenalectomy to treat the insulinoma.

Alopecia without pruritus

Male, or female without vulval swelling

- If resolves on its own, possibly seasonal alopecia.
- If progresses or remains, check for parasites or fungal infestation.
- If tests negative, do adrenal ultrasound. If adrenals enlarged, check plasma steroid levels. If elevated, proceed to adrenalectomy. (Unilateral adrenalectomy if only one adrenal gland is affected. If both glands are affected, bilateral adrenalectomy can be performed, or unilateral and subtotal adrenalectomy of less diseased gland.)

Female with vulval swelling

- Give two doses of human chorionic gonadotropin.
- If swelling decreases, neuter or check for ovarian remnants.
- If no decrease in swelling, ultrasound adrenal glands. If enlarged, check plasma steroid levels. If raised, adrenalectomy.

Pruritus

Pruritic diseases in ferrets are most likely to be caused by parasites.

Pruritus

- If lesions present, do skin scrapes. If positive, treat. If negative, do fungal culture.
- If ear exudate, examine exudate for *Otodectes*. Treat if positive. Clean ears.
- If systemic involvement indicated (e.g. pyrexia) check vaccination status. Investigate possible distemper.
- If alopecia, but no other lesions, do endocrine work-up. (Ultrasound adrenals, check plasma steroid levels.)
- If no alopecia or any other lesions, treat empirically for ectoparasitic infestation.

Ectoparasites

The most common parasitic infestation is with *Otodectes cynotis*. This is communicated via direct contact with other infected animals. Clinical signs include head shaking, scratching at the ears, an inflamed external ear canal and a brown, waxy exudate. The level of pruritus with this infestation can vary but extremely itchy animals will create self-trauma lesions of excoriation. On the other hand, some carriers can be asymptomatic. To confuse the picture further, a brown, waxy exudate can often occur in parasite-free ferrets. Therefore, diagnostic testing is called for and empirical treatment is not advised. A simple ear swab spread thinly onto a slide can determine whether or not mites are present. If mites are identified, the ear should be cleaned with a proprietary cleaner and miticidal drops applied twice daily for 1 week. Treatment should be repeated at the third week to eliminate all stages of the mite's life cycle. If mites are not identified, ear cleaning is still recommended. All in-contact pets should be treated and environmental control is useful in preventing future infestations.

The ferret's ear canal is quite narrow, making topical ear treatment a bit of a challenge. Additionally, the pinnae are very delicate and must be handled carefully. If miticidal drops are not proving effective an injection of ivermectin at 200–400 micrograms/kg, given subcutaneously, can be used. The injection will need to be repeated every 2 weeks for a total of 4 weeks until the ears are completely clear of infestation.

Various *Ctenocephalides* species can affect the ferret, especially if there are other animals in the household. Infested ferrets will exhibit mild to intense pruritus, especially at the nape of the neck. Heavy infestations can contribute to alopecia in the dorsal cervical and thoracic regions. Fleas are identified via coat brushings or by collecting flea faeces in a tape strip. Treatments licensed for cats are generally safe to use on ferrets. Organophosphates should be avoided in ferrets. The modern chemicals (e.g.

fipronil) are safe, albeit not licensed. If using a spray, the ingredient can be sprayed onto a cloth and then rubbed into the ferret's coat.

Ticks also occur on ferrets and can be treated with the same medications as used for flea treatment. Removal of the tick is recommended, as with any species.

Sarcoptes scabiei can infest ferrets via fomites or direct contact with an infested animal. Clinical signs include focal to general alopecia with severe pruritus. Focal infestations occur on the paws, which will become swollen, erythematous and crusty. Nail deformity will develop and entire nails can be sloughed off. The layman's term for this type of infestation is 'foot rot' as a ferret can actually lose its foot due to self-trauma and secondary infection instigated by the mite infestation. Diagnosis is via skin scrapes. Ivermectin at 200–400 micrograms/kg every 7–14 days until skin scrapings are negative has been the treatment of choice. The use of selamectin has not been documented but anecdotal reports are positive. Two doses, 1 month apart, should be given with the appropriate strength for the weight of the ferret.

Cutaneous myiasis can occur in ferrets kept outdoors during the summer months. Young kits are particularly susceptible. *Dipterid* fly larvae of the *Cuterebra* species tend to deposit eggs on the face, neck and flanks of ferrets. These hatch subcutaneously and the larvae create nodular swellings that are not unlike abscesses. There is an air hole present in each swelling, which can be enlarged to remove the larva intact. Removal of the entire larva is the goal, as remnants left behind can become a nidus for infection. Antimicrobial topical treatment is a good idea and in some cases systemic antimicrobials are required. The lesions can be left to heal by second intention.

Dermatophytosis

Fungal infections in ferrets are not common. If they do occur the responsible organism is usually *T. mentagrophytes*. This is a zoonotic infection so diagnosis and treatment are required, although the disease usually infects only young ferrets and is self-limiting in nature. The clinical picture is of small papules that spread peripherally to a large, circumscribed lesion of alopecia with inflammation and crust. Thickening of the skin will occur at the site. It the lesion is pruritic, this is usually due to a secondary pyoderma that has developed opportunistically. If pyoderma occurs, secondary lesions due to self-trauma will complicate the picture.

T. mentagrophytes does not fluoresce, so a fungal culture is the only worthwhile diagnostic test to perform for dermatophytosis in the ferret. Once identified, clipping around the lesion is indicated and antifungal topicals can be used on the site (for examination, Daktarin cream, Janssen-Cilag or Malaseb Shampoo, Leo Laboratories). Systemic treatment is not always necessary but if used, griseofulvin at 25 mg/kg per os, once daily with a fatty acid supplement can be given for 21–30 days. Griseofulvin, aside from being teratogenic, can cause leucopoenia, anaemia, lethargy, anorexia, ataxia and depression. The owner must be reminded to disinfect the environment with a bleach solution or enilconazole. All in-contact pets will require treatment as well.

Cutaneous bacterial infections

Bacterial infections in ferrets are often due to bite wounds. Abscesses or cellulitis may form. The causative bacteria are usually staphylococcal or streptococcal species, although *Corynebacterium* spp, *Pasteurella* spp, *Aetinomyce* spp and haemolytic *E. coli* have been identified. Usually the infection is localised and treatment by lancing and flushing is most helpful. A swab for culture and sensitivity can be taken from the discharge obtained if that is deemed necessary. If needed a drain can be exploited to manage the situation. Systemic antibiotics can be chosen empirically or via results from culture and sensitivity.

'Lumpy jaw' is a condition caused by an infection with the relatively rare *Actinomyces* spp, a Gram-positive bacterium that enters wounds in the mouth or is ingested. The resultant cervical mass can be drained of a yellow to green purulent exudate. The area should be thoroughly debrided and a drain placed. Culture should be peformed to identify the microorganism exactly or, alternatively, a high dose of a penicillin-family drug can be given. This condition can lead to dyspnoea so should be treated aggressively.

Neoplasm

Any mass which is not identified as an abscess should be biopsied as a possible neoplasm. A variety of malignant and benign tumours occur in ferrets. Adenocarcinomas are rare tumours of the adnexa, primarily the sweat glands. Metastasis and recurrence is possible with adenocarcinomas. Most tumours of this type are located in the perineal area.

Cutaneous mast cell tumours in the ferret are usually benign. The average age of onset is 4 years and there is no sex predilection. Tumours can appear on the neck, shoulders or trunk as single growths or multiple, well-circumscribed, alopecic nodules. The tumours are usually unpigmented and can ulcerate if pruritic, leading to a dark, crusty exudate. Fine-needle aspirates will give a diagnosis and excisional biopsy will remove the problem.

Sebaceous epitheliomas appear on the head, neck, shoulders and feet. The average afflicted ferret is 5 years of age and 70% are female. The growths are pendunculated or plaque-like. Metastasis and reoccurrence are rare. Although benign, these tumours can be fast-growing and tend to ulcerate. Surgical excision is recommended.

Squamous cell carcinomas occur on the head, lips, digits, tarsi and footpads. These are firm, well vascularised masses that do tend to ulcerate. Metastasis to the lymph node can occur. Recurrence is also possible. Surgical excision is the best therapeutic option.

Cutaneous lymphoma, haemangioma, fibroma and fibrosarcoma have all been reported in ferrets.

Viral disease

The primary viral disease that can stimulate skin lesions in the ferret is canine distemper. In an ideal world all ferrets would be vaccinated against this disease. In the real world unvaccinated ferrets fall prey to the virus via direct contact, fomite contact or aerosol spray. The incubation period is 7 days. Infected ferrets will have mucopurulent nasal and ocular discharges. An erythematous skin rash under the chin and in the inguinal and perineal regions will manifest 10–15 days post-exposure. A general orange tinge to the skin can develop and pruritus and secondary pyoderma are also possible. Brown crusts will appear on the face, chin, lips and eyelids, accompanied by oedema. Hyperkeratosis occurs on the footpads.

A conjunctival swab or a blood smear prepared on the ninth day of infection may capture the shedding virus. Treatment is only supportive. The prognosis is guarded and death usually occurs between the 12th and 22nd day of infection.

GUINEA PIGS

Ectoparasites

Ectoparasites affecting guinea pigs include fleas, lice and mites. *C. felis* is the flea that affects guinea pigs most often. Treatments used in the elimination of fleas in rabbits are used with guinea pigs, although there is nothing actually licensed for flea treatment in guinea pigs. Environmental treatment is always recommended to prevent re-infestation.

Guinea pig lice are the species *Gliricola porcelli* and *Gyropus ovalis*. These are both biting lice that feed on epithelial debris. *G. porcellis* is found more commonly. This is a slender, yellow to grey louse of about 1.5 mm in length. *G. ovalis* is less elongated and has a wider head. Clinical signs relate to the level of infestation. A light infestation will lead to mild pruritus, especially behind the ears. A heavy infestation can lead to alopecia. Lice and their eggs are sampled via coat brushings or tape strippings. Treatment with ivermectin at 200–400 micrograms/kg per os or subcutaneously is usually practised. Dosing needs to be repeated in 10 days time. Alternatively, the guinea pig can be bathed in a selenium sulphide shampoo (Seleen, Sanofi) three times at weekly intervals. A 10-minute contact time is required and combing out the nits enhances treatment. Unfortunately, guinea pig lice have a more than passing resemblance to human head lice, which may worry many owners. Lice are host specific, however, so owners should not be concerned about zoonosis.

The most frequently observed parasite in guinea pigs is the mite *Trixicarus caviae* (Fig. 13.2). It is a burrowing sarcoptid mite that causes intense pruritus. Excoriations, induced by self-trauma, and secondary infection often accompany infestation. Severely affected guinea pigs can suffer from seizure-like episodes. Lesions occur first on the back and shoulders and can become generalised. Humans can be transiently infected.

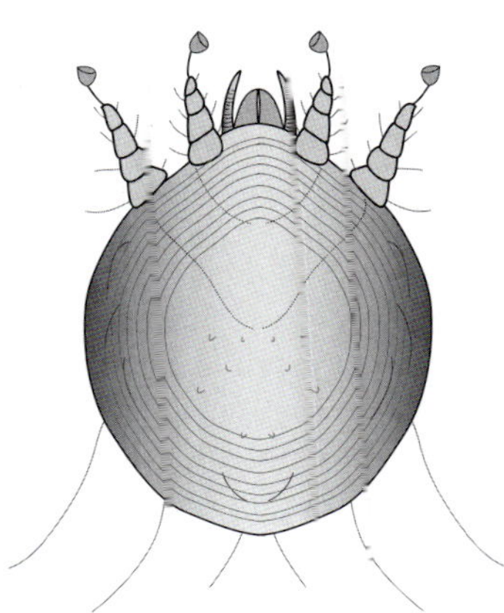

Figure 13.2 Fur mite of the guinea pig (*Trixicarus caviae*). Notice the concentric circles on the body.

T. caviae is diagnosed via skin scrapings. Treatment is with ivermectin at 200–400 micrograms per kilogram per os or subcutaneously repeated twice at 7-day intervals. The environment should be thoroughly cleansed and all in-contact pets should be treated. Bathing with a soothing shampoo, for example with a colloidal oatmeal (Episoothe, Virbac), can help to ease the pruritus and cleanse the secondary lesions. Guinea pigs which experience pruritic seizures can be treated with diazepam at 1–2 mg/kg. Steroids are contraindicated.

Chirodiscoides caviae is a fur mite that affects guinea pigs. As it is not a burrowing mite it does not create the same level of pruritus as *T. caviae*. Identification of *C. caviae* is established by gathering coat brushing or tape strip samples. Treatment with ivermectin at 300 to 400 micrograms/kg twice, with a 10-day interval, is suggested. Environmental elimination is also required, as well as treatment of other in-contact pets.

Demodectic mange is not common in the guinea pig but can occur, causing alopecia at the head and forelegs. Pruritus is absent. Diagnosis is achieved via skin scrapes and treatment is given with ivermectin, three times at 2-week intervals.

Myiasis occurs rarely in the guinea pig; if it does, this species is less susceptible to the toxic shock that rabbits experience with fly strike. The same method of treatment (i.e. cleaning and cleansing the area) is used for guinea pigs. Again, the owners need education on appropriate husbandry.

Dermatophytosis

Dermatophytosis in the guinea pig is primarily a *Trichophyton mentagrophytes* infection, although *M. canis* has been observed. Ringworm in guinea pigs usually occurs secondarily to overcrowding and poor husbandry. Deficiencies of vitamin C may predispose an animal to infection. Young guinea pigs are most susceptible. Transmission between small mammals contained together occurs easily and environmental contamination doubles the opportunity for infection.

Focal areas of alopecia and crusting typically begin at the face, forehead and ears, spreading back to the trunk and limbs. Diagnosis is obtained via a fungal culture. The affected pet and all in-contact pets should be treated topically with enilconazole 0.2% rinse (Imaverol, Janssen-Cilag) or miconazole (Daktarin ointment, Janssen-Cilag). Treatment should be applied every third day for a minimum of 3 weeks, or until a negative fungal culture is achieved. Antifungal shampoo (e.g. Malaseb, Leo Laboratories) can be used as adjunctive treatment. Alternatively, griseofulvin can be given at 25 mg/kg per os, once daily or in divided doses for 3–5 weeks. This drug should be given with an essential fatty acid supplement to enhance absorption. Griseofulvin is contraindicated in pregnant sows and pigs less than 3 months old. Itraconazole oral drops (Itrafungol, Janssen) is another treatment option, although not yet licensed for use in guinea pigs.

Problems with husbandry

There are numerous dermatological problems which can be traced to problems with husbandry. Abscesses can occur due to fight wounds. It is inadvisable to keep two intact boars in the same pen as fights can result. Similarly, guinea pigs should never be kept with rabbits as rabbits are much larger and stronger and can do fatal damage to guinea pigs. Abscesses in guinea pigs are treated the same as in other species: lance, drain, flush and give systemic antibiotics. Topical antibiotics at the site are recommended by some practitioners. Guinea pigs tend to heal from abscesses somewhat better than rabbits.

Anal fold dermatitis can occasionally occur, especially in overweight guinea pigs. The area should be cleansed with dilute chlorhexidine and topical antibiotic cream applied twice daily till the erythema subsides.

Alopecia that is not due to parasites or dermatophytes can be the result of fur chewing. Samples of the hair will show fractured shafts. Guinea pigs will chew their own fur or their hutch mates' fur. This behaviour can be related to dominance, lack of roughage in the diet or boredom. Improving the diet can be tried and if that is not successful, guinea pigs should be separated. Sows with pups may show alopecia due to the pups chewing at the sow's fur. Chew toys can be provided to enrich the environment.

Diets low in vitamin C can lead to scurvy in the vitamin C-dependent guinea pig. Alopecia is one of the clinical signs, along with lethargy, lameness and bleeding gums. Sows late in pregnancy may lose fur that grows back after parturition, and with the assistance of vitamin B supplements. Other sows lose fur after parturition, probably due to the stress that pregnancy puts on the body. High-level nutrition and avoiding frequent pregnancies can bring the coat back into condition.

'Broken back' is a condition of hair loss along the dorsum. The area can fissure and crust over. Reportedly, this condition is due to pregnancy or stress. The affected area should be bathed with warm salt water and a topical antibiotic cream applied three times daily. Light-coloured guinea pigs seem particularly susceptible to this condition. Improved nutrition can speed recovery.

Pododermatitis is sometimes called 'bumble foot'. It is a common disorder among obese guinea pigs kept in wire-floored hutches. Rough flooring is abrasive to the feet and hyperkeratosis evolves. Ulceration can follow, allowing microbes (usually *S. aureus*) to enter. In the worst-case scenario, osteomyelitis develops. Clinically, the guinea pig will appear very lame and will vocalise in pain. Treatment requires debridement of the area and soaks in a warm saline solution. Some feet may require bandaging. If bone involvement is suspected radiographs are indicated. The flooring of the hutch should be changed and the guinea pig provided with dry, soft bedding. Weight reduction should be advised.

Post-natal sores occur especially after a long labour. Fluids caking on the ventral abdomen and rump irritate the skin. The sow may later rip out the fur to ease the irritation. The area should be gently cleansed with saline.

Scent glands exist at the base of the spine. These glands can create a greasy exudate at the site, especially in sows. This is perfectly normal but can be wiped away if it is offensive to the owners.

Urine scald can be caused by polyuria or incontinence. Identifying the exact condition and diagnosing the cause is essential to resolve the problem. The area should be cleansed with saline and protected with petroleum jelly.

Other dermatological conditions affecting guinea pigs

There are a variety of other conditions which can affect guinea pigs and which are not necessarily related to husbandry issues. Cervical lymphadenitis can be caused when some rough feed injures the mouth, allowing commensal bacteria to enter the bloodstream. Nodules develop in the cervical region, coalescing into a pus-filled mass. The abscess should be lanced and culture and sensitivity performed to identify the causative agent. *Streptococcus zooepidemicus* is often the instigating microbe. The area should be drained and flushed copiously and the guinea pig should be treated with systemic antimicrobials. Isolation is recommended. If the disease becomes systemic septicaemia or pneumonia can result.

Endocrine alopecia manifests as bilateral, symmetrical flank alopecia with hyperpigmentation. This condition is seen only in the sow as it is caused by ovarian cysts. Diagnosis is by clinical history, palpation of the cysts in the abdomen or ultrasonography. The cysts can be deflated via aspiration or by surgical excision. Alternatively, human chorion gonadotropin injections can be given once or twice, 7–10 days apart.

Epidermoid sebaceous cysts usually occur on the dorsum. These can be removed if the guinea pig finds them irritating but surgical excision is not necessary otherwise. A fine-needle aspirate will assist diagnosis.

Basal cell tumours also occur on the dorsum. These tumours are oval, well circumscribed and mobile. Metastasis is rare but recurrence is not. The tumours are usually benign but warrant excision as they usually do ulcerate.

Trichofolliculoma is the most common skin tumour in the guinea pig. This is a benign, basal cell epithelioma. The mass is solid and usually occurs at the lumbosacral area. Fine-needle aspiration will reveal that the mass is comprised of sebum, hair and keratinous debris. Surgical excision is recommended as the neoplasms often become infected. Some clinicians opt to send samples for biopsy.

OTHER SMALL MAMMALS

The other small mammals – hamsters, chinchillas, gerbils, rats and mice – suffer from many of the same conditions that rabbits and guinea pigs do, to a lesser or greater degree. Treatment of wounds and abscesses is primarily the same for any of these species. Diagnostic testing for parasites remains the same and treatment for ectoparasites still relies heavily on the use of ivermectin, although selamectin is now being used by some practitioners. Again, husbandry problems can predispose an animal to skin disorders. There are some particular dermatological conditions that are more specific to these smaller species.

Hamsters

Hamsters have two anatomical aspects that often cause owners to worry. Cheek pouches can become impacted if the animal is fed the wrong type of food. While hamsters are omnivores, their diverse tastes should not be too widely encouraged. A bit of meat and vegetables alongside the hamster mix is fine but hamsters should really stay out of the chocolate box! Chocolate can cause terribly impacted cheek pouches which some owners do mistake for tumours. The pouches need to be cleaned out thoroughly so the animal can eat again properly.

The other confusing part of the hamster's anatomy are the scent glands located on each flank. In male hamsters, the area of the gland can become alopecic and hyperpigmented. Owners fear that their pet has bilateral tumours. Unfortunately, hamsters can get bilateral, symmetrical alopecia for pathological reasons as well. Hyperadrenocorticoidism does occur in hamsters. The dermatological signs are non-pruritic and accompanied by polyuria, polydipsia and polyphagia. Hyperadrenocorticoidism can be diagnosed via an ultrasound of the adrenal glands or an ACTH stimulation test. However, these are very difficult procedures in such small animals. Some clinicians feel that diagnosing by the clinical signs is more appropriate. Lysodren is the usual treatment given but the prognosis is guarded.

When hyperadrenocorticoidism is suspected, *Demodex criceti* should be ruled out via a skin scraping and/or a biopsy. Hamsters are more prone to demodectic mange than are other small furries and will exhibit variable pruritus with *D. criceti* infestation. If the mite is identified, ivermectin is given at 0.2–0.4 mg/kg subcutaneously every 5–7 days until two negative skin scrapes are achieved. Amitraz (Aludex, Intervet) washes can also be used at dose rates of 250 parts per million, once weekly until negative skin scrapes are obtained for two consecutive weeks (Scott, et al 2001).

Epitheliotrophic lymphoma is one other condition that should be included in the differential list with hyperadrenocorticoidism. Diagnosis is via biopsy. Treatment is not offered, as chemotherapy is impractical in an animal this small.

An additional dermatological problem for hamsters is trichoepithelioma. This is a benign tumour of the hair follicle. While the tumours are not life threatening, they can grow in locations that cause discomfort to the hamster and, in those cases, should be removed. Any hamster with a trichoepithelioma should be assessed for polyoma virus, which is often the underlying cause of trichoepithelioma in the hamster. Polyoma virus is easily passed between hamsters via urine and is considered a major problem in this species.

Chinchillas

Chinchillas can get fleas if they are exposed; however, they are not particularly prone to parasites. Obviously, the environment and the pet sharing its fleas will need treatment. Chinchillas themselves can be treated with ivermectin. There are no studies supporting the use of other flea treatment such as fipronil, imadicloprid or selamectin. However, anecdotal reports support efficacy and safety with these products if given at the appropriate dose for the animal's weight. Using fipronil spray on a cloth, rubbed into the animal's fur can be a safer method of application for this species.

Chinchillas are susceptible to dermatophyte infections. Loss of fur at the nose, behind the ears and on the forefeet is strongly indicative of a ringworm infection. If the case is severe, the area of infection will become inflamed and crusty. *T. mentagrophytes* is usually the species responsible. Fungal cultures are used for diagnosis, and treatment is the same as for guinea pigs.

Dust baths are essential to a chinchilla's wellbeing. A dish of dust should be provided daily for 30 minutes. If the dust is left too long the chinchilla may over do it and develop conjunctivitis. Without a dust bath, chinchilla fur becomes matted. Over-warm or overly humid enclosures can also lead to matting of the fur. Fur slip, leading to patches of alopecia, occurs when chinchillas are handled roughly.

Gerbils

Nasal dermatitis is a particular problem in gerbils. Gerbils, which bang their noses against their cages, stimulate secretion of porphyrins from the harderinan gland near the nares. This secretion is irritating and can contribute to moist dermatitis, manifesting as erythema around the nares and often complicated by a secondary bacterial infection. Stress, over crowding and a humidity level higher than 50% can contribute to the onset of nasal dermatitis. The face should be cleaned daily and the gerbil removed to a dry, spacious environment with sand or soft clay as bedding. Topical and/or systemic antibiotics should be given if the secondary infection is severe. Infecting bacteria are usually *S. aureus* or *S. xylosus*.

Reducing crowding is also helpful for reducing the number of fight wounds a gerbil encounters, as this species is prone to aggressive encounters.

Like the hamster, gerbils also have glands which can be mistaken for tumours. Gerbils have large scent glands on their ventral abdomen. Occasionally these glands become infected or become sites for neoplasia. Debriding and topical therapy are recommended.

A final note on gerbils. If picked up by the tail, the gerbil will extricate itself from its own tail. This leaves a de-gloving injury which quickly becomes necrotic. Amputation is the most usual treatment.

Mice and rats

Mice and rats are prone to pelage (fur) mites. These are long-legged surface mites. The clinical signs are thinning of fur and variable pruritus. The mice mites are *Mycoptes musculinus* and *Psoregates simplex*. The rat mite is *Ornithonyssus bacoti*. As these are surface dwellers, ivermectin is not an efficient means of elimination. Topical treatment, in the form of a selenium sulphide shampoo, is preferred. Baths should be once every 7–10 days, for a total of three treatments, to eliminate all life stages of the mite.

Cheyletiellid mites also affect rodents. *Myobia musculi* and *Radfordia affinis* are of the long-legged cheyletiellids. Ivermectin given as subcutaneous injections at a dose rate of 200–400 micrograms/kg given three times at 2-week intervals, along with selenium sulphide washes, have been recommended for the treatment of these surface mites.

Sarcoptid mites are burrowing and thus cause far more irritation. Pruritus will lead to secondary lesions such as excoriations and even ulcers. The nails should be clipped to limit self-trauma and secondary bacterial infections should be treated with topical ointments. *Sarcoptes scabiei* can affect rats, although rodents have their own sarcoptid mite in the form of *Notoedres mores*. As these are burrowing mites, ivermectin is a good choice of treatment, at 200–400 micrograms/kg given subcutaneously. Alternatively, the ivermectin can be diluted 1:100 with water and mixed with propylene glycol. This mixture can then be used as a spot-on at the back of the head. Ingestion of the mixture is not harmful and actually enhances treatment. Three doses should be given at 2-week intervals. Diagnostic tests for all of these mites would be tape strips and coat brushings for the surface mites, hair plucks and skin scrapings for the burrowing mites.

Seborrhoea can affect older rats, especially male rats. An anti-seborrhoeic shampoo that has been licensed for cats is usually mild enough for rodents.

Castration is another treatment modality. 'Ring tail', avascular necrosis of the tail, is another rat problem but occurs less often in pets than in laboratory rats.

Mice are known to barber each other; the actual barbering is carried out by the dominant mouse. Dominant females often barber and hoard the fur for nests. Males are more likely to fight rather than barber. Alopecia on the muzzle can also be caused by trauma against the side of the enclosure. Enrichment of the environment can help to decrease this behaviour. Alopecia of the ventral abdomen and thorax in the female is related to nursing.

Both mice and rats are prone to tumours and abscesses. Diagnosis of a lump should be by fine-needle aspirate. *S. aureus, Pasteurella pneumotropica* and *Streptococcus pyogenes* are opportunistic pathogens that will cause abscesses given the chance. Lancing, flushing, debriding and systemic antibiotics are the treatment required.

The tumours most likely to appear are mammary adenocarcinomas, fibrosarcomas and fibroadenomas. Malignant tumours number about 10% and frequently recur after excision. As mammary tissue is extensive, especially in the rat, lumps can progress from the neck to the inguinal region. The prognosis is generally poor if the tumour is malignant. Spayed rats tend to have a lower incidence of malignant tumours.

REPTILES

Reptile skin is protected by overlapping scales in some but not all reptilian species. Scales in themselves are extremely keratinised epithelium. Beneath the scales lies the epidermis consisting of a stratum germinativum, stratum spinosum and a stratum corneum. The dermis layer rests under the epidermis and consists of connective tissue. Some species of reptile have osteoderms within the dermis, for example, tortoises. This does make radiography complicated. The skin is directly connected to muscle and bone as there is no hypodermis. Instead, fat is stored in the abdomen. Modifications of the epidermis include adornments such as crests, horns, spines and dewlaps. Chelonians, of course, have their shells, made up of bone and epithelial elements.

Reptile skin has very few glands. There is a nuchal gland at the neck and a cloacal gland at the caudal ventrum. However, reptiles do have sensory receptors, such as heat pits in snakes, which help them to gravitate towards sources of warmth. Additionally, reptiles have chromatophores in their skin. These are areas of pigmentation that can take on different shades (think of a chameleon changing its colour.) Chromatophores are governed by hormones and may also have a neurological component. There are five different possible pigmentations, including melanin, erythrin (red and orange), xanthus (yellow), carontenoids (orange) and guanins. A change in colour may occur as camouflage or to ward off predators. Pathological changes in colour can be caused by injury, which may lead to hypo- or hyperpigmentation at the site of insult. Albinism is not normal in the wild but has been cultivated through breeding programmes.

Ecdysis, or skin shed, is a normal process in the reptile. Ecdysis is continuous in the crocodilian and chelonian families, while it is periodic in the squamata (snake) family. Complete or partial shed occurs depending on the species. Juvenile squamata shed every 1–2 weeks, while adults shed two to four times per year. Prior to shed, more epithelial cells are produced. Lymphatic fluid infiltrates between the old and new epithelial cells, forcing away the old cells. Clinically, the animal develops a lack-lustre hue to its skin and the eyes develop a blueish tinge about 10 days before beginning to shed. Hyperkeratosis is apparent as the old cells peel away and the skin is sloughed off. Snakes need something to rub their noses against to begin the shed, peeling away the old layer from nose to tail in one piece. Some species eat the shed skin.

Initial examination

Getting a good history. Husbandry and nutritional problems are major factors in reptile skin disease. A host of problems can be prevented by good husbandry and sound nutrition – basically, owners who have done their homework have healthier pets. As with any dermatological case, a thorough history is necessary to get to the bottom of the problem. To examine a reptile fully, one must be well aware of its living conditions and the level of nutrition it is receiving. Providing owners with a questionnaire to fill out in the waiting room or prior to the visit can be helpful. Even if the owner does not know what the temperature and humidity of the vivarium are, that lack of knowledge in itself is a significant point. Be sure to ask the following questions:

- What type of vivarium is being used?
- What sort of light is provided?
- What heating system are you using?
- What kind of substrate is provided?
- What sort of hidey-holes have you created for your pet?
- What is the temperature and humidity in the vivarium?
- How often is the enclosure cleaned and with what cleaning product?

As you begin the physical examination of a reptile it is important to know what type of animal you are handling. Sadly, many owners do not even realise when they have a dangerous pet. Just because the owner is happily handling the animal does not mean that it is safe. If you do not recognise the species as a harmless pet look it up in a reference text. If you are at all unsure, DO NOT HANDLE THE ANIMAL. Unfortunately, there are some unscrupulous animal dealers who will sell anything if people will pay for it. Deadly rattlesnakes and cobras are available to the general public.

Once you have identified the species do make sure that you are comfortable handling that type of reptile. Snakes should be restrained behind the head and handled very gently as they can bruise and scales are easily damaged. Do not drape a constrictor over your shoulders, no matter how heavy it is. If it constricts, that will be your neck getting squeezed. Most lizards are best restrained at the shoulders and just above the hind legs. Large lizards have quite powerful tails, which can give you a painful lashing if you get in the way.

Conditions related to husbandry

Burns are serious injuries that are caused primarily by poor heating arrangements. Snakes are known to wrap around bulbs and develop full-thickness ventral burns. Hot rocks are used in many vivariums and scorch many a reptile that falls asleep on them. Full-thickness burns can become necrotic all the way to the body wall. This carries a poor prognosis. Secondary infection with *Pseudomonas* spp is common. Supportive treatment should be given in the form of gentle cleansing, fluids and systemic antibiotics.

Rostral lesions are much less serious but very common problems, especially in nervous lizards and snakes without hidey-holes. All vivariums should have private places where the reptile can retreat to rest unseen. A glass vivarium should be tinted so that the animal is aware of an obstruction and will not repeatedly bang itself against the glass sides. Topical treatment can be given to aid healing of these injuries. Betadine solution applied once daily is recommended.

Skin lacerations and *bite wounds* can occur due to inter-species or same-species aggression or even from prey. The wound can be cleansed with warm saline, or if very infected with 50% dextrose, flushed away 2–4 hours later with saline. Betadine or chlorohexidine solution can be used for daily cleaning before applying betadine ointment or silver sulfadiazine as topical treatments to the wound. An adhesive drape dressing should be adhered to protect the wound. Healing is temperature-dependent in the reptile, so great attention should be paid to the environment. A preferred optimal temperature zone and/or a temperature gradient should be provided in the vivarium.

If an abscess develops due to an injury it is usually capsular in nature. The abscess can be lanced and the caseous material within curetted out. If you are lucky, the entire abscess will pop out as a whole unit. Systemic antibiotics are required in the case of abscesses. When choosing an antibiotic empirically, it should be kept in mind that reptiles are more prone to Gram-negative infections than other types of pets. Bacterial species affecting reptiles include: *E. coli, Klebsiella, Proteus, Pseudomonas* and *Salmonella*, to name a few. Fluoroquinolines are usually chosen.

Chelonians can inflict shell damage to each other (especially during mating). However, nutritional, metabolic and genetic factors can also contribute to shell damage. Any shell fracture over 6 hours old should be considered contaminated and warrants broad-spectrum systemic antibiotics. A culture and sensitivity test should be performed in case fine-tuning of the antibiotics are needed later. The devitalised tissue should be removed and the wound flushed with warmed saline solution. Wet to dry bandaging should be used till fracture reduction takes place. Epoxy resin used to be used for shell repair but it apparently gets quite hot and can cause additional problems. Acrylic polymer is less damaging. Cerclage wire, plates or braces can be utilised to reduce shell fracture in the same way they are used in other bony areas. Full healing can take 6–30 months.

Dysecdysis is a difficult or incomplete shed. Often, dysecdysis is caused by a relative lack of humidity in the reptile's environment. A desert species should have a humidity of 30–50%, subtropical species should be kept in 50–80% humidity and tropical species need 70–90% humidity. However, a nutritional protein deficiency, bruising, parasites and disease can also cause problems with shedding. Age, size, gender and species are all factors in a reptile's ability to shed easily, or not. It is usually snakes that suffer from dysecdysis and this will be a common problem presented at the veterinary surgery. Snakes can be assisted with shedding by soaking them in warm water (26.5–28.8°C) for 15–30 minutes. Manual assistance may also be required. Care must be taken at the spectacles, which are the unique shaped scales that cover the snake's eyes. Rough handling can damage the eyes, and retention of spectacles can lead to subspectacle abscesses.

Necrotizing dermatitis, also known as skin-blistering disease, occurs in snakes kept in damp, dirty vivariums. Initially vesicles appear on the ventrum, but as secondary bacterial infection sets in the lesions become pustular. Initial treatment involves cleansing of the environment. The snake is given dry newspaper as a substrate and water is offered only twice weekly for a few hours at a time. Betadine solution can be used to bathe the skin and systemic antibiotics are required in severe cases. At the next shed the lesions should resolve, provided the husbandry has improved markedly.

Septicaemic cutaneous ulcerative disease (SCUD) occurs in freshwater turtles that have been forced to survive in poor-quality water conditions. Ulcers appear on the turtle's shell. Generally, the causative bacteria are opportunistic Gram-negative microbes. The turtle needs to be 'dry-docked' on a soft surface until the lesions improve. Necrotic tissue should be debrided and the wounds flushed with saline or 50% dextrose. The dextrose needs to be flushed out with saline 2–4 hours later. Topical antibacterial agents, such as silver sulfadiazine, should be applied to the wounds. Systemic antibiotics need to be used only if the condition has generalised.

Nutritional disorders

There are a variety of nutritional disorders which plague captive reptiles.

Hypovitaminosis A occurs among chelonians and presents as a disorder with hyperkeratosis of the epidermis and scute loss. Other clinical signs include blepharoedema (swollen eyelids) pharyngitis and pneumonia. Clinical signs and history can help with a diagnosis, although a plasma retinol level is needed for a definitive diagnosis. Vitamin A injections at 1500–2000 iu/kg subcutaneously can be given once weekly for 2–4 weeks.

Hypervitaminosis A is an iatrogenic disease caused by overdosing with vitamin A. Vesicles develop subepidermally and the epidermis becomes excessively dry. Secondary infection can occur, as can dehydration. A definitive diagnosis of hypovitaminosis A should be gained before beginning injections because overdosing has such serious consequences.

Fish-eating reptiles, such as crocodilians, can develop a *vitamin E deficiency* when fed a fish diet high in polyunsaturated fatty acids. Subcutaneous nodules of fat will form in the reptile and give a yellow to orange tinge to the skin. The diet should be changed to leaner forms of fish.

A poor balance of calcium and phosphorus, with the ratio being in favour of the phosphorus, can lead to secondary *hyperparathyroidism*. Young chelonians will show shell deformities and fast-growing lizards can also be affected. Radiographs will reveal poor bone density. Oral calcium glubinonate given at the dose rate of one millilitre (1 ml) per kilogram once to twice daily is the treatment protocol. The animal may also need a period of supportive care, including fluid therapy. Dietary changes should be reviewed with the owner.

Snakes with easily torn skin can suffer from manual restraint. They can also experience splitting when they have eaten a large meal. Skin this fragile and inelastic may be due to a *vitamin C deficiency* or *hypoproteinaemia*. Diet and history should be reviewed carefully in order to ascertain the cause and treat the problem.

Parasites

Reptiles can have parasite problems too! The *snake mite*, *Ophysioyssus natricis*, looks like tiny brown dots between the scales. *Hirstiella* species are orange. Both types of mite are very mobile. The head is particularly favoured by snake mites. The rims of the eyes will swell as mites become embedded in them. Snake mites feed on blood and can be a vector for blood parasites or bacteria, even leading to fatal septicaemia. Less drastically, the mites can cause anaemia and dermatitis.

Acetate tape strips are probably the most comfortable method of gathering samples for identification, although skin scrapes can be utilised. Once an infestation is diagnosed the snake itself can be treated with fipronil spray. The spray should be applied to a cloth, which is then rubbed onto the snake. Ivermectin at 0.2 mg/kg per os or subcutaneously every 14 days, for 6 weeks, is an alternative method of treatment. Additionally, the vivarium should be completely emptied and then cleaned with a 3% bleach solution. All furnishings and substrate should be thrown away and new ones purchased. The outside of the vivarium walls can be wiped down with fipronil. Plastic pest strips (dichlorovinyl dimethyphosphate) can be placed in a container with holes so that the chemicals can leech out but the snake cannot come into contact with the pest strips. The pest strip should remain in the vivarium with the snake for 24 hours. If any mites are still seen moving on the snake the strip should be left in place for a further 24 hours. If strips are not used, pyrethrin, permethrin or pyrethroid sprays are acceptable means of environmental control. The owner needs to be reminded to change the substrate and disinfect the vivarium regularly.

Ticks can also be found on reptiles. Fipronil should be applied to the tick to relax its mouthparts and then it should be promptly removed. Maggots are another nasty parasite that find their way onto reptiles that live outdoors. Infestation usually occurs around the cloaca. Manual removal is recommended, followed by flushing the area with an iodine solution or warm, soapy water.

Aquatic pets can be parasitised by *leeches*. The leech should be removed with forceps and the site of attachment washed with 2% chlorhexidine. Leeches can be vectors for disease so they should always be removed as soon as identified. Dilute iodine baths can be used to cleanse aquatic pets of other ectoparasites. Ivermectin should never be used in turtles as it can prove fatal.

Internal parasites such as trematodes, cestodes and nematodes can have dermatological manifestations. The parasites may encyst in the skin and blood vessels, leading to tissue necrosis and oedema. Pustular dermatitis is also a consequence. Surgical excision of the encysted parasite is advised. Care should be taken as many of these parasites are potentially zoonotic.

Fungal infections

Fungal infections in reptiles can be caused by *Aspergillus*, *Candida* and *Trichophyton*, among other opportunistic species. Fungal infections are usually due to poor husbandry. The temperature and humidity should be adjusted to the needs of the enclosed reptile. Good ventilation is essential. The infection itself can appear as erosions, ulcers, vesicles or crust. Frequently, pododermatitis occurs. A sample should be taken for fungal culture; this will need to be incubated at 28°C. Positive cultures indicate the need for long-term treatment. Antifungal creams such as miconazole (Daktarin, Janssen-Cilag) or 2% chlorhexidine can be used topically. If the infection is severe, itraconazole (Itrafungol, Janssen) at 5–10 mg/kg can be administered.

Viral infections

Viral infections in reptiles are rare in captivity but occur more often in the wild. Thus, a wild caught pet may be affected with a virus. Papillomavirus, poxvirus and herpes virus can affect reptiles. Diagnosis has improved with improved blood assays for reptiles but few treatment options are available. Debulking of papillomas and supportive therapy can be offered.

Neoplasia

Neoplasia is not prevalent in reptiles; however, fibrosarcomas, squamous cell carcinomas, melanomas and lipomas can occur. Diagnosis is achieved via biopsy. Treatment should be surgical excision or cryotherapy. A complete blood cell count can indicate whether metastasis has occurred. If metastasis has already taken place the prognosis is grave.

BIRDS

Because most birds fly, the less they weigh the better. Therefore, the skin is extremely thin and delicate to save on weight. At feathered regions, the skin may be only ten cell layers thick, so it is important to remember this when giving birds subcutaneous injections. A parallel angle should be adopted with the needle or the subcutaneous tissue will be bypassed and the injection will reach deeper regions. The epidermis consists of a stratum corneum and three germinal layers – basal, intermediate and transitional. New cells are produced at the basal level. Under these layers lay slender slices of dermis and subcutaneous tissue. Feather follicles, blood vessels and nerves are found in the dermis, along with the smooth muscles that control feather movement. The subcutaneous tissue consists of striated muscle and fat. Bird skin is mostly attached to bone and tends to be dry and inelastic. The most significant gland is the uropygial (preening) gland at the dorsal tail base. The secretions from this gland assist in waterproofing the bird. Other glands include mucus glands at the vent and meibomian glands in the eyelids.

The beak is formed from modified epithelial tissue. The stratum corneum layer is extremely thick, creating a horny, firm beak in some types of bird or a soft, pliable beak for other species. A bird's diet is dependent on the type of beak it has. Phosphate, hydroxyapatite, phospholipids, calcium and keratin contribute to the composition of a good beak. Beaks grow continuously through life. Wear and tear keeps a beak trim in the wild but pet birds often need their beaks trimmed. Overgrown beaks can inhibit feeding and lead to starvation. Monthly clipping can be carried out at home or veterinary clipping can be done every 3–4 months. Beaks can bleed, so haemostatic powder should be at hand when clipping. The cere is the thickly keratinised area of skin at the base of the beak. In some species the cere is a different colour according to the bird's sex – for example, in budgies the female has a brown cere while the male has a blue cere.

The feathered part of a bird is referred to as the pterylae, while the unfeathered body is the apteria. A feather consists of a central shaft known as a 'rachis', with barbs to either side of the rachis. Barbules extend from each barb and interlock with each other to create the plume of the feather. Each growing feather has an artery and a vein, which is why bleeding occurs when such 'blood' feathers are lost. Mature feathers do not bleed.

The main types of feather are:

Contour. These are the wing and tail flight and body feathers. Wing feathers are separated into primary and secondary feathers. The ten primary feathers are strongly attached to the metacarpals via muscle. Primary feathers enable forward flight. The ten secondaries attach to the ulna and provide lift in flight.

Covert. These cover the bases of the flight feathers.

Semiplumes These are insulating feathers with very long shafts. Mostly, they are located along the tracts of contour feathers.

Down. These are small, fluffy feathers with short or non-existent shafts; they are the first feathers to appear on a chick and serve to insulate the adult bird.

Powder down. These are specialised down feathers that disintegrate into a powdery dust. The dust is used for waterproofing.

Bristles. These are bristly feathers which have a very stiff rachis and hardly any barbules. They act as eyelashes and vibrissae.

Filoplumes. These are similar to bristle feathers but have a finer shaft with a tuft of barbs at the tip.

Moulting is the complete or partial replacement of feathers. All birds moult at least once a year. Moulting and feather growth are affected by age, gender, body weight, body temperature, metabolic rate and the surface area of the bird. External factors affecting moult are nutrition, the season of the year, and whether or not the bird is breeding. Juvenile feathers moult just before the bird reaches maturity. New feather growth takes a lot of energy. Birds need improved nutrition and care during the 6 weeks of moult.

Examination

When examining the bird remember that these animals frighten easily. Owners should be warned that some birds can die of shock just from being handled. Whenever possible, the owner should handle the bird. Some birds can be dangerous to the handler. Wearing gauntlets and protective eye gear is necessary. Remember that talons can be far more painful than beaks. However, a large parrot can easily break your fingers with its beak.

A questionnaire to get a full history is also important with birds. A modified version of the earlier questionnaires can be used. Specific questions to ask about birds are:

- What kind of cage is used? (Some cages are made of toxic material!)
- What type of perches does the bird have?
- How much time does the bird exercise out of the cage?
- Does the bird live indoors or out? If outdoors, is there any contact with wild birds?
- If indoors, which room in the house? How close is the bird to the kitchen? (Some cooking vapours can be very dangerous for birds.)
- Does anyone in the household smoke?
- Is the bird covered at night? At what time of day is the bird covered?
- How much sleep does the bird get each day?
- For how long each day is the bird left alone?
- Does the bird have a mate?

Describe the diet in detail, including fresh foods, treats and supplements.

Pathology

Beak disorders

Beak disorders are quite serious because they affect a bird's ability to feed. Soft-beaked birds such as pigeons and doves can experience demineralisation of their beaks. This can be due to malnutrition or hyperparathyroidism. Calcium and vitamins should be added to the diet and the bird may need a beak splint to aid healing. If demineralisation is generalised, the ribs and sternum will become too weak for adequate respiration to occur and the bird will need to be euthanised.

Trauma to the beak can occur through accidents or by acts of aggression from larger birds. Repair of beaks can be carried out with the use of epoxy resin or wire. Prosthetic beaks can be made from dental acrylics and attached with wire. Regardless of the repair method, the bird, at first, will not be able to feed naturally and will need assisted nutrition in order to survive.

Beak overgrowth results because the beak grows continuously and needs maintenance. Grinding down the beak is safer than cutting it as overzealous trimming can lead to haemorrhage. Beak clipping should take place two to four times per year. Mite infestations can also lead to overgrown beaks. Antiparasitic measures should be taken if mites are contributing to beak deformities.

Hypertrophy of the cere can affect older, female budgies. The cere becomes a darker brown and hyperkeratinised. Skin overgrowth can block the nares – so should be scraped off. Moisturising cream can be applied to aid treatment. Hyperkeratinisation often recurs and is probably hormonal in origin.

Overgrown claws

Claws are also modified, heavily keratinised epithelium. Claw overgrowth is another problem in captive birds. Claws should be trimmed regularly as overgrown nails prevent perching behaviour. Bricks can be placed in the cage to help wear down nails. Sandpaper on perches does not help to wear down claws but can traumatise feet and lead to bumble foot, a staphylococcal based infection of the feet.

Feather disorders

Feather disorders are easily noted by the owner and are thus a frequent reason for avian veterinary visits. Preening is essential to a bird's wellbeing. During preening, secretions from the uropygial gland are spread to give the plumage its glossy, water-resistant look. The hooks of the barbules are lined up tidily to keep the feathers watertight and ready for flight. If a bird is unable to preen due to a beak deformity, or an Elizabethan collar, other birds should be allowed to do the preening for the affected bird. Over-preening can occur, however, leading to the loss of blood feathers and thus haemorrhage. Bleeding can be stopped with pressure. Underlying causes for over-preening should be investigated.

Blocked uropygial glands prevent preening. Blockage can be caused by a build-up of secretions in the gland. This condition is likely in the budgie, finch or canary. The bird will experience discomfort, which results in self-trauma. The gland must be expressed or lanced to be emptied of its contents. Antiseptic cream or solution should be applied after flushing the gland clear.

Stress can initiate feather loss in birds. Poor nutrition, over breeding and irregular photoperiods can wreak havoc on a bird's health. Opportunistic microbes then overpopulate when the bird's defences are low, leading to feather loss. Stressed birds may show 'fret' lines along their feathers. These lines will be in the same place on all the feathers and indicate a period of stress during the growing phase of the feather. Feathers are weaker along fret lines and can break at those points. Fret lines should be a major warning signal that motivates a change in husbandry measures.

Canary dysplastic feather syndrome, also known as 'straw feather', can affect canaries. This is a genetic condition in which the barbs and barbules are deformed at the first moult. Dorsally, the bird will appear glossy but ventrally the feathers will be dull. The bird cannot maintain its body heat so it dies.

Hypothyroidism affects budgies and cockatiels, leading to elongated down feathers. The pattern of feather change occurs bilaterally and symmetrically on the body under the wing. Advanced cases show generalised feather loss with unruly down feathers protruding over the body. Secondary bacterial and fungal infections ensue, along with lethargy, depression, lowered body temperature, obesity and bradycardia. Diagnosis is reached via blood testing to ascertain whether thyroxine (T4) levels are low and thyroid-stimulating hormone (T4/TSH) levels are high. Biochemistry will also show hypercholesterolaemia. Treatment is oral thyroxine. The down feathers should be plucked out. If they regrow at odd angles the dose of thyroxine needs to be increased. Iodine (in the form of 5% Lugol's solution) can be added to the drinking water. Monitoring should occur every 4–5 months. Indications of iodine overdosing are weight loss, diarrhoea, vomiting and hyperactivity.

Feather picking is a common disorder in psittacines. The underlying causes are legion. Biological causes should be eliminated before attributing the behaviour to some form of psychological motive. A thorough examination (including full history and extensive diagnostic tests) is required to come up with a definitive diagnosis for feather picking. Owners should be questioned about the length of time the bird has been picking and exactly when the behaviour started. If the behaviour is seasonal in nature an allergic component might be part of the problem. Pruritus would be another significant clinical sign. The time of day the bird picks, and whether or not it picks when the owner is present, are facts that need to be established. Vocalisation while picking could indicate pain, which points more towards a physical problem. The room the bird lives in should be smoke-free and the humidity level ascertained. The bird's enclosure must be discussed in detail, as must the bird's sleeping arrangements and general lifestyle. Nutrition is a leading cause of feather picking, so the bird's feeding regime must be discussed in detail. Peanut- and seed-based diets, common among parrots, can lead to hypovitaminosis A, exhibited by dry, flaky skin and poor wound healing. Psittacines should have a varied diet of sprouted seed, highly coloured vegetables, rice, sweet corn, apricots, etc. Complete pelleted diets are much healthier than seed mixes.

Pathological conditions to test for in a feather-picking examination include the following:

1. Feather plucks and skin scrapes should be taken to test for ectoparasites.
2. Faecal examination can indicate the presence of endoparasites or internal infections. (*Giardia* spp can cause gut pain, which leads to self-trauma.)
3. Feather pulp cytology involves squashing fresh feather pulp and staining it with Diff-Quik. Bacteria and yeast can be identified via this method and the pulp can also be utilised for culture and sensitivity testing. Folliculitis, demonstrated by erythema, swelling and exudate at the flight feathers is one cause of feather picking.
4. Swabs for fungal culture can be taken from the cloaca and head region if there are white crusts

visible or patchy feather loss. *Candida* or *Aspergillus* fungi may be causing these lesions.

5. Viral testing of the feather pulp can be performed for Psittiacine Beak and Feather Disease and polyoma virus.
6. Bloods should be taken to test for heavy metal levels and *Chlamydia psittaci* (the causative organism of the disease psittacosis).

If all biological pathology has been eliminated, then feather picking can be diagnosed as psychological in origin. With this scenario, the bird's lifestyle needs to be examined and adjusted to make the bird feel more secure and less bored. If the picking is related to moulting or sexual behaviour, these are relevant points. Birds need an area of privacy – a box can satisfy this need. Nine to twelve hours of sleep should be assured nightly. If the bird is living in a busy intersection of the home, it should be moved to a quiet, dark room in the early evening and left to rest till the early morning. Some birds need their cage to be covered to enhance rest and privacy.

To prevent boredom the bird should be provided with plenty of interactive toys and lots of time out of the cage to exercise. Some psittacines, such as parrots, are extremely intelligent pets. Their IQ has been likened to that of a 3-year-old. This sort of pet cannot be left alone in a cage all day. They need stimulation and interaction. If a person is away from home for long stretches of the day perhaps a parrot is not the best choice of pet. Companionship of another bird may help in some instances, but if the birds do not get along, further feather loss can take place in a dominant–submissive relationship.

Interim measures to use in order to decrease the level of self-mutilation include the use of Elizabethan collars and pharmaceuticals. Antidepressants have also been used with some success. Fluoxetine (Prozac, Eli Lilly) at 0.4 mg/kg per os, twice daily, is an effective therapy. Alternatively, diazepam can be used, given per os at 2.5–4 mg/kg as needed. Hormonal drugs, such as human chorionic gonadotrophin, can be useful, especially in cases where aggression or sexual frustration play a part. However, injections must be given on a frequent basis, making this treatment less convenient.

Ectoparasites

Clinical signs which indicate that there is an ectoparasite infestation present include frantic preening, feather picking, pruritus, alopecia, erythema and generally poor body condition. Beak and leg mites (primarily *Knemidokoptes laevis spp*) create a characteristic honeycomb pattern with excessive scale. Many parasites are vectors for other disease so infestations should be eradicated promptly and thoroughly.

Flies are usually transitory irritants; however, they can transmit other organisms such as mites and lice, although lice are more often transmitted via wild birds. Lice lay eggs on the flight feathers and feed on down feathers. The bird itself can often control a lice infestation via preening. Plucking a mature flight feather will harvest louse nits for diagnosis if diagnosis cannot be made by observing lice quickly moving between the feathers of the bird. Biting and sucking varieties of lice can infest birds. A permethrin powder designed for use on avians is the treatment of choice. The powder should be applied every 2 weeks until the infestation is cleared.

Mosquitoes are another transitory pest that may alight on birds. The bites are very painful to avians and may form focal lesions. Mosquitoes usually attack around the bird's face. Mosquitoes are dangerous because they are intermediate hosts for other parasites and can also transmit poxvirus.

The ubiquitous *flea* can also infest birds, particularly if the birds are exposed to mammalian pets or wild birds. Affected cage birds will show signs of pruritus, weakness and irritability. The face, head and neck are the areas most likely to be affected. Treatment of the entire environment (not just the cage) is necessary for control of the infestation. However, the bird must be removed when premise spray is being used. The bird itself can be treated with a permethrin powder. Flea infestations affect nestlings significantly, so control should be initiated as soon as an infestation is identified.

Ixodid ticks, i.e. hard ticks, can attach themselves to birds and present a serious risk to the bird's health. These ticks emit toxins during their attachment and can cause sudden death in a bird. Research is currently being undertaken on tick-induced fatalities in birds. Any tick found on a bird should be removed immediately. If the bird is showing systemic signs, supportive treatment such as fluids, warmth and improved nutrition are advised. Antimicrobial therapy should be administered according to the condition of the bird.

Feather, nest and skin mites affect birds. The feather mites *Protolichus* spp and *Dubinina* spp among others scavenge on feathers, scale and epithelial lipids. Usually these mites do not create any problems. Debilitated birds may suffer from the mites taking advantage of the situation and overpopulating. In such cases, the underlying cause of poor condition needs to be addressed and the mite infestation should be treated with permethrin powder.

Quill mites, such as *Syrigophilus spp, Dermatoglyphus spp,* and *Ascouridus* spp. attach are the primary mites which feed on fluids within the quill. Their activities can lead to broken feathers, feather loss, self trauma and eventually secondary infection. Diagnosis is made by squeezing the mite out from the quill and onto a slide with mineral oil. Miticidal dusting powder is used to remove these mites. Fipronil can also be used.

Nest mites feed on litter in the nest and food debris found in the cage or aviary. *Dermanyssus gallinae,* or 'red mite', is the most common of these mites and can cause anaemia. Affected birds will have poor feather condition and will be weak, itchy and irritable. Over-preening is another clinical sign. Collecting samples of these mites is done by placing a white sheet over the cage, or on the floor of the cage at night. First thing in the morning, the sheet should be examined for what look like moving grains of sand. The bird itself can be treated with permethrin or carbaryl powder. The nesting material should be burned and the cage or aviary thoroughly cleaned. The mites can live in the environment for up to 30 weeks so environmental elimination is essential. *Ornithonyssus* spp is another environmental mite that can cause anaemia. It is transmitted via wild birds so is more likely in outdoor aviaries.

The skin or cere mite is *Knemidokoptes* (Fig. 13.3). These mites are transmitted from hen to chick as commensal mites that become pathological only when stress or illness lowers the bird's immunity. *Knemidokoptes* mites cause proliferative honeycomb-like lesions on the cere, base of beak and feet, thus the common names 'scaly face', and 'scaly leg'. Extensive infestations can lead to deformed beaks that inhibit feeding. Identification of the mite is achieved by skin scrapings. The mite is spherical with stubby legs, the female mite being twice the size of the male mite. These are burrowing mites so the use of systemic treatment is worthwhile. Ivermectin can be diluted into a spray form by mixing 0.5 ml of 1% ivermectin in 1.1 litres of water. The bird should then be sprayed from head to toe every 2–3 weeks until the infestation has cleared. The nests should also be treated to eliminate recurrence via the environment. Some clinicians prefer intramuscular injections of ivermectin, not to exceed a dose rate of 200 micrograms/kilogram. A further method of application is to dilute the dose of ivermectin 1:10 with propylene glycol and apply it as a spot-on at the featherless area over the jugular furrow. Apply this solution sparingly or the waterproofing of the feathers can be affected. The dose should be given 3 times at one week intervals. Subcutaneous mites from the families *Laminosioptidae* and *Hypoderatidae* can cause firm nodules in the breast tissue, as well as other areas. In pisttacines, these mites can prove fatal. Systemic treatment with ivermectin is effective.

Internal parasites can cause dermatological symptoms as well. *Giardia*, a protozoal internal parasite, affects budgies and cockatiels particularly. Clinical signs include soft, green droppings, weight loss, dry, flaky skin, and self-trauma to the axillae, mid-dorsum and lateral body under the wings. Self-inflicted damage can range from feather picking to ulceration of the skin. Faeces must be collected for diagnostic testing and it must be examined on a wet-mount slide within 5–10 minutes. Several

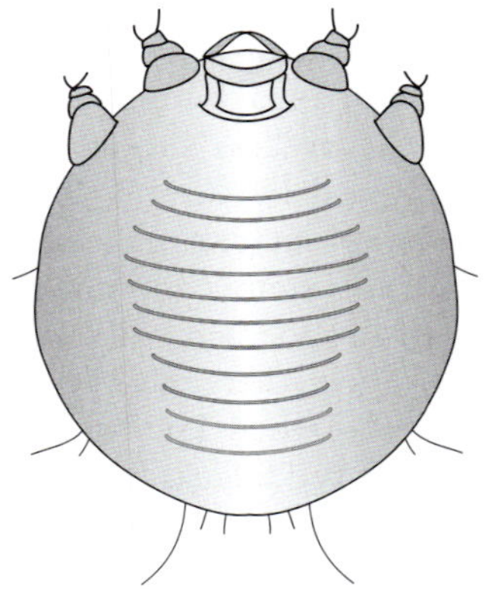

Figure 13.3 *Knemidokoptes* spp. A bird mite that causes scaly beak and scaly leg.

samples may need to be tested over a period of days as the protozoan is not shed continuously and false negatives are common. As this is a zoonotic disease, gloves should be worn and health and safety precautions adhered to strictly.

Blood samples for haematology will indicate a parasitic infection with basophilia and eosinophilia. However, these are not specific enough signs with which to make a diagnosis. Faecal sampling is required. Once diagnosed, *Giardia* can be treated with metronidazole at 25–35 mg/kg t.i.d. intramuscularly for 2–5 days. Self-trauma should be limited via an Elizabethan collar and secondary infections should be treated accordingly.

Trichomonas affects raptors, pigeons, canaries, finches and budgies. Most common in the pigeon, the disease manifests with caseous lesions of the mouth, oesophagus and crop. Occasionally, these lesions spread to the beak and face. The bird is anorexic and loses weight. A swab taken from a lesion can be spread onto a slide and the motile, flagellated protozoa can be seen swimming around. Treatment of the lesions can be with an iodine solution once daily. Systemic treatment is with metronidazole at 10 mg/kg once daily for 5 days. The bird should be supported with improved nutrition and vitamin and mineral supplementation.

Bacterial and fungal disease

Microbial disease is not that common in birds due to the birds' high natural body temperature. *Subcutaneous abscesses* do occur, but they are caseous in nature and thus difficult to aspirate. Abscesses usually appear at sites of feather loss and can be caused by a damaged follicle, a feather cyst, a wound or foreign body. The periocular region and the uropygial gland are common sites for abscesses.

Diagnosis is by observation of a lump which yields pus on aspiration. The abscess should be lanced and the exudate removed by curette. Five percent Lugol's iodine or antibiotic cream should be applied to the cleared area. Systemic antibiotics may be given, along with an Elizabethan collar.

Folliculitis can present when there has been damage to an immature blood feather. The feather should be plucked from the infected follicle and sent for culture and sensitivity. The appropriate treatment should be given for a minimum of 3 weeks.

Granulomatous dermatitis appears as single to multiple nodules on the head or cere. Histology is the means of diagnosis. The granuloma(s) should be excised and the bird given systemic antimicrobial therapy.

Pododermatitis is commonly known as 'bumble foot' and does afflict birds frequently. Overweight birds, arthritic birds and birds with bad perching material are predisposed to pododermatitis. A puncture wound to the foot and hypovitaminosis A can also predispose a bird to this condition. Diagnosis is made by observation of lameness and inflammation of the foot or feet. The foot should be surgically debrided and the bird placed on long-term antibiotic therapy. A culture and sensitivity test is recommended to aid in accuracy of treatment.

Gout can easily be mistaken for pododermatitis as both diseases cause a similar sort of lameness. Gout, however, is due to the body's inability to eliminate nitrogenous wastes. Urates are thus deposited at the joints, especially in the feet and legs. Nodular swelling occurs at the affected joints. If the nodules are removed, uric acid crystals can be identified in the diseased tissue. The bird should have its diet altered completely. The level of protein should be reduced markedly and vitamin A levels increased. Fruits and vegetables should be added to the food plan. Antibiotics can be given for secondary infection and allopurinol can be administered, but generally speaking, the kidney damage is permanent.

Secondary bacterial infection occurs with *leg band constriction*. As the bird grows, skin layers grow over the identification band and swelling and infection develop. Gangrene often follows. If observed early enough, the band can be removed and the leg will heal with appropriate treatment, otherwise, amputation is the only option.

Staphylococcal infections in birds can appear as yellowish vesicles and crust under the wings. The lesions later spread to the breast and abdomen. Cytological examination can confirm a bacterial infection. Clavanulate-potentiated amoxicillin (Synulox, Pfizer) is the treatment of choice for these infections.

Chronic skin and respiratory problems in a bird are strongly indicative of a fungal infection. *Candida*, *Aspergillus*, *Malassezia*, *Microsporum*, *Trichophyton* and *Penicillium* are among the many species of fungi found in birds. Hypovitaminosis A predisposes birds to fungal infections. Birds with combs or wattles are more likely to become afflicted with fungi, especially if their environment is wet and dirty. Clinical signs include feather loss, skin thickening and crusts encircling feather follicles. Diagnosis is made by skin scrapes and microscopic examination for hyphae. Fungal culture should also be carried out. Topical antifungals can be used to treat the condition. Enilconazole (Imaverol, Janssen-Cilag) can be used diluted 1:50 or 1:100 depending on the size of the bird. Application should be twice weekly until negative fungal cultures are attained. Systemically, fluconazole can be given at 20 mg/kg once every 48 hours for 14–60 days (NB Itraconozole cannot be given to African Greys) or itraconazole at 10 mg/kg b.i.d. Cage conditions and nutrition should be improved to enhance recovery.

Viral disease

Avian pox creates intracytoplasmic inclusion bodies in the epithelium. This is a hardy virus that is resistant to light, humidity and dryness. It is viable in the soil for 18 months. Mosquitoes are a vector for this virus. Avian pox spreads quickly and there is a high mortality rate, especially among canaries.

The dermatological features of the dry form of avian pox are yellow papules which appear at the beak, nostrils, eyes, lower legs and feet. Later the papules become vesicles or pustules. The lesions take on a brown colour and become crusted. Pruritus exists, leading to self-trauma and secondary infection. Wound healing is very slow. If the bird survives, scars will remain at the sites of the papules.

The wet form of the disease manifests with papules of the oral mucosa, larynx and tongue. The papules become caseous and secrete a fibrinous exudate. The lesions can become quite large but are difficult to remove without causing severe haemorrhage. Due to the location of the lesions, dyspnoea can result, leading to death.

Diagnosis of avian pox is performed via histology coupled with the clinical signs. Because the virus is easily passed between birds in the cage, via food and through social interaction, the treatment is to cull the affected birds. The cage or aviary must be thoroughly disinfected with quaternary ammonium compounds. Valuable/beloved birds can be treated with vitamins A and C, and antibiotics should be given for the secondary infection. Tincture of iodine should be applied to the lesions. The prognosis is guarded.

Psittacine beak and feather disease (PBFD) has the clinical signs of beak, nail and feather deformities. Hyperkeratosis of all of these regions results in a shiny beak that can easily break and haemorrhage. Feathers may show symmetrical loss. Although re-growth is possible, the feathers will grow in twisted and moult easily. Clinical signs can be acute or progressive. The acute stage usually occurs at the first moult when feather fracture, loss of pigmentation, haemorrhage and necrosis can all occur. Secondary infection is the usual cause of death. PBFD, caused by a circovirus, affects 35 species of psitticines. Birds can be asymptomatic carriers for a long time before outside stressors promote the onset of clinical signs.

PBFD is diagnosed by sampling the deformed feathers and preserving them in formalin. A laboratory will examine the feathers for evidence of the virus. Some laboratories prefer the feather plus a biopsy of the follicle as well. Whole blood collected in an EDTA tube can be used for viral assay. The disease cannot be cured. The bird is treated supportively with antibiotics, vitamins and fluid therapy. Quarantine of affected birds is essential and the enclosure will need to be disinfected with a quaternary ammonium or iodophor disinfectant. Any equipment used to collect samples from the bird should be disinfected as well because the virus is shed via beak and nail dust. The survival rate is low.

Papovavirus has different forms. Papillomas (wart-like lesions) can occur on the legs, head and eyelids. The lesions can become ulcerated and crusty over time. Different species of bird are affected more significantly in one area rather than another; for example, African Greys tend to have lesions on their head and eyelids, finches on their legs. The lesions can be removed for biopsy. Once identified, the disease can be treated with an autogenous vaccine (these are vaccines created from material harvested from the affected bird's lesions).

Papovavirus Adult budgies can be asymptomatic carriers of papovavirus, causing budgerigar fledgeling disease in their chicks. A malformation of their down feathers will occur, along with retarded growth of tail and body feathers. The skin takes on a reddish tone and secondary infection is very likely to occur. Fatality rates are high. Unfortunately, diagnosis is usually made at post-mortem examination, although histopathology can be used if the disease is caught early enough. Cloacal swabs or faeces are useful for diagnosis if the virus is being shed at the time of collection. Otherwise, false-negative results will occur. Culling of affected birds is recommended along with stringent disinfection protocols for the cage or aviary. The virus is shed in feather dander and via the urinary and gastrointestinal tract, making the presence of the virus prevalent and quite a difficult job to eliminate.

French moult is a multifactorial disease that develops when the bird is also afflicted with other stressors such as parasites, poor nutrition, bad genes or an inappropriate environment. Viral infection with PBFD or papovavirus may also contribute to the disease. Budgerigars are the species most affected. Clinical signs show breakage of tail and wing feathers, often very close to the skin. Severely affected birds never grow normal feathers but some birds do outgrow the condition in 2–3 months. Diagnosis is established via clinical signs. Affected birds should be removed from a breeding programme.

Abnormal masses

Benign fibromas and malignant fibrosarcomas can occur on the wings, legs, beak and uropygial area. Fibrosarcoma are firm, oval in shape and frequently have necrotic centres. While locally invasive, these tumours rarely metastasise. Treatment and diagnosis is by surgical excision and biopsy.

Haemangiomas and haemangiosarcomas are rare in birds. These growths appear as red to black subcutaneous swellings, usually at follicles. Sarcomas can be invasive and metastasise. Diagnosis and treatment is by surgical excision and biopsy.

Benign lipomas and malignant liposarcomas affect budgerigars in particular. Growths can appear on the sternum, wing and abdomen. Overweight budgies are particularly affected by lipomas. Lipomas enlarge and fat necrosis begins centrally. The lesion should be surgically excised and the budgie put on a diet. Lipomas are single or multiple and encapsulated. Liposarcomas are firm and vascularised. Both should be excised and biopsied for diagnosis.

Papillomas can be finger-like, wart-like or crusty growths. They often occur at the feet, leg, neck, wing, eyelids and uropygial gland. Papillomas are usually benign but will bleed if self-trauma takes place so removal is recommended.

Cloacal papillomas can also occur and appear as cauliflower like proliferations of tissue at the cloaca. They are often misdiagnosed as cloacal prolapse. The growth can inhibit defecation. Human haemorrhoid treatments can be used to decrease the size of the mass but excision is a more permanent solution.

Squamous cell carcinomas affect budgerigars at the neck and uropygial glands. Suspicious growths should be removed for biopsy. Wide margins or excision can make the diagnostic procedure the treatment as well.

Xanthoma and xanthomatosis occurs in cockatiels and, less often, in budgerigars. Due to an alteration of lipid metabolism, lobular masses occur on the wingtips. The thick, yellowish masses can progress down the wing towards the body. The weight of the masses prevents flight. The bird's attempt to pick at the masses results in haemorrhage. If the growths are extensive, treatment is amputation of the wing.

Cysts are not uncommon in birds. Canaries are prone to epidermal cysts, which usually appear on the head. The cyst is filled with a brownish fluid and will collapse on puncture. Budgerigars suffer from inclusion cysts at the uropygial gland and mucus cysts on the sternum. Both should be removed.

Feather cysts are the result of ingrown feathers that gather necrotic feather material. Single or multiple cysts can be observed. Feather cysts tend to affect long wing feathers, with canaries being genetically predisposed. A subcutaneous white swelling gradually increases in size and causes the bird to practice self-trauma. The cyst should be incised and the caseous material within removed with a curette. The area should be infused with antibiotic ointment as infection can easily develop. If possible, the base of the feather should be left to grow in later.

EXOTICS FORMULARY

The BSAVA formulary and/or an exotics formulary should be consulted for dose rates for specific species. There are almost no drug therapies licensed for use in exotics.

Antiparasitics

Carnidazole is used for the treatment of trichomoniasis and giardiasis in birds.

Cyromazine (Rearguard, Novartis) is licensed for use in rabbits for the prevention of myiasis.

Fipronil (Frontline, Merial) has been used in reptiles and birds. The preferred method of application is to spray the solution onto a cloth and rub it into the animal.

Imidacloprid (Advantage, Bayer) is licensed for use in rabbits for the treatment of fleas.

Ivermectin (Panomec, Merial) is widely used in exotic pets. Dose rates, as prescribed by appropriate formularies, should be adhered to carefully as most exotics are easily overdosed. Ivermectin cannot be used in turtles.

Metronidazole is used for the treatment of giardiasis in birds.

Permethrin (various formats) can be used as a powder on birds and small mammals. It can also be used as an environmental spray, provided the animals have temporarily been removed to another location.

Selamectin (Stronghold, Pfizer) has been used in a variety of exotic species. To date, there is not enough information to advise regarding dose rates and safety for particular species.

Antimicrobials

Amoxicillin and amoxicillin/clavulanate can be used for birds. Cefalexin, clindamycin, doxycycline, enrofloxacin and trimethoprim are all used successfully in birds.

Enrofloxacin, trimethoprim-sulphonamide, tetracycline HCl and chloramphenicol can be used in small mammals. In rabbits, penicillin can also be used. The health and safety risks to humans must be considered when using chloramphenicol (humans handling chloramphenicol may increase their risk of developing fatal aplastic anaemia); gloves must be worn when handling this drug.

Enrofloxacin tends to be used most often in the treatment of antimicrobial infections in reptiles.

Topical antimicrobials

Birds and reptiles respond well to iodine and betadine solutions or ointments. Chlorhexidine can also be used. Small mammals can be cleansed with chlorhexidine solutions and treated with most antibacterial ointments. Guinea pigs and birds should never be given any creams or ointments that also include steroids as these animals do not do well with steroid treatment.

Fungal treatments

Itraconazole, fluconazole and griseofulvin can be used in exotic species although intraconazole should be avoided in African Grey Parrots. Enilconazole solution is a useful topical treatment in birds and small mammals. Chlorhexidine has antifungal properties and is used in all exotic species. Miconazole ointments can be used in reptiles and small mammals.

There are very few drugs that are licensed for use in exotic species. Dose ranges can vary widely. A standard formulary, along with an exotics manual, should be consulted for correct dosages for each species.

References and Further Reading

Axelson R, Dean D V M 1997 Avian dermatology. In: Hoefer Heidi (ed) Practical avian medicine. Veterinary Learning Systems, Trenton, NJ, p 186–208

Campbell Terry W 1995 Common parasites of exotic pets, Part I. Exotic animals, a veterinary handbook. Veterinary Learning Systems, Trenton, NJ, p201

Cooper John E 2003 Skin diseases of reptiles. Veterinary Times 23 June:12

De Vosjoli Phillipe 1991 General care and maintenance of Burmese pythons. Advanced Vivarium Systems, Inc. Lakeside, CA, p 34–36

De Vosjoli Phillipe 1994 The lizard keeper's handbook. Advanced Vivarium Systems, Inc. Lakeside, CA, p 130–133

Forbes Neil A 2002 Birds. In: Foil C, Foster A (eds) BSAVA Manual of small animal dermatology. BSAVA Publications, Gloucester, p 256–268

Hillyer Elizabeth V 1997 Dermatological disease. In: Hillyer E, Quesenberry K E (eds) Ferrets, rabbits and rodents. W B Saunders, New York, p 212–219

Malley A Dermod 1996 Feather and skin problems. In: Benyon P H (ed) BSAVA Manual of psittacine birds. BSAVA Publications, Gloucester, p 96–104

Mc Tier T, Hair H, Walstrom D, Thompson L 2003 Efficacy and safety of topical administration of selamectin for treatment of ear mite infestation in rabbits. JAVMA 223(3):322–324

Mitchell Mark, Colombini Sarah 2002 Reptiles. In: Foil C, Foster A (eds) BSAVA Manual of small animal dermatology. BSAVA Publications, Gloucester, p 269–275

Orcutt Connie 1997 Dermatological disease. In: Hillyer E, Quesenberry K E (eds) Ferrits, rabbits and rodents. W B Saunders, New York, p 115–130

Richardson V C G 2000 The skin. Diseases of domestic guinea pigs. Blackwell Science, Oxford, p 1–13

Rosenthal Karen 1997 Unique features of the avian integumentary. In: Hoefer Heidi (ed) Practical avian medicine. Veterinary Learning Systems, Trenton, NJ, p 180–185

Rosenthal Karen L 2002 Ferrets. In: Foil C, Foster A (eds) BSAVA Manual of small animal dermatology. BSAVA Publications, Gloucester, p 252–255

Scarff David H 2002 Rats and rodents. In: Foil C, Foster A (eds) BSAVA Manual of small animal dermatology. BSAVA Publications, Gloucester, p 242–251

Schaeffer Dorcas O, Donnelly Thomas M 1997 Diseases of domestic guinea pigs. In: Hillyer E, Quesenberry K E (eds) Ferrets, rabbits and rodents. W B Saunders, New York, p 266–268, 274–275

Scott D W, Miller W H, Griffin C E 2001 Dermatoses of pet rodents, rabbits and ferrets. Muller and Kirk's Small animal dermatology, 6th edn. W B Saunders, London, p 1439–1440

Wall Richard, Shearer David 2001 Veterinary ectoparasites. Blackwell Science, Oxford, p 171, 227–235

CASE STUDY 1

Ectoparasitic infestations in a rabbit

Signalment

One-year-old entire male rabbit. English crossbred. Black and white. Weight 3 kg.

Problem

Generalised pruritus and crusts noted in the inside of the pinnae of both ears. Patch of hair loss noted on dorsal spine. Animal inappetant and less active than usual.

History

The rabbit lived with one other rabbit and a guinea pig in an indoor hutch. There were also eight dogs, numerous birds and a cat living at the premises, along with four adult humans. The rabbit was fed a rabbit mix and hay, with occasional fresh vegetables. The owner had recently purchased a new bag of hay.

Physical examination

On examination, the inside of both pinnae were encrusted with debris. The alopecic patch on the dorsal, thoracic spine was oval in shape and surrounded by white, flaking tissue debris. The rabbit was lethargic and did not resist examination. Temperature, pulse and respiration were within the normal range. There were no apparent ocular or dental problems and the rabbit was not exhibiting signs of diarrhoea at this time.

Differential diagnosis

- *Cheyletiella* parasitovorax infestation
- *Psoroptes cuniculi* infestation
- Flea infestation
- Dermatophytosis (most likely to be *Trichophyton mentagrophytes*)
- Otitis due to pasteurellosis syndrome
- Bacterial dermatitis (*Staphylococcus* spp or *Pseudomonas*)

Laboratory and other diagnostic tests

- Acetate tape strip at area of hair loss on dorsum
- Skin scrapings at same area
- Swabs of ear crusts

The tape strip was mounted on a slide and examined under low magnification. Nothing was discovered. The skin scrapings were mounted in liquid paraffin and examined under low magnification. Again, nothing was identified. However, the clinical symptoms along the dorsal spine were indicative of *C. parasitovorax* and the veterinarian felt that empirical treatment for that infestation was warranted.

The swab from the ear was broken up to improve visibility and this sample was mounted in liquid paraffin. A 40× magnification revealed large numbers of adult mites, eggs and deutonymph/male adult attachments. The observed mites were revealed to be the species *P. cuniculi*.

Diagnosis and prognosis

Surface infestation – possible infestation with *Cheyletiella parasitovorax*. Figure 13.4 shows *Cheyletiella* infestation.

Ear infestation: *Psoroptes cuniculi*.

The prognosis was guarded as severe mite infestations of the ear can be a causative factor in ear infections. Infections in the rabbit can be frustrating problems to treat and success is not always assured.

Treatment

The owner was advised to thoroughly cleanse and disinfect the rabbit's hutch and bring in the two other hutch mates for treatment. A premises treatment for the home was also strongly suggested as *Cheyletiella* spp can live off the host for up to 1 month. The current supply of hay was to be burned and a new supply purchased. A consent form was signed to allow the rabbit to have a general anaesthetic. Although not always recommended, it was decided that it would be best to anaesthetise this rabbit and remove the otic debris in order to better examine the ear.

Propofol (Rapinovet, Coopers Pitman-Moore) was given at a dose rate of 10 mg/kg intravenously into the marginal ear vein. Unfortunately, intravenous access was not attained. As a result, the patient was masked down with 3% isoflurane (IsoFlo, Mallinckrodt Veterinary Ltd) and oxygen at a flow rate of 1.2 litres/minute. This is not the best method to anaesthetise a rabbit as it is very stressful for the animal. Using forceps, the otic crusts were plucked out and then the ear was examined with an otoscope. A purulent infection was observed in the left ear, probably secondary to the mite infestation. The ears were cleaned with a ceruminolytic (Epiotic, Virbac) and then medicated topically with an anti-infective, anti-inflammatory agent (Canaural, Leo Laboratories). The rabbit was also injected with ivermectin (Panomec, Merial) at a dose rate of 200–400 micrograms/kg subcutaneously for the *C. parasitovorax* and *P. cuniculi* infestations. Florfenical (Nuflor, Schering-Plough) was given as an intramuscular injection at a dose of 0.3 mg/kg. The florfenical would need to be given for 5 days in total and the ivermectin would need to be given

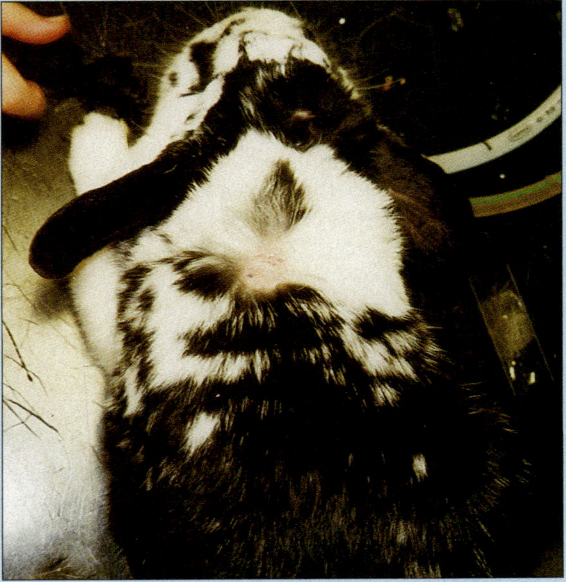

Figure 13.4 *Cheyletiella* infestation in the rabbit. Dorsal scaling and alopecia are typical clinical signs of *Cheyletiella* infestation in the rabbit.

three times, at 2-week intervals. The Canaural was to be applied twice daily for 3 weeks. The rabbit was hospitalised overnight and discharged the next day, when his hutch mates were brought in for treatment.

Re-inspection and final outcome

It was necessary to see the rabbit daily for three additional days for his florfenical injections. One week after the beginning of treatment, the rabbit developed diarrhoea. He was re-hospitalised and placed on a hay-only diet for 2 days, at which point the diarrhoea had resolved. An examination 1 week later showed that he was healthy with normal appetite and activity levels. The treatments were continued until the 6-week period had passed and the rabbit was deemed fully recovered from his ear and fur mites, as well as the ear infection.

Discussion

C. parasitovorax lives all of its life stages on the host, generally in the back and shoulder region – demonstrated in this rabbit with the area of alopecia at the dorsal thoracic region. Causing exfoliative dermatitis, the mites' progress through this sea of scurf, agitates the debris – thus the term 'walking dandruff'. There is a 3–5-week life cycle involving an egg, pre-larval (legless sac with a mouth), larval, nymph I and II and adult stages, thus requiring the above mentioned 6 weeks of treatment. Larvae have three pairs of legs and the adults (the only sexually dimorphic state) have four pairs of legs.

Aside from acetate tape strips and skin scrapes, vacuuming is another method of mite collection (Flecknell 1996). Rabbits apparently enjoy the sensation. Ivermectin at a dose rate of 200–400 micrograms/kg is the most often used treatment for *C. parasitovorax* and was chosen in this case, despite the use being extra-license. Three subcutaneous injections, 2 weeks apart, are essential to prevent the immature life stages from developing into viable adults. Although *C. parasitovorax* rarely causes the rabbit distress it can be a vector for myxomatosis and can also transiently infect humans, so treatment is essential (Flecknell 1996). A very mobile mite, *C. parasitovorax* can easily infest hutch mates, which is why treatment was required for the patient's hutch mates in this case.

P. cuniculi is the most common mite of the rabbit ear canal (Flecknell 1996). This mite feeds on the tissue and fluid of the canal, forming crusts of serum, mites, mite exoskeletons and desquamated epithelial cells. As the crusts are adherent, removal can be exceedingly painful and cause bleeding. Most clinicians do not remove the crusts and begin treatment with an acaricide instead. Then, when the crusts have softened, a general anaesthetic can be undertaken and the crusts removed (Flecknell 1991). However, the policy of this practice to remove the debris from the ear canal at the outset so that a full otoscopic examination can be performed. It is often found that an ear mite infestation can lead to secondary infection of the ear canal, which cannot be diagnosed without first clearing away the occluding debris. In this case, an ear infection was identified after clearing the debris so the use of anaesthetic at this point was warranted.

P. cuniculi has a 3-week life cycle Ivermectin, although not licensed for use in rabbits, is commonly used. Treatments can be given three times at 8-day intervals or twice, 18 days apart, at a dose rate of 400 micrograms/kg (Hillyer 1997). Alternatively, topical acaracidals can be used for 3 weeks, twice daily (omitting treatment during the second week). It is sometimes necessary to use the topical acaricide below the ear and down the neck region as *P. cuniculi* can live outside the ear canal (Ayers & Romich 1994). In the case of this rabbit, the topical acaricide was used liberally, but only within the ear itself.

REFERENCES

(for Case Study 1)

Ayers Laura, Romich Janet A 1994 Husbandry of the rabbit, Part II Exotic animals – a veterinary handbook. Veterinary Learning Systems, Trenton, NJ, p 74

Flecknell Paul 1991 Rabbits. In: Benyon P H, Cooper J E (eds) Manual of exotic pets. British Small Animal Association, Gloucestershire, p 75, 80

Stein S, Walshaw S 1996 Diseases of rabbits. In: Laber-Laird K, Swindle M M, Flecknell P (eds) Handbook of rodent and rabbit medicine. Pergamon Press, London, p 202–204

Hillyer Elizabeth 1997 Dermatological diseases. In: Hillyer E, Quesenberry K E (eds) Ferrits, rabbits and rodents. W B Saunders, Philadelphia, PA, p 215–216

CASE STUDY 2

Trixicarus caviae in a guinea pig

Signalment

- Species: guinea pig
- Breed: English Self (Smooth-coated)
- Age: 11 months
- Sex: female, entire
- Weight: 500 grams

Problem

Severe pruritus and hyperkeratinisation, weight loss.

History

The guinea pig lived with one other guinea pig and two rabbits in an outdoor hutch. The animals were rarely taken indoors and did not have free access to the garden. The caretakers were two young boys and their mother. The sleeping material in the hutch was hay, which the owner had recently begun purchasing from another outlet rather than from her usual pet store. The guinea pig had been scratching at herself for 1 week and had now gone off her food. The owner reported significant weight loss. Clinical signs were not observed in the other in-contact pets or the owners.

Physical examination

On examination, the guinea pig was indeed too thin. Throughout the examination, the guinea pig continued to scratch obsessively. The skin along her flanks showed much dry scaling and was erythematous, probably due to self-trauma. The guinea pig was tachycardic and displayed tachypnoea (heart rate greater than 130–190 beats per minute and respiratory rate greater than 90–150 breaths per minute). Her temperature was not taken as she showed hypersensitive nervous signs and was deemed too fragile for invasive investigation.

Differential diagnosis

- *Trixicarus caviae* infestation
- *Chirodiscoides caviae* infestation
- *Gliricola porcelli* infestation
- *Gyropus ovalis* infestation
- *Ctenocephalides felis* infestation
- Dermatophytosis (most likely *Trichophyton mentagrophytes*)

Laboratory and other diagnostic tests

The hair coat was thoroughly examined and no parasites were identified grossly. Pluckings and skin scrapings were then taken while the owner restrained the guinea pig. The collected hair and squames were mounted on two different slides in liquid paraffin, and then examined under a microscope at low magnification. Numerous eggs were identified in the squame sample, along with an adult mite *Trixicarus caviae*. Adult mites were also discovered in the hair pluckings.

Diagnosis and prognosis

Trixicarus caviae infestation. A moderately positive prognosis was given rather than a positive prognosis due to the guinea pig's debilitated state. It was considered that the anorexia could be caused by impacted hair in the oral cavity due to the self-trauma and barbering associated with the pruritus. *T. caviae* infestation is shown in Figure 13.5.

Treatment

Three subcutaneous injections of ivermectin (Panomec, Merial) at a dose rate of 0.4 mg/kg were given 8 days apart. The owner was advised to dispose of her current supply of hay and to clean and disinfect the hutch thoroughly. It was requested that all in-contact animals be brought in for examination and possible treatment. The owner was advised to separate the infested guinea pig until the infestation was resolved. It was also noted that *T. caviae* can transiently infect humans so the young boys were asked to avoid contact with their guinea pig until she had recovered.

Re-inspection and final outcome

After 1 week, the guinea pig was much less agitated and was markedly less pruritic. She had also put on some weight. However, there was severe scaling occurring and the owner requested a solution to bathe the pet in to clear away some of the debris. Epi-soothe shampoo (Virbac) was chosen for its emollient qualities and the pet owner was directed to bathe the guinea pig once or twice a week, depending on the scale build-up. A contact time of 5–10 minutes was recommended for epidermal hydration.

As the pruritus had nearly ceased, the guinea pig was given a good prognosis. On clinical examination her hutch mates seemed free of disease, probably due to the owner's prompt quarantine measures and thorough hygiene procedures. The owner opted against prophylactic treatment for the hutch mates. A week later, the patient was given her third ivermectin injection. She had gained weight and scaling was no longer occurring. She was given a clean bill of health.

Discussion

T. caviae, a sarcoptid mite of the suborder *Astigmata*, is the more common of the guinea pig mites, causing extreme pruritus and lesions along the dorsum and hips (Flecknell 1991). *Chirodiscoides caviae*, while difficult to distinguish from *T. caviae* microscopically, shows different lesion patterns and much less acute symptoms. Dermatophyte infestations present on the face, forehead and ears, so can be distinguished on clinical examination from *T. caviae* (Schaeffer & Donnelly 1997).

The life cycle of *T. caviae* is 14–17 days. Pruritus is evident 8 days post-exposure and alopecia will occur after 2 weeks (Flecknell 1996). *T. caviae* can cause such severe pruritus as to involve the nervous system. In such cases, diazepam at 1–2 mg/kg may be administered (Flecknell 1991). Luckily, in this case, nervous system involvement was avoided just in the nick of time. Secondary keratinisation disorders, e.g. excessive scaling, as occurred in this case, are not uncommon with mite infestations (Ackerman 1993). As excessive dry seborrhoea is an ideal climate for bacteria and yeast overgrowth (Tilley & Smith 1997) some method of removal of the scale is recommended. In this case the owner requested shampooing and that was deemed an appropriate method for dealing with the scaly debris.

T. caviae is a burrowing mite and is spread by direct contact. Generally, it is recommended that all in-contact animals be treated. However, the owner refused treatment on the grounds of cost because none of her other pets showed obvious infestation. Infestation can result in leukocytosis, monocytosis, eosinophilia and basophilia (Schaeffer & Donnelly 1997). However, blood sampling from a debilitated guinea pig is ill advised. As an obligate parasite, sarcoptid mites are best treated systemically so ivermectin is the choice of treatment, although it is not licensed for treatment of small animals. Due to the life cycle of sarcoptid mites, three treatments, 7–8 days apart, are essential to eradicate the infestation completely – a protocol that was followed in this case and resulted in a satisfactory resolution.

REFERENCES

(for Case Study 2)

Ackerman Lowell 1993 Pet skin and hair coat problems. Veterinary Learning Systems, Trenton, NJ, p 7

Flecknell Paul 1991 Guinea pigs. In: Benyon P H, Cooper J E (eds) Manual of exotic pets. British Small Animal Association, Gloucestershire, p 55–56

Flecknell Paul 1996 Diseases of guinea pigs. In: Laber-Laird K, Swincle M M, Flecknell P (eds) Handbook of rodent and rabbit medicine.Pergamon Press, London, p 120–121

Schaeffer Dorcas O, Donnelly Thomas M 1997 Disease problems of guinea pigs and chinchillas. In: Hillyer E, Quesenberry K E (eds) Ferrets, rabbits and rodents. W B Saunders, Philadelphia, PA, p 244–245, 266–267

Tilley Larry P, Smith Francis W K Jr 1997 Dermatoses. The five minute veterinary consult. Williams & Wilkins, Baltimore, MD, p 40–41

Index

C

D

E

F

G

R

S

T